Thread Lifting Techniques for Facial Rejuvenation and Recontouring

Souphiyeh Samizadeh

Editor

Thread Lifting Techniques for Facial Rejuvenation and Recontouring

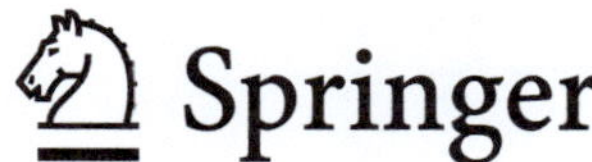 Springer

Editor
Souphiyeh Samizadeh
University College London-Division of Surgery &
Interventional Science
London, UK

King's College London-Dentistry, Oral & Craniofacial Sciences
London, UK

ISBN 978-3-031-47956-4   ISBN 978-3-031-47954-0   (eBook)
https://doi.org/10.1007/978-3-031-47954-0

This Springer imprint is published by the registered company Springer Nature Switzerland AG
The registered company address is: Gewerbestrasse 11, 6330 Cham, Switzerland

Paper in this product is recyclable

To my family and husband: Your love, support, and unwavering belief have been my pillars, enabling me to navigate the demands of research and practice. Your patience and understanding, especially during periods of intense dedication to our field, have been my constant source of strength.

To my mentors, educators, and the medical community: Your guidance has been instrumental in shaping my approach to aesthetic medicine. Your wisdom and encouragement have inspired continuous improvement and innovation.

To the patients and dedicated professionals I work with: The trust you place in me and the daily lessons of resilience and compassion you provide are invaluable. Your experiences enrich my practice and this field immeasurably.

To my colleagues and contributors to this book: Your collaboration has been essential. The insights, critiques, and shared knowledge have not only enhanced this work but also underscored the collaborative spirit of our community.

This book is a tribute to each of you, a reflection of our shared journey in advancing aesthetic medicine. Thank you for being my inspiration, my challenge, and my support.

—Souphi Samizadeh

Foreword

In the early 1990s, a new branch of minimally invasive aesthetic surgery began to flourish, evolving from traditional plastic and aesthetic surgery. This marked a significant shift, making aesthetic enhancements more accessible and appealing to a broader audience. It was during this transformative era that thread lifting methods, aimed at correcting facial deformities, started gaining traction. These innovative techniques rapidly caught the attention of the medical community, sparking a wave of scientific exploration and discussion in professional circles.

Tracing the roots of thread lifting, we find the origins in the mid-1950s with Buttkewitz's pioneering work. The field has since been enriched by the contributions of esteemed colleagues like Guillemain, Mario Gonzales Ulloa, Sergio Capurro, Sassaki, and others. Among them, Pierre Fournier of France stands out for his instrumental role in propelling thread lifting to global recognition through his extensive publications and lectures.

A landmark moment in the evolution of thread lifting was the introduction of barbed threads in 1996, a concept inspired by an intriguing discovery—the presence of golden threads beneath the skin of an Egyptian mummy. This revelation, combined with the known benefits of gold for human tissues, led to the innovative practice of implanting fine gold threads for skin rejuvenation. However, the smooth surface of gold threads limited their effectiveness in lifting sagging skin. Addressing this challenge, the mid-1990s saw the advent of threads designed with protrusions, leading to a surge in the development of varied thread designs over the past quarter century.

As a forerunner in the field of minimally invasive and nonsurgical thread lifting, I have witnessed and contributed to the remarkable evolution of these techniques. The advancements in technology and methods have not only enhanced patient outcomes but have also expanded the toolkit of surgical and nonsurgical practitioners alike. Reflecting on this journey, it is gratifying to see the growth of our company, which now offers an extensive range of thread products, finding applications beyond aesthetic surgery, in areas like general surgery for the face, body, breasts, and intimate areas.

Dr. Souphi Samizadeh, a respected academic and clinician, recognized the gap in comprehensive literature on thread lifting. This book, bridging expertise from East and West, is a testament to her commitment to advancing the field and enhancing patient safety through education.

Therefore, this book is more than just a valuable resource; it is a pivotal contribution to the fields of dermatology, plastic and aesthetic surgery, and related specialties in aesthetic medicine. Its rich content and insights make it an indispensable guide for practitioners striving to excel in this dynamic area of medical science.

Marlen Sulamanidze
Plastic, Reconstructive and Aesthetic Surgeon
Tbilisi, Georgia

Preface

In the ever-evolving world of aesthetic medicine, our pursuit of groundbreaking techniques for rejuvenation and recontouring is relentless. This book represents a collective endeavour, drawing on the vast expertise of scientists, plastic surgeons, dermatologists, dental surgeons, and many more, highlighting the interdisciplinary essence of our field. Our commitment extends beyond merely adopting new procedures; it encompasses a dedication to evidence-based practice and patient-centred care, ensuring our interventions are not only effective but also tailored to the unique needs of each individual. *Thread Lifting Techniques for Facial Rejuvenation and Recontouring* emerges from this commitment to scientific rigour and patient welfare.

Thread lifting has undergone significant advancements and refinements, particularly in Asia and certain European countries, renowned for their pioneering practices and extensive expertise. Recognising this, I have engaged with leading experts from these regions and around the world, who have contributed their invaluable insights, thus merging the best of Eastern and Western practices.

This book is more than a collection of techniques; it is a dedicated effort to illuminate the nuanced world of thread lifting—a subject that, despite its controversy, is increasingly in demand. Our mission is clear: to prioritise knowledge, skill, evidence-based practice, and, above all, patient safety.

Tailored for aesthetic practitioners at every level—from those newly initiated into the field to the most seasoned professionals—we begin with the foundational principles of material science, and then advance to explore more sophisticated thread-lifting techniques. Emphasising both preventive strategies and the management of complications, this book integrates empirical case studies with thorough scientific analyses.

The field of aesthetic medicine is in constant flux, with thread lifting undergoing significant transformation. This book captures a detailed view of the latest advancements, enriched by the collective wisdom of a diverse group of global experts.

I extend an invitation to you, the reader: immerse yourself, absorb the knowledge, and become part of this dynamic conversation. Together, let's push the boundaries of safe and informed aesthetic practice.

Warm regards,

London, UK   Souphiyeh (Souphi) Samizadeh

Terminology

Understanding the terminology associated with suture-based minimally invasive procedures for soft tissue repositioning and realignment is essential for effective communication in the scientific community and in educating patients.

Synonyms

Barbs = hooks = cogs (While "barbs," "hooks," and "cogs" can be considered similar in function (they all are used to engage tissue for lift or anchorage), the exact terminology can vary based on the specific design and function of the thread lift product. It's essential to be precise, as each term might refer to a slightly different mechanism of action or design feature.

Sutures = threads sutures, thread(s) (In the context of aesthetic procedures, "sutures" and "threads" can be used interchangeably when referring to thread lifting. However, "sutures" is a broader term also used in general surgery and other medical fields, not just for cosmetic procedures.)

Glossary of Terms

APTOS Threads
Articulus 400 = Version of Contour Threads
Contour Threads
Hyaluronic acid (HA)
Polylactic-co-glycolic acid (PLGA)
Polylactic acid-caprolactone (PLACL)
Poly-caprolactone (PCL)
Polydioxanone (PDO)
Polyester (Polyethylene terephthalate—PET)
Polylactic acid (PLA)
Polypropylene
Silhouette Soft Threads
Silicone (solid and from medical grade)
United States Pharmacopeia (USP)
Woffles Lift
Woffle Wu Threads

Acknowledgment

Embarking on a pioneering endeavor such as this, especially in a field as intricate and evolving as aesthetic medicine, is not a journey undertaken alone. The creation of this book is a testament to the collective wisdom, experience, and dedication of many, and it is with profound gratitude that I acknowledge their invaluable contributions.

First and foremost, I am deeply indebted to my family and husband for their steadfast presence and unwavering support throughout this journey. Their understanding, love, and the sacrifices made for my vision and work have been the cornerstone of all my endeavors.

I owe an immense debt of gratitude to my mentors and trainers, who have shaped my thinking, refined my skills, and instilled in me the values and principles that underpin my professional life. Your influence extends beyond my personal growth, fostering a culture of knowledge sharing and innovation. To the aspiring professionals I've been fortunate enough to teach, your unending curiosity and commitment to the field have constantly reminded me of the importance of sharing knowledge and fostering growth in the next generation.

A heartfelt thank you to all the experts who generously contributed their insights and expertise to this book. Without your willingness to share, discuss, and collaborate, this work would not have reached its current depth and breadth. Your dedication to the field and commitment to advancing our collective understanding has made this book a true reflection of international collaboration and shared knowledge.

To my colleagues worldwide, your passion and dedication continue to inspire me. This book stands as a testament to what we can achieve together in the spirit of progress and shared knowledge.

In essence, while my name appears on the cover, this book embodies the collective voice and experience of our community. My deepest thanks to each of you for making this vision a reality.

Warm regards,

Souphi Samizadeh

Contents

Part I

Foundations of Facial Aesthetics

History of Thread Lifting

Souphiyeh Samizadeh

Abstract

The evolution of thread lifting techniques within aesthetic medicine has been both dynamic and complex, provoking profound discussions and analysis among scholars and industry experts alike, particularly those specializing in minimally invasive treatments. This chapter explores the history of thread lifting, from its origins to its development, and looks ahead to its potential future directions. With a rapidly expanding repository of techniques and associated tools, the field is marked by an accelerated pace of innovation. However, a critical examination reveals a significant gap in the rigorous scientific study of many of these devices, tools and the techniques employed. The appeal of nonsurgical and minimally invasive cosmetic procedures, including thread lifting, lies in their promise of a swift recovery, immediately visible results, minor side effects, overall aesthetic enhancement, and relatively long-lasting effects. Nevertheless, the fulfillment of these promises hinges on the proper application of quality threads and scientifically validated techniques. This chapter aims to provide a comprehensive understanding of the history of thread lifting, its current state, and future prospects, emphasizing the importance of evidence-based practice in achieving optimal outcomes in aesthetic medicine.

S. Samizadeh (✉)
University College London, London, UK

King's College London, London, UK

Great British Academy of Aesthetic Medicine, London, UK
e-mail: info@baamed.co.uk

© Springer Nature Switzerland AG 2024
S. Samizadeh (ed.), *Thread Lifting Techniques for Facial Rejuvenation and Recontouring*, https://doi.org/10.1007/978-3-031-47954-0_1

Keywords

Aging · Facial aging · Thread lifting · Thread lift · Facial rejuvenation · Nonsurgical · APTOS · PDO · Silhouette soft · Woffles threads · Nonsurgical facelift · Facial thread lift

Thread lifting, an increasingly popular technique in aesthetic medicine, has a rich and fascinating history that is inextricably tied to the evolution of materials science, technological innovations, and changing societal attitudes toward beauty and aging. This procedure, which uses sutures or "threads" to lift and tighten sagging skin, has undergone significant developments since its inception.

Over the years, society's perception of cosmetic treatments has undergone a transformative shift. Once considered a luxury reserved for the affluent and famous, these treatments have become increasingly democratized. The pursuit of health, well-being, and aesthetic enhancement is no longer confined to a select few but has become a global phenomenon. This transformation has been fueled by increased accessibility to both surgical and nonsurgical cosmetic procedures, competitive pricing, and substantial investment in the development of new nonsurgical techniques and technologies.

The past few decades have witnessed a significant evolution in nonsurgical aesthetic medicine. Innovations and advancements have democratized access to safe and effective rejuvenation and enhancement of the face and body. Aided by increased media attention and societal acceptance, the willingness of individuals to undergo such procedures has grown exponentially. The present-day aesthetic landscape is characterized by a preference for nonsurgical, quick, noninvasive, and natural modalities [1–4] A noteworthy trend is the increasing demand for cosmetic and antiaging treatments among younger patients [3]. This shift in demographic interest is evidenced by the reported doubling of millennials' usage of injectable cosmetic products from 2014 to 2020 [3].

Moreover, it is becoming internationally acceptable to have more frequent noninvasive or minimally invasive treatments over time for enhancement and antiaging, than extensive surgical procedures with an extended downtime [3].

This has spurred the development and popularization of various techniques and technologies aimed at mitigating and potentially reversing age-related changes. Among these, the use of absorbable sutures, or "thread lift" techniques, has seen a resurgence. These techniques leverage use of suture (threads) with various characteristics as a biostimulant and to enable soft tissue repositioning [5, 6].

The utilization of sutures is not a recent phenomenon; their application in facial and plastic surgery has a rich historical background. Some report the use of gold threads for facial rejuvenation as far back as ancient Egypt, though not proven [7]. Furthermore, in Asia, gold thread embedding acupuncture has been practiced, and its use for tightening facial tissues has become once more widespread. This process triggers a mild inflammatory response, resulting in collagen deposition around the threads and subsequent tissue contraction and tightening [7–9]. One of the earliest threads used for lifting were the "gold/golden threads." However, these lacked an anchoring function, negating the "lifting" effect and leading to their eventual decline in popularity. These threads can be detected on radiographic head and neck scans such as Orthopantomogram (OPG) often leading to much confusion [9, 10]. This critical information should be incorporated into the training curricula for healthcare professionals, including dental surgeons.

Surgical sutures for facial tissue repositioning and hence rejuvenation go back to the 1950s (Dr Buttkewitz). In 1970, Rene Guillemain used special needles for thread implantation and presented the "Curl lift" technique in Paris. This technique is becoming popular once more, with studies reporting "long-lasting result procedure to elevate the eyebrows" [11].

In 1964, Dr. John Alcamo, a general surgeon, patented the use of his barbed sutures, and this was the first time this concept of the use of sutures without knots was first described. His sutures' patent was on barbed and unidirectional sutures (Fig. 1.1) [7, 12]. Soon afterwards, Dr. Alan McKenzie, an orthopedic surgeon,

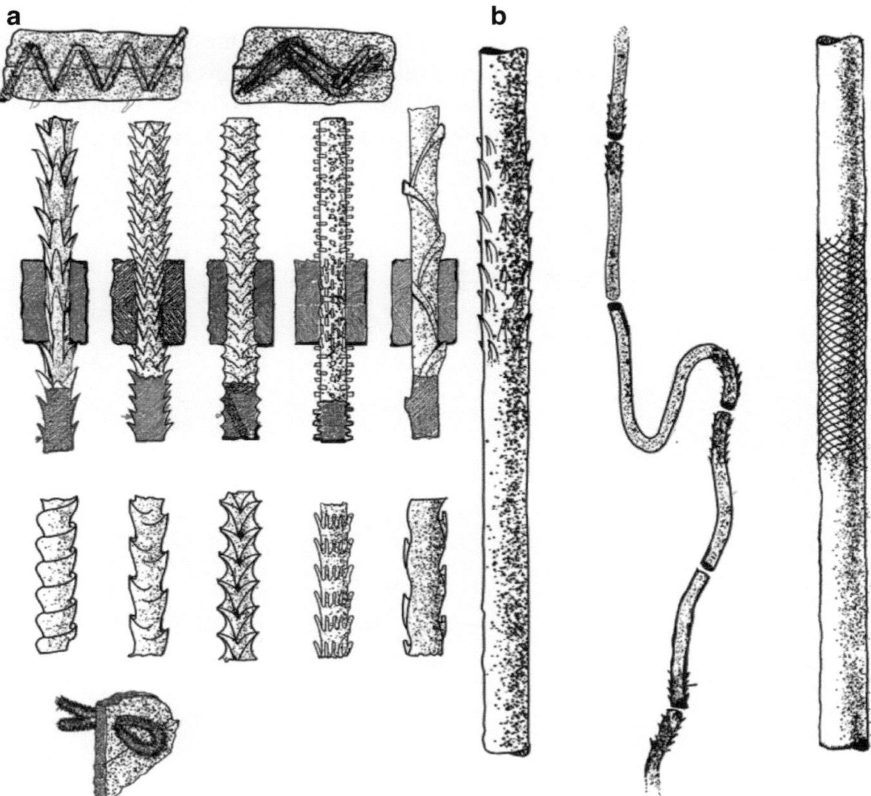

Fig. 1.1 Original drawings for barbed sutures (**a** and **b**). Reproduced from Alcamo JH. US Patent 3,123,077, 1964 [17]. Obtained from USPTO.gov websites

developed a device with several barbs extending in both directions to improve tendon restoration. However, he abandoned this due to technical difficulties [13]. In 1972, an American inventor, named Tanner, patented a device with barbs in two directions, only at the terminal ends [13]. The concept was further advanced in 1984 by Dr. Fukuda and later by Dr. Ruff in 1994 [14–16]. Dr. Gregory Ruff sought patents in 1993 for a cannulated device designed for single-direction insertion and a bidirectional design, which were granted in 1994 and 2001, respectively. In 1986, Drs. Akira Yahai, Osama Fukuda, and Sinichi Hiribayashi from Japan introduced a technique using a curved double-edged needle with a fastener running through its center.

In 1997, Dr. Buncke applied for patents covering a range of suture designs, both unidirectional and bidirectional, intended for uses including wound closure, tendon repair, and internal tissue repair. These designs were described as providing 'lines of tissue support beneath the skin' (Fig. 1.2). Interestingly, Dr. Buncke's inspiration came from the sticktight seeds found near his cottage in the Sierra Nevada, demonstrating nature's influence on medical innovation. His patent was granted in 1999, after which Dr. Buncke transferred his patent rights to Quill Medical, a company associated with Dr. Ruff.

1968 marked a significant year when German specialists patented a thread with barbs, initially aimed at treating acute Achilles' tendon ruptures. This development was paralleled by efforts in the United States, where surgeons experimented with connecting wound edges using transverse single sutures and threads equipped with barbs [19]. However, it was not until 1998 that the concept of barbed threads took a

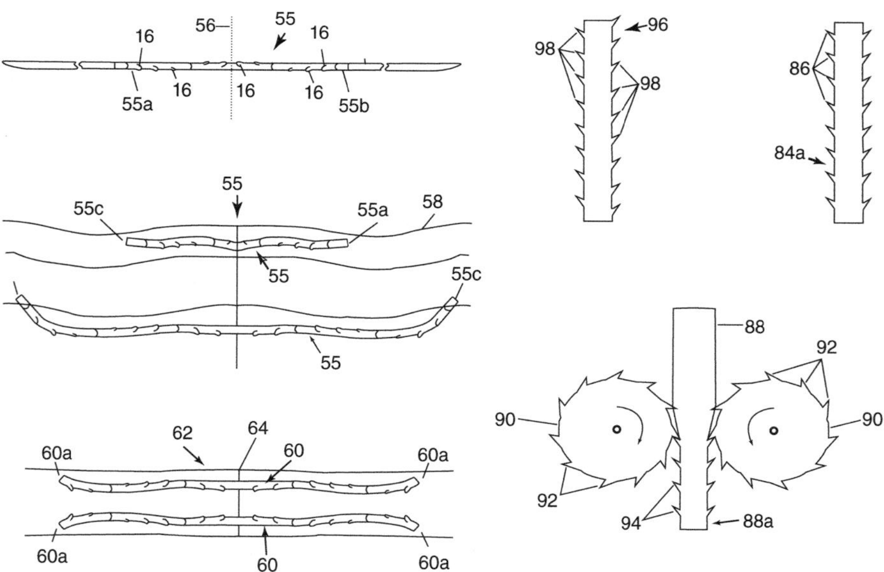

Fig. 1.2 Original drawings for barbed sutures. Reproduced from Buncke, US Patent 5,931,855, 1999 [18]. Obtained from USPTO.gov websites

significant turn towards cosmetic applications, thanks to the pioneering work of Georgian plastic surgeons M. and G. Sulamanidze. [20, 21]. They introduced the first barbed threads for cosmetic surgery, branded as 'antiptosis' or APTOS threads—a name derived from the Greek words for 'against' and 'sagging.' Their innovation laid the groundwork for soft tissue thread lifting, which they had been presenting worldwide since 1996, thereby popularizing thread use for anti-aging and rejuvenation purposes [19].

Dr. Woffles Wu from Singapore envisioned and developed a barbed suture sling in 2002 (Woffles Threads). He combined the properties of a suture suspension sling with the self-retaining properties of the barbed threads. The Woffles thread is a blue Prolene 2.0 suture, 60 cm in length with bidirectional barbs on either side of a 4 cm clear (non-barbed) zone at the midpoint of the thread enabling the thread to be folded at this point into a U-shaped sling. Clinical application of the Woffles Lift began in late 2002. He published nonsurgical "Woffles Lift," using long, barbed self-retaining slings which get inserted via a needle introducer to suspend loose, mobile and ptotic facial tissue (skin, subcutaneous fat, and SMAS of the lower face) to the dense tissue of the scalp (thick and immobile temporal fascia) [22].

In 2002, Drs Sassaki and Cohen used two needles with nylon thread combined with a surgical face lift [21, 23, 24]. Dr. Mathay, an expert from the Philippines, reported utilizing hypodermic sutures to reduce his patients' nose tips. Nikolai Serdev, a professor at the New Bulgarian University, demonstrated comparable techniques with a cannula. Apart from moving various layers of soft face tissues, these procedures can secure the thread to the anchor zones, including fascia and periosteum, resulting in a long-lasting effect. The French surgeon Pierre Fournier's lectures and scholarly papers presented at numerous congresses and scientific conferences aided in the development of thread lifting techniques [19].

In 2003, Dr. Isse was inspired by Woffles Wu and APTOS threads and developed "Isse Endo Progressive Facelift Sutures" and consequently Silhouette Suture®

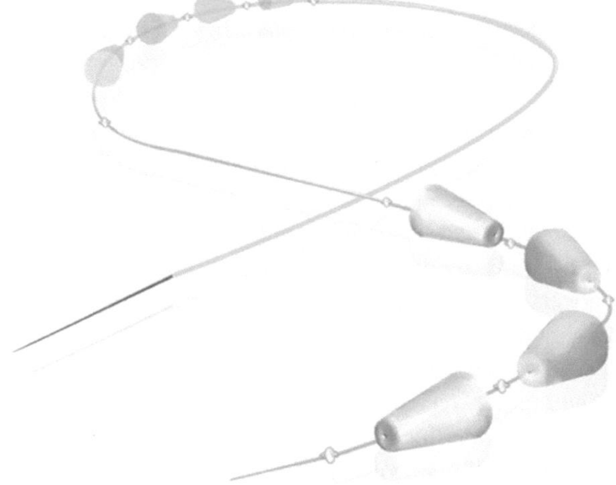

Fig. 1.3 Silhouette Suture® threads with "cones" throughout the threads

threads with "cones" along the threads (Fig. 1.3). These cones were placed on the threads to help increase the "holding" power of the threads on placement and resorption (8 months post-placement). This would produce an enhanced inflammatory response, causing new collagen formation and increasing the longevity of the effects [7, 25, 26].

Taking inspiration from Dr Fernandes and the APTOS suture, Wu developed Woffles lift and threads (60-cm length of 2–0 Prolene with two long barbed sections) and presented successful results in 2003 [7, 14].

Dr. Gregory Ruff designed Contour Threads, now known as Articulus, with opposing barbs and straight needles. It received FDA clearance in 2004. In his words: "Inspired by the quill of the North American porcupine, I envisioned a bidirectional array of barbs that could secure tissue without relying on constricting loops. One set of barbs could anchor the other." Knotless, strong, and "easy to place", barbed sutures (bidirectional and unidirectional formations) offered the potential to suspend ptotic tissues with no surgical intervention [13].

The primary objective of these sutures, also known as threads, was to realign the ptotic subcutaneous tissues, thereby creating a "lift" effect. Given their diverse material composition, lengths, sizes, and surface characteristics, these threads can be adapted for a multitude of applications. These include rejuvenating the face, neck, and body through strategic repositioning of soft tissues, wrinkle reduction, and volume enhancement [27, 28].

The rise of synthetic materials in the twentieth century catalyzed a revolution in thread lifting procedures. Threads were developed from a variety of materials, including polydioxanone (PDO), polycaprolactone (PCL), and poly-L-lactic acid (PLLA), each with distinct advantages and uses. These threads are absorbable, minimally invasive, and have helped improve the longevity and outcomes of thread lifting procedures.

The evolution of thread lifting has not been limited to materials alone. Over time, threads have been designed in various lengths, sizes, and with different surface characteristics to cater to the diverse aesthetic needs of patients. Modern threads often feature barbs, cogs, or cones that aid in anchoring to the subcutaneous tissues, enhancing the lifting effect and tissue repositioning.

The application of thread lifting has also expanded beyond facial rejuvenation to include neck and body treatments. The ability to strategically reposition soft tissues, reduce rhytids, and enhance volume has made thread lifting a versatile tool in aesthetic medicine.

Today, thread lifting is considered a minimally invasive, in-office procedure that can be performed under local anesthesia. The procedure offers a relatively quick recovery time with immediate visible results, making it a popular choice for patients seeking nonsurgical cosmetic treatments.

The success of thread lifting procedures is influenced by a myriad of factors, including the type, quality, biocompatibility, and the mechanical, physical, and chemical properties of the threads used. The production process of these threads is equally crucial, playing a pivotal role in their clinical effectiveness and safety. Despite technological advancements, it's essential to recognise that thread lifting is a techniquesensitive procedure. Outcomes depend on precise patient selection, the correct thread choice for each case, and the application of skilled techniques. The training and expertise of the medical professional performing the procedure are fundamental to achieving optimal aesthetic results, underscoring the need for comprehensive education and an in-depth understanding of facial anatomy and thread lifting mechanics. Additionally, adherence to aftercare instructions is crucial, as it significantly influences the longevity and success of the treatment.

Looking forward, the future of thread lifting in aesthetic medicine appears promising. The continual advancements in material science and technology, alongside growing patient demand for minimally invasive aesthetic procedures, suggest that thread lifting will remain a vital tool in the aesthetic medicine arsenal. As we further our understanding and refine techniques, the potential for thread lifting to deliver safe, effective, and long-lasting aesthetic enhancements continues to grow.

Conclusion

The trajectory of thread lifting techniques in aesthetic medicine has been a dynamic one, marked by continuous evolution and innovation. The increasing popularity of these minimally invasive procedures in recent years has spurred a surge in the development and refinement of thread systems and techniques. This trend has concurrently driven an increase in academic inquiry and clinical trials, thereby enriching our understanding of thread lifting procedures and enhancing the techniques employed.

The body of scientific and clinical evidence surrounding thread lifting is gradually building, contributing to the establishment of more effective and safer practices in aesthetic medicine. However, it is crucial to acknowledge that there remains a significant opportunity for further research, particularly in the areas of long-term effects and comparative studies with other minimally invasive procedures.

As we look toward the future, it is anticipated that the continued growth and development of thread lifting will be propelled by advances in material science, technological innovations, and the ongoing quest for improved patient outcomes. The coming years will likely see an increased focus on standardizing procedures, optimizing patient selection criteria, and establishing best practices based on evidence-based medicine.

Consequently, the history of thread lifting serves not only as a reflection of past progress but also as a roadmap for future directions in aesthetic medicine, underscoring the importance of scientific rigor, clinical validation, and patient safety in shaping the evolution of this dynamic field.

References

1. Samizadeh S. The ideals of facial beauty among Chinese aesthetic practitioners: results from a large national survey. Aesthet Plast Surg. 2018;43:1–13.
2. Samizadeh S, Wu W. Ideals of facial beauty amongst the Chinese population: results from a large national survey. Aesthet Plast Surg. 2018;43:1–11.

3. McClean ME, et al. Suture lifting: a review of the literature and our experiences. Dermatol Surg. 2020;46(8):1068–77.
4. Yun Y, Choi I. Effect of thread embedding acupuncture for facial wrinkles and laxity: a single-arm, prospective, open-label study. Integr Med Res. 2017;6(4):418–26.
5. Villa MT, et al. Barbed sutures: a review of the literature. Plast Reconstr Surg. 2008;121(3):102e–8e.
6. Savoia A, et al. Outcomes in thread lift for facial rejuvenation: a study performed with happy lift™ revitalizing. Dermatol Ther. 2014;4(1):103–14.
7. Kress D. The history of barbed suture suspension: applications, and visions for the future. In: Simplified facial rejuvenation. Springer; 2008. p. 247–56.
8. Rondo W Jr, Vidarte GD, Michalany N. HISTOLOGIC STUDY OF THE SKIN WITH GOLD THREAD IMPLANTATION. Plast Reconstr Surg. 1996;97(1):256–8.
9. Moulonguet I, et al. Histopathologic and ultrastructural features of gold thread implanted in the skin for facial rejuvenation. Am J Dermatopathol. 2015;37(10):773–7.
10. Garg R, Fernandes B, Sunil MK. Unusual radiopacities spotted in a dental radiograph: case report. J Indian Acad Oral Med Radiol. 2017;29(2)
11. De Paola DQ, De Paola Neto D. Abstract: eyebrows elevation—a new, easy and cheap trick. Plast Reconstr Surg Glob Open. 2017;5(9 Suppl):74–5.
12. Yousif NJ, Summers A. The midface sling: a new technique to rejuvenate the midface. Plast Reconstr Surg. 2002;110(6):1541–53; discussion 1554.
13. Cui H. Aesthethic thread REJUVENATION IN ASIANS chapter: Gregory L. Ruff: several viewpoints on thread rejuvenation. 2019.
14. Wu WT. Barbed sutures in facial rejuvenation. Aesthet Surg J. 2004;24(6):582–7.
15. Ruff G. Technique and uses for absorbable barbed sutures. Aesthet Surg J. 2006;26(5):620–8.
16. de Pinho TJ, et al. Facial thread lifting with suture suspension. Braz J Otorhinolaryngol. 2017;83(6):712–9.
17. Alcamo J. Surgical suture United States Patent. 1956. p. 3.
18. Buncke HJ. Surgical methods using one-way suture. Google Patents. 1999.
19. Cui H. AESTHETIC HREAD REJUVENATION IN ASIANS chapter: sulamanidze:several viewpoints on thread rejuvenation. Peking University Medical Press; 2019.
20. Sulamanidze M, et al. Facial lifting with "APTOS" threads: featherlift. Otolaryngol Clin N Am. 2005;38(5):1109–17.
21. Sulamanidze M, et al. Removal of facial soft tissue ptosis with special threads. Dermatol Surg. 2002;28(5):367–71.
22. Cui H. Aesthethic thread REJUVENATION IN ASIANS chapter Woffles Wu: several viewpoints on thread rejuvenation. Peking University Medical Press; 2019.
23. Pierre A, et al. Soft tissue lifting by suspension sutures chapter from Cosmetic Medicine & Surgery book. 2017.
24. Fournier PF. Reflexions sur les fils tuteurs APTOS de Sulamanidze. La revue de chirurgie esthetique de langue Francaise. 2001;25(104):23–7.
25. Isse N, Lee S. Barbed polypropylene sutures for midface elevation. Arch Facial Plast Surg. 2005;7:55–61.
26. Isse NG. Endoscopic forehead lift: evolution and update. Clin Plast Surg. 1995;22(4):661–73.
27. Gold MH, Sundaram H. The use of absorbable sutures for suspension and volumising.
28. Kim B, Oh S, Jung W. Wrinkles around the eyes. In: The art and science of thread lifting: based on pinch anatomy. Singapore: Springer Singapore; 2019. p. 179–83.

Clinical Anatomy of the Face for Minimally Invasive Cosmetic Interventions

2

Souphiyeh Samizadeh

Abstract

A comprehensive and nuanced understanding of facial anatomy, with its intricate structures and layered complexity, is fundamental for practitioners in aesthetic medicine. The efficacy of treatments and the avoidance of complications are correlated with the depth of anatomical knowledge and the ability to apply it in practice. In an era of rapidly advancing scientific discovery, it is incumbent upon practitioners to remain abreast of emerging research and newly published studies. This continual learning process fortifies the foundational knowledge that underpins their practice. Recognising the inherent variations across the general population is critical. Furthermore, an evolving body of research is shedding light on ethnic disparities in facial anatomy, thereby necessitating a nuanced, individualised approach to aesthetic treatments. This chapter aims to illuminate the three-dimensional architecture of facial anatomy, dissecting it layer by layer. Each section will explore into the specifics of key structures, their interrelationships, and relevance to aesthetic procedures. Emphasis will be placed on the anatomical considerations pertinent to thread lifting procedures. By providing a detailed exploration of facial anatomy, this chapter will equip practitioners with the knowledge required to optimise outcomes and minimise potential complications in their aesthetic practice.

S. Samizadeh (✉)
King's College London, London, UK

University College London, London, UK

Great British Academy of Aesthetic Medicine, London, UK
e-mail: info@baamed.co.uk

© Springer Nature Switzerland AG 2024

S. Samizadeh (ed.), *Thread Lifting Techniques for Facial Rejuvenation and Recontouring*, https://doi.org/10.1007/978-3-031-47954-0_2

Keywords

Ageing · Facial ageing · Thread lifting · Thread lift · Facial rejuvenation · Anatomy · Facial layers · Facial threads

Introduction

A comprehensive and profound understanding of facial anatomy is the cornerstone for the safe and efficacious execution of both surgical and non-surgical facial rejuvenation procedures. The landscape of non-surgical aesthetic interventions is rapidly evolving, becoming increasingly diverse, intricate, and sophisticated. Despite this growing complexity, patients' expectations remain constant. They seek procedures that maintain a high degree of non-invasiveness while minimising side effects and downtime. Consequently, the practitioner's challenge lies in aligning these evolving techniques and technologies with the patient's expectations, underpinning the importance of continual learning and skill development in this dynamic field of aesthetic medicine.

Amid this context of evolving aesthetic interventions and patient expectations, understanding facial anatomy becomes paramount, particularly in the realm of rejuvenation treatments. These techniques aim to counteract the changes occurring at various layers and components of the facial structure, restoring disrupted facial contours to their original state.

The complexity of facial anatomy demands a precise and detailed understanding for safe and effective implementation of thread lifting procedures. In the subsequent sections of this chapter, we will delve into an in-depth exploration of facial anatomy, with a specific focus on the anatomical considerations pertinent to thread lifting procedures. Through this focused exploration, we aim to equip practitioners with the knowledge and understanding required to optimise outcomes and minimise potential complications in their aesthetic practice.

The face holds significant value from multifaceted perspectives, including function, aesthetics, psychology, identity, and social interaction. Consequently, any alteration, whether through surgical or non-surgical interventions, carries profound implications. These changes can have positive or negative ramifications on an individual's quality of life, contingent upon the circumstances. It is essential to consider the psychological repercussions of facial ageing and rejuvenation treatments in addition to their physical impact.

The detailed analysis of regional facial anatomy warrants an extensive understanding of its key elements. These foundational structures encompass the supportive skeletal foundation, diverse facial layers, intricate innervation, comprehensive vascular system, distinctive musculature, supportive ligaments, and the strategically placed adipose tissue. A concise summary of these structural components will be provided subsequently. Nevertheless, while these elements are delineated individually, it is essential to consider the complex interconnections and functional interplay amongst them. These sophisticated spatial relationships and synergistic interactions significantly influence the overall form and function of the face. Thus, it is vital not to oversimplify this intricate network in the process of understanding each component in isolation. A holistic understanding, acknowledging the dynamic equilibrium of these structures, is imperative to fully comprehend the complex anatomy of the face.

The skeletal structure of the face provides the foundation of the soft tissues and is fundamental for facial appearance. The underlying bones of the face determine the overall facial appearance [1]. The individuality of the face is determined by the convexities and concavities of these bones, in addition to the presence/absence of fat, colour, effects of ageing on the skin, and facial hair [2, 3]. Ageing affects all facial layers. Increasing and collective changes with time in all structural components of the face lead to a change in the morphology of the whole face in terms of topography, shape, and proportions [4].

Facial Skeleton

The facial skeleton, an integral component of the skull, collaboratively forms a structure known as the cranium. Encompassing the oral and nasal cavities, along with the ocular structures, the facial skeleton, or the viscerocranium, provides a robust and intricate framework for the face. The viscerocranium comprises a total of 15 bones, with three existing as singular, unpaired entities, and six presenting in symmetrical pairs. This complex skeletal construct underpins the physical characteristics of the face and offers a foundational understanding for aesthetic procedures and interventions [2]. Apart from the mandible, every bone within the skull structure is interconnected through sutures, also known as synarthrodial joints (Fig. 2.1). These fibrous connective tissues offer both structural integrity and flexibility to the skull, contributing to its resilience and function.

Facial bones:
- Zygomatic
- Nasal
- Platine
- Maxilla
- Mandible
- Inferior nasal concha
- Lacrimal
- Vomer

Unpaired bones:
- Mandible
- Ethmoid
- Vomer

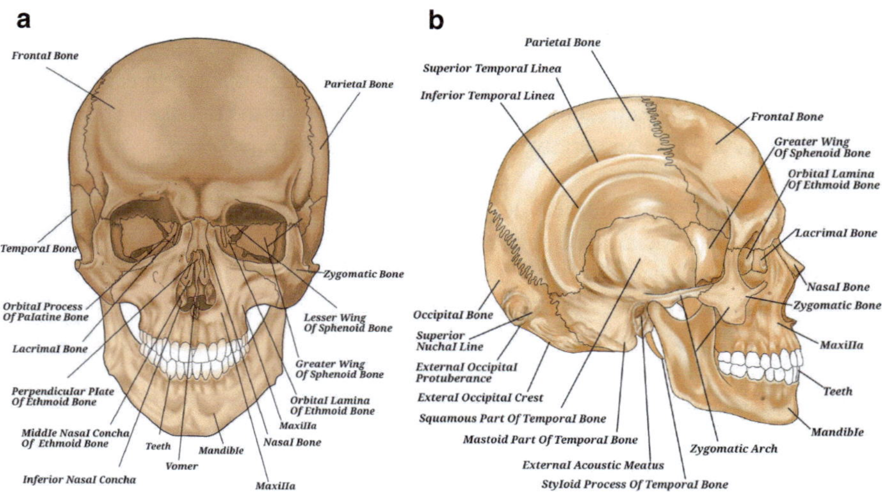

Fig. 2.1 The skull (**a**) front, (**b**) side. The neurocranium consists of eight parts: frontal, sphenoid, ethmoid, occipital, two temporal, and two parietal bones. Viscerocranium: two nasal, two lacrimal, two palatine, two inferior nasal concha, two zygomatic, two maxilla, one mandible, and one vomer

Paired bones:
- Maxillae
- Inferior nasal conchae
- Zygomatic bones
- Palatine bones
- Nasal bones
- Lacrimal bones

A comprehensive understanding of the foramina and their respective locations in the maxillofacial region is critical for safe and effective aesthetic procedures. These foramina serve as conduits for vital neurovascular bundles, constituting an integral part of facial anatomy. Each side of the face comprises four distinctive foramina, as depicted in Fig. 2.2. These structures and their contained elements play significant roles in facial sensation, movement, and vascular supply, underscoring the importance of their identification in surgical planning and procedure execution. These include:

1. *Supraorbital foramen*
    (a) It is present in the supraorbital margin of the frontal bone and provides passage of supraorbital nerve and vessels.
2. *Infraorbital foramen*
    (a) It is present in the infraorbital margin formed by the maxillary bones with the connection of the zygomatic bone. It provides passage to the infraorbital vessels and nerves [2].

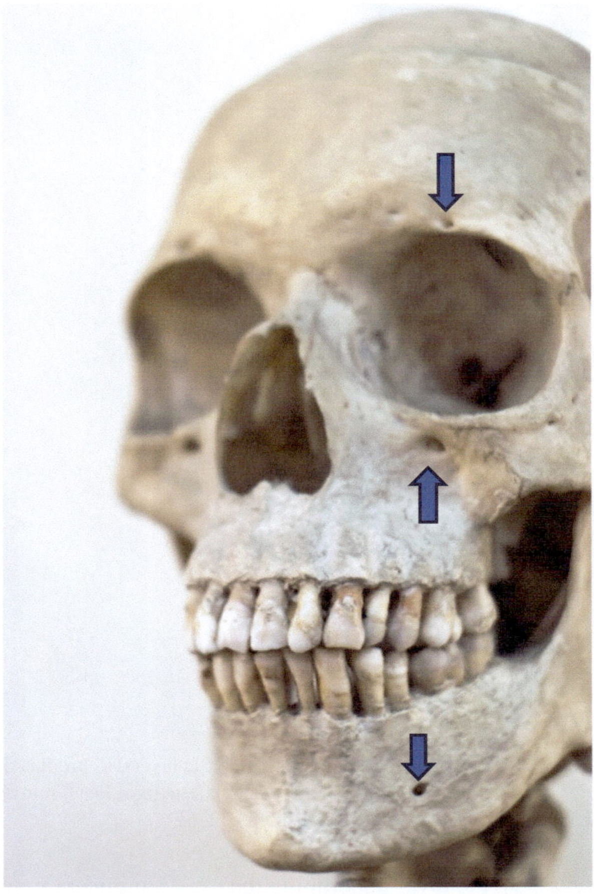

Fig. 2.2 Foramina: *Supraorbital, infraorbital, zygomaticofacial and mental. Image Credit: Shutterstock*

3. *Zygomaticofacial foramen*
    (a) It is present in the lateral wall of the zygomatic bone on each side and transmits the zygomaticofacial nerve.
4. *Mental foramen*
    (a) It is present inferior to the second premolar on the mandible and provides passage to the mental nerves and vessels [1].

Soft Tissue Layers

The facial structure can be characterised by five basic layers, most prominently observed in the scalp region (Fig. 2.3). These layers extend across the facial expanse, with noticeable modifications and compaction in various facial regions, serving functional adaptations (Fig. 2.4). Notably, the retaining ligaments and facial spaces

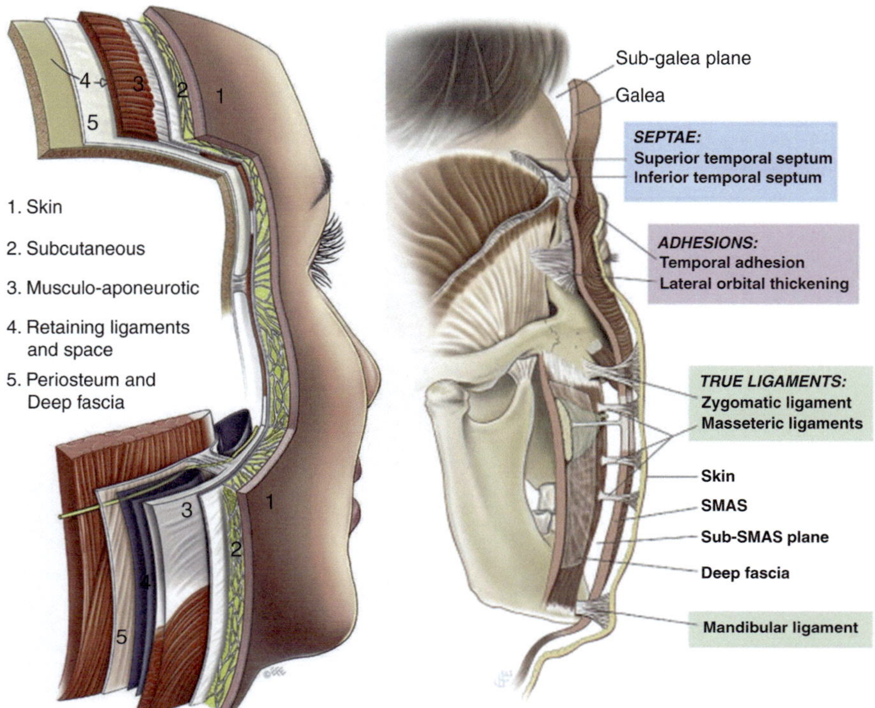

Fig. 2.3 The face is constructed of five basic layers. Reproduced with permission from Fitzgerald R, Carqueville J, Yang PT. An approach to structural facial rejuvenation with fillers in women. Int J Womens Dermatol. 2018 Dec 13;5(1):52–67

represent the layer undergoing the most significant modifications. These alterations underscore the dynamic nature of facial anatomy and the adaptability of its structures to fulfil their specific roles and requirements [4]. The primary five layers include [4]:

Facial layers can further be seen as (Fig. 2.4):

1. Skin
2. Superficial fat layer
3. Superficial musculoaponeurotic system (SMAS)
4. Retaining ligaments and spaces
5. Deep fat layer
6. Periosteum/deep fascia
7. Bone

Facial Anatomy Layers

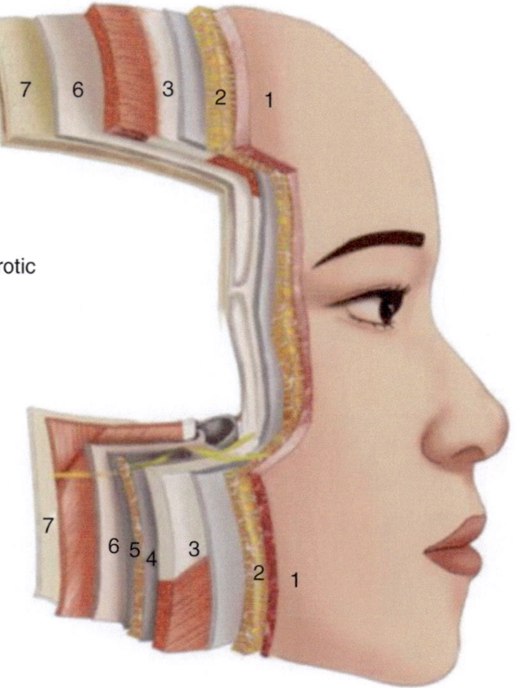

1. Skin

2. Superficial fat

3. SMAS [superficial musculoaponeurotic system]

4. Retaining ligaments and spaces

5. Deep fat layer

6. Periosteum, deep fascia

7. Bones

Fig. 2.4 Facial layers. There is significant modification and compaction of these layers in different parts of the face for functional adaptation

A recent study has reported a new layered arrangement for the forehead (Fig. 2.5) [5]:

- Layer 1: Skin
- Layer 2: Superficial fatty layer (superficial fat compartments)
- Layer 3: Suprafrontalis fascia
- Layer 4: Frontalis muscle
- Layer 5: A homogeneous layer of fat separated by the orbicularis retaining ligament and supraorbital ligamentous adhesion into three parts:
  - Preseptal fat
  - Retro-orbicularis fat
  - Retrofrontalis fat
- Layer 6: Subfrontalis fascia
- Layer 7: A supraperiosteal plane containing loose areolar connective tissue separated into compartments and deep fat
- Layer 8: Periosteum

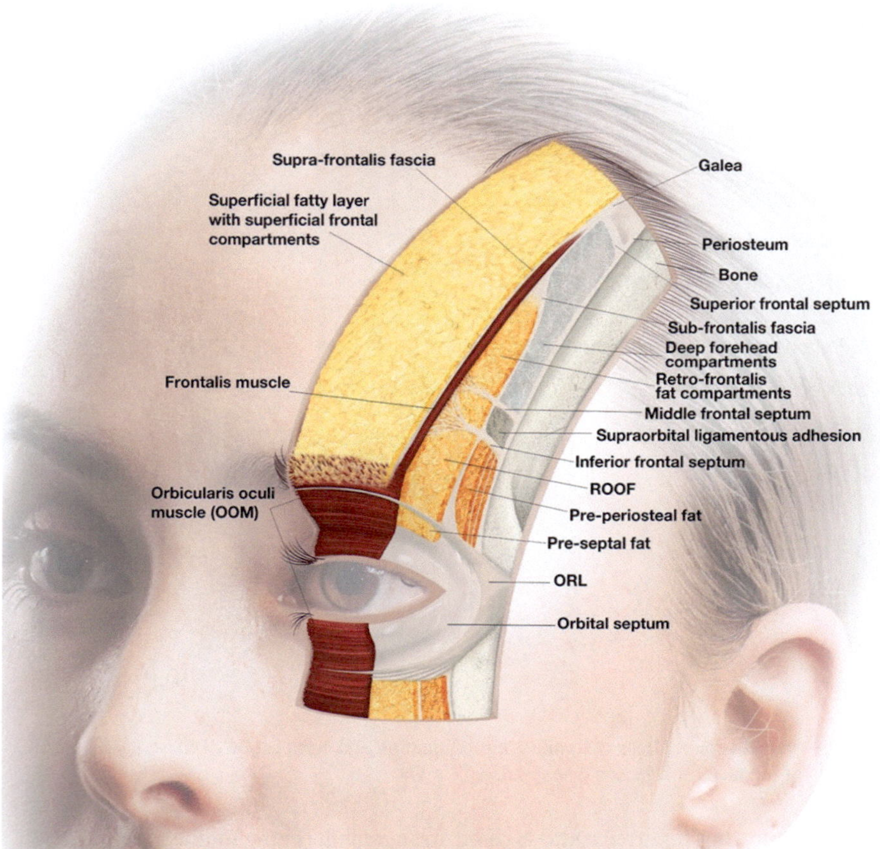

Fig. 2.5 Schematic drawing showing the layered arrangement of the forehead from an oblique frontal view. The fascial layers have been exposed in a stepwise approach starting from the skin (medially) and moving deeper until reaching the bone (laterally, temporal crest). The depth of each respective structure can also be appreciated in relation to the colour of the adjacent fat. The superficial fatty layer is lightest in colour (yellow), whereas the retrofrontalis fat is slightly darker in colour (bright orange), and the preperiosteal fat is darkest (dark orange). Note how the orbicularis retaining ligament and the supraorbital ligamentous adhesion transition into more superficial layers and form boundaries for compartments located cranially and caudally. Reproduced with permission from Reevaluation of the Layered Anatomy of the Forehead: Introducing the Subfrontalis Fascia and the Retrofrontalis Fat Compartments Plastic and Reconstructive Surgery 149(3):587–595, March 2022 [5]

Skin

The skin, as a highly complex organ, comprises two primary layers—the superficial epidermis and the underlying dermis, both of which contribute to sensation and protection (Fig. 2.6). A thorough understanding of the skin's anatomical and

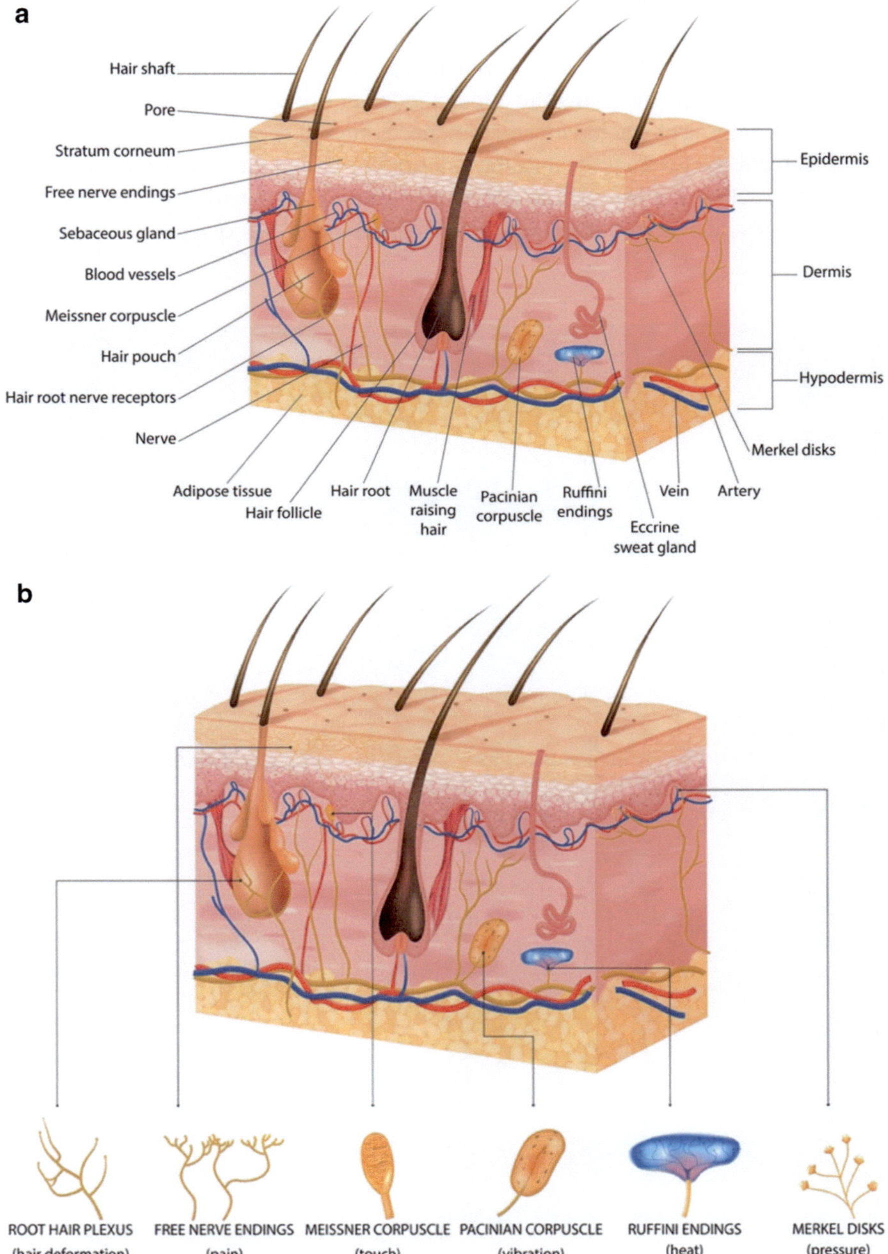

Fig. 2.6 (**a**) Epidermis, dermis, and subcutaneous connective tissue layers. (**b**) Skin sensory receptors. Image Credit: Shutterstock

physiological properties is paramount, as these factors directly impact the final aesthetic outcome of any cosmetic procedure. Specifically, the topographic thickness of the skin plays a crucial role in surgical procedures and in the administration of injectables. The skin overlying the upper and lower eyelids, the glabellar areas, and the nasal regions is characteristically thin, necessitating special care during an intervention. Conversely, areas such as the anterior cheek and the mental region boast a relatively thicker skin layer (Fig. 2.7). Understanding these variances in skin thickness and structure across different facial regions ensures more precise, safe, and

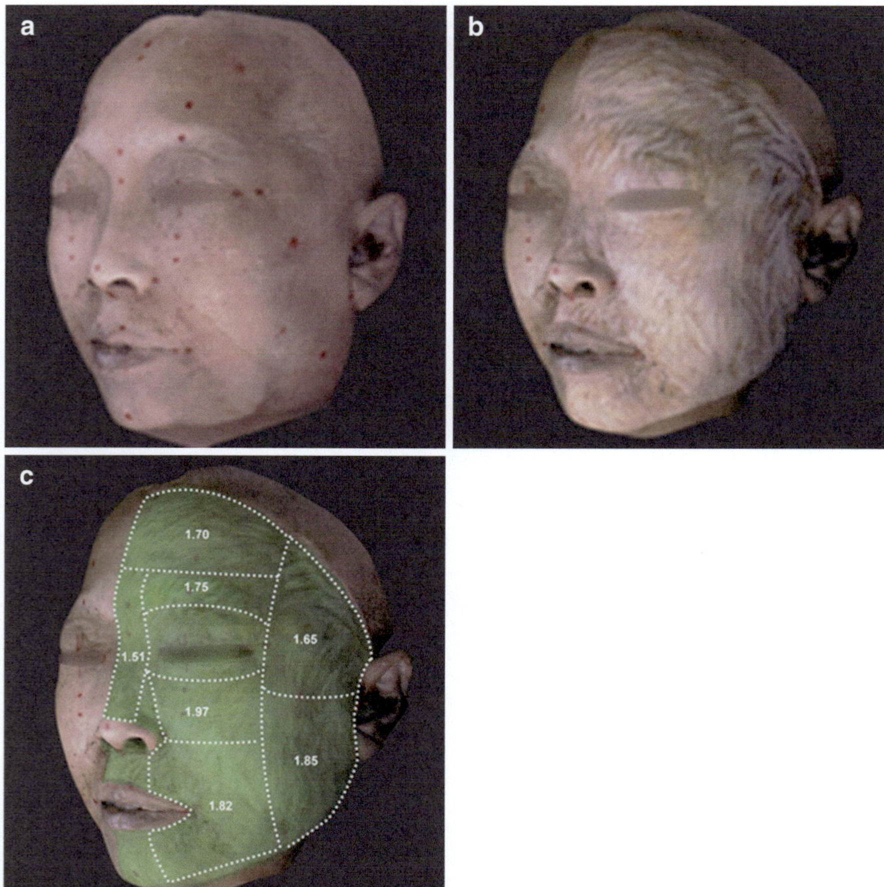

Fig. 2.7 Superimposed 3D image reconstructed from two different layers of the faces. Undissected (Scan 1, **a**) and dissected 3D scanned image after removal of the facial skin (Scan 2, **b**) were superimposed using MDS 3.0 program (**c**). Based on the anatomical regions of the face, the mean value of skin thickness is shown (mm). Reproduced with permission from Kim, You-Soo, Kang-Woo Lee, Ji-Soo Kim, Young-Chun Gil, Tansatit Tanvaa, Dong Hoon Shin, and Hee-Jin Kim. "Regional thickness of facial skin and superficial fat: application to the minimally invasive procedures." Clinical Anatomy 32, no. 8 (2019): 1008–1018 [8]

effective aesthetic interventions [6]. Gender-based differences exist within the integumentary system, where males typically exhibit marginally thicker skin than their female counterparts. Ethnic differences in skin characteristics are observed and documented. These disparities range from the skin's structural composition to its physiological responses. Variations in skin thickness, melanin content, lipid composition, and hydration levels have been reported across different ethnic groups, leading to differences in skin ageing, pigmentation, and sensitivity to environmental factors. As such, acknowledging these variations is essential in the field of aesthetic medicine to ensure personalised and effective treatment strategies.

The thickness of the skin is not uniform across the facial topography, exhibiting significant variations across different regions (Figs. 2.7 and 2.8). This discrepancy is influenced by individual-specific factors, including age, ethnicity, and gender, thus contributing to the overall diversity in skin characteristics.

For instance, a comparative evaluation of dermal thickness between Koreans and Caucasians reveals similar measurements. However, Koreans exhibit a distinctly thicker epidermis compared to their Caucasian counterparts (Fig. 2.7) [7].

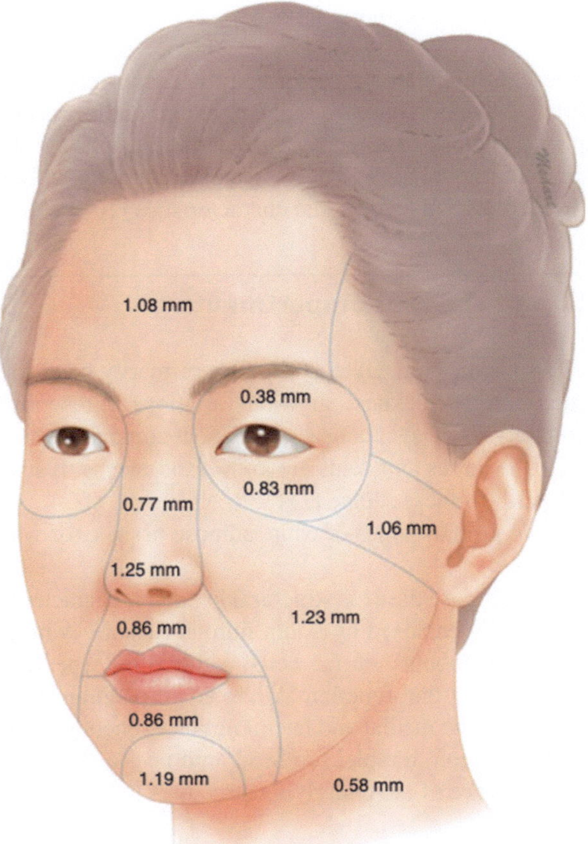

Fig. 2.8 Average skin thickness of the face. Reproduced with permission from Kim, H.J., Seo, K.K., Lee, H.K. and Kim, J., 2016. General Anatomy of the Face and Neck. In Clinical Anatomy of the Face for Filler and Botulinum Toxin Injection (pp. 1–53). Springer, Singapore

Fat Pads

Facial adipose tissue, a key component in the aesthetic and functional aspects of the face, is organised into three distinct categories based on their anatomical location. These include the superficial and deep fat pads, along with the buccal and temporal deep fat pads, which represent the deepest facial fat compartments [9, 10]. This trichotomy underscores the structural complexity and functional diversity of facial adipose tissue, emphasising the need for a nuanced understanding of these structures in aesthetic medicine [10]:

- Superficial: Dermal white adipose tissue
- Deep: Subcutaneous white adipose tissue
  - Fibrous
       Perioral region
  - Structural
       Major parts of the midface
  - Deposit
       Buccal fat pad
       Deep temporal fat pad

These differentiated types of adipose tissue exhibit diversity not only in their anatomical location but also in their cellular and extracellular compositions. They display variations in adipocyte size and the composition of their extracellular matrix, particularly collagen. These disparities subsequently contribute to differing functional roles and mechanical characteristics [10].

Superficial Fat Compartments

The subcutaneous layer of the face primarily comprises dermal white adipose tissue, with its thickness showing variations in response to factors such as age and ethnicity. This layer consists of distinct compartments demarcated by fibrous septae [9, 10]. Nerves and veins are known to traverse this plane, typically located within the walls of these septae [11].

Two primary types of white adipose tissue exist within the subcutaneous layer:

Type 1 adipose tissue is structural in nature, characterised by larger adipocytes individually enclosed by a thin fibrous capsule. A meshwork of fibrous septae surrounds lobules of fat cells within this type, imparting unique viscoelastic properties that function akin to small padding. Predominantly found in regions such as the medial and lateral midface (encompassing certain areas of the periorbital region, temple, forehead, and neck), this type is characterised by a loose adherence of the underlying structures to the skin [10, 12]

Type 2 adipose tissue, in contrast, is fibrous and contains smaller adipocytes, each enclosed by a thick fibrous capsule. This type can further be subdivided into lobular and non-lobular subtypes. This tissue type displays a complex meshwork of collagenous and elastic fibres, along with muscle fibres. In areas where type 2 adipose tissue is present, facial muscles, the collagenous network surrounding the adipocytes, and the skin are closely adhered to one another. Collagenous and muscular fibres insert into the skin, thus anchoring the skin to the underlying facial expression muscles. These muscle fibres, in turn, insert into the dermis, creating an integrated network of collagen fibre and muscle. Interposed within this network are fat cells. Type 2 adipose tissue is predominantly found in the perioral and nasal areas, as well as the periorbital region (eyebrows) [10, 12].

The most distinguishable demarcation lines between these two subcutaneous arrangements include [10]:

- The nasolabial sulcus
- The labiomandibular sulcus
- The submental sulcus

The superficial fat compartments of the face (Table 2.1, Fig. 2.9) along with their boundaries are as follows [13–17].

Table 2.1 Names and boundaries of the superficial facial fat compartments. Reproduced with permission from Cotofana S, Lachman N. Anatomy of the Facial Fat Compartments and their Relevance in Aesthetic Surgery. J Dtsch Dermatol Ges. 2019 Apr;17(4):399–413 [13]

	Superior border	Inferior border	Medial/anterior border	Lateral/posterior border	Floor	Roof
Superficial lateral forehead compartment	Superior frontal septum	Cutaneous insertion of orbicularis oculi muscle complex	Superficial central forehead compartment	Superior temporal septum	Frontalis muscle	Skin
Superficial central forehead compartment	Superior frontal septum	Cutaneous insertion of orbicularis oculi muscle complex and procerus muscle	–	Superficial lateral forehead compartment	Frontalis muscle	Skin
Superficial upper temporal compartment	Superior temporal septum	Inferior temporal septum	Superior temporal septum	Superior temporal septum	Superficial temporal fascia	Skin
Superficial lower temporal compartment	Inferior temporal septum	Adhesions to the zygomatic bone	Cutaneous insertion of lateral orbital thickening (LOT)	Inferior temporal septum	Superficial temporal fascia	Skin
Superficial nasolabial fat compartment	Tear trough	Nasolabial sulcus	Lateral side and ala of nose	Superficial medial cheek and jowl fat compartment	Orbital part of the orbicularis oculi muscle (in its superior part) and by the midcheek superficial musculo-aponeurotic system (in its lower part)	Skin
Superficial medial cheek fat compartment	Cutaneous insertion of orbicularis retaining ligament	Jowl fat compartment	Tear trough and superficial nasolabial fat compartment	Superficial middle cheek fat compartment	Orbital part of the orbicularis oculi muscle (in its superior part) and by the midcheek superficial musculo-aponeurotic system (in its lower part)	Skin

	Superior border	Inferior border	Medial/anterior border	Lateral/posterior border	Floor	Roof
Superficial middle cheek fat compartment	Adhesions of zygomatic bone	Cutaneous adhesions to the platysma	Superficial medial cheek and jowl fat compartment	Superficial lateral cheek fat compartment	Orbital part of the orbicularis oculi muscle (in its superior part) and by the midcheek superficial musculo-aponeurotic system (in its lower part)	Skin
Superficial lateral cheek fat compartment	Adhesions to the zygomatic bone	Cutaneous adhesions to the platysma	Superficial middle cheek fat compartment	Auricle	Superficial musculo-aponeurotic system	Skin
Jowl fat compartment	Superficial medial cheek fat compartment	Cutaneous adhesions to the platysma	Labiomandibular sulcus	Superficial medial cheek fat compartment	Midfacial superficial musculo-aponeurotic system (in its upper part) and platysma (in its lower part)	Skin

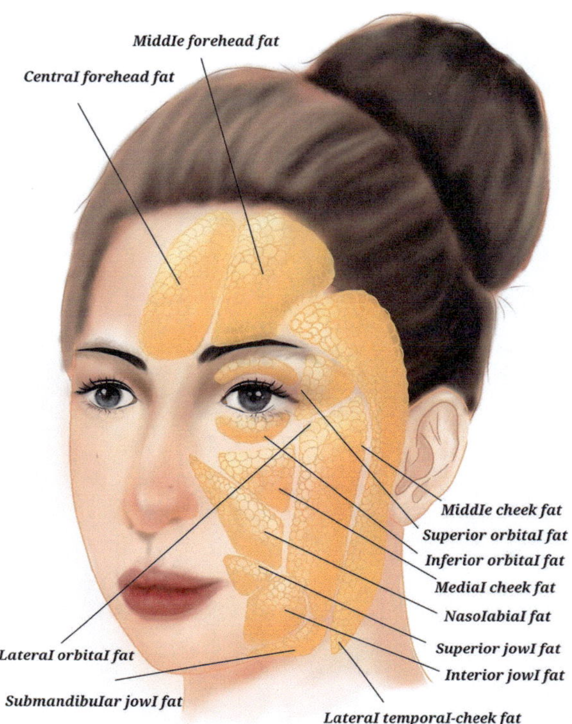

Fig. 2.9 Superficial fat pads of the face

Deep Fat Pads of the Face

The deep fat layer of the face predominantly consists of subcutaneous white adipose tissue, segmented into individual compartments by fibrous septae (Table 2.2, Fig. 2.9). Serving as conduits for branches of the facial nerve and for branches of the facial artery and vein, these septae play crucial roles in the facial structural framework [10, 18–20]. Various structural elements demarcate this layer from the superficial layer (dermal white adipose tissue) across different facial regions. These include [10]:

- Temple: Superficial temporal fascia
- Midface: SMAS
- Neck: Platysma

Certain fat pad boundaries may be defined by the origins of facial expression muscles and their corresponding bony origins [10, 21]. Deep facial fat compartments (Table 2.2, Fig. 2.10) are typically located beneath the mimetic muscles and overlay the deep fascia of the face [13, 15, 17].

Table 2.2 Names and boundaries of the deep facial fat compartments when viewed from the anterior aspect of the face. Reproduced with permission from Cotofana S, Lachman N. Anatomy of the Facial Fat Compartments and their Relevance in Aesthetic Surgery. J Dtsch Dermatol Ges. 2019 Apr;17(4):399–413 [13]

	Superior border	Inferior border	Medial border	Lateral border	Floor	Roof
Deep lateral forehead compartments	Superior frontal septum	Middle frontal septum	Fibrous envelope of the supraorbital neurovascular structures	Temporal ligamentous adhesion	Periosteum	Fibrous sheet covering the underside of the frontalis muscle
Deep central forehead compartment	Superior frontal septum	Middle frontal septum	–	Supraorbital neurovascular structures travelling in a longitudinal orientation	Periosteum	Fibrous sheet covering the underside of the frontalis muscle
Retro-orbicularis oculi fat compartment	Middle frontal septum	Orbicularis retaining ligament	Supraorbital neuro-vascular bundle	Open and connected via the superior interval to the inferior temporal compartment	Periosteum of the frontal bone	Underlying fascia of frontalis muscle
Medial sub-orbicularis oculi fat compartment	Orbicularis retaining ligament	Zygomatico-cutaneous ligament	Angular vein	Lateral SOOF	Midfacial extension of the superficial lamina of the deep temporal fascia	Orbicularis oculi muscle
Lateral sub-orbicularis oculi fat compartment	Orbicularis retaining ligament	Zygomatico-cutaneous ligament	Medial SOOF	Open and connected via the temporal tunnel to the inferior temporal compartment	Midfacial extension of the superficial lamina of the deep temporal fascia	Orbicularis oculi muscle
Premaxillary space	Angular vein	Fascial fusion of the midcheek SMAS and the levator labii superioris alaeque nasi muscle	Lateral nasal wall and lateral nasal vein	Angular vein	Levator labii superioris alaeque nasi muscle	Orbital part of the orbicularis oculi muscle (in its superior part) and by the midcheek superficial musculo-aponeurotic system (in its lower part)

(continued)

Table 2.2 (continued)

	Superior border	Inferior border	Medial border	Lateral border	Floor	Roof
Deep pyriform space	Bony attachment of the levator labii superioris alaeque nasi muscle	Levator anguli oris muscle	Lateral nasal wall and depressor septi nasi muscle	Infraorbital neurovascular bundle	Levator anguli oris muscle and periostium of maxilla	Levator labii superioris alaeque nasi muscle
Deep medial cheek fat compartment	Bony attachment of the levator labii superioris alaeque nasi muscle	Fusion of the levator anguli oris and the levator labii superioris alaeque nasi muscle in its medial part and by the zygomaticus major and the transverse facial septum in its lateral part	Infraorbital neurovascular bundle	Angular vein and deep lateral cheek fat	Periosteum of the maxilla	Levator labii superioris alaeque nasi muscle
Deep lateral cheek fat compartment	Zygomatico-cutaneous ligament and/or zygomaticus minor muscle	Zygomaticus major muscle and transverse facial septum	Angular vein and deep medial cheek fat	Zygomaticus major muscle and transverse facial septum	Periosteum of the maxilla	Orbicularis oculi muscle and the midcheek SMAS

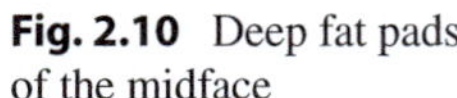

Fig. 2.10 Deep fat pads of the midface

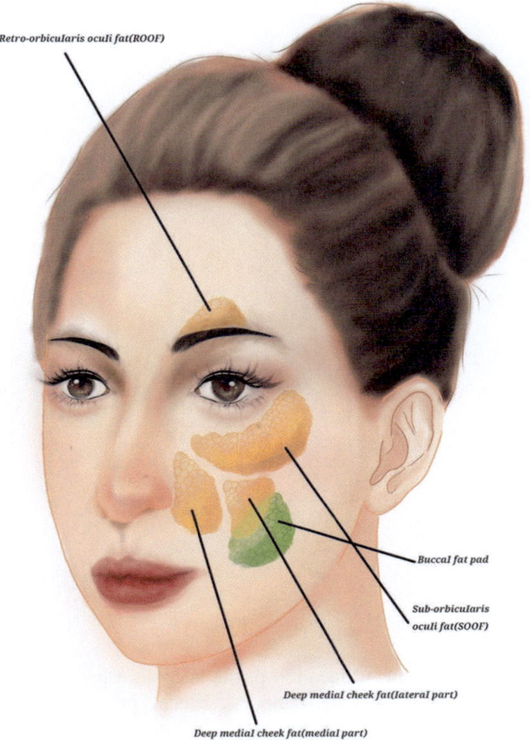

The Deepest Fat Pads of the Face

The buccal fat pad, characterised by the presence of deposit or metabolic type white adipose tissue, comprises large adipocytes that are marked by an exceedingly sparse or absent collagen network devoid of individual adipocyte encapsulation (Fig. 2.11) [12]. Occupying the buccotemporal space sandwiched between the buccinator muscle and the masseter muscle fascia, it holds a central position in the midface [10, 22, 23]. This fat pad exhibits four distinct extensions [10, 23]:

- Buccal
- Pterygoid
- Pterygopalatine
- Temporal (superficial and deep)

The superficial and deep temporal projections of the buccal fat pad are delineated by the temporal fascia, thus establishing a distinct separation from the temporal fat pad [23, 24].

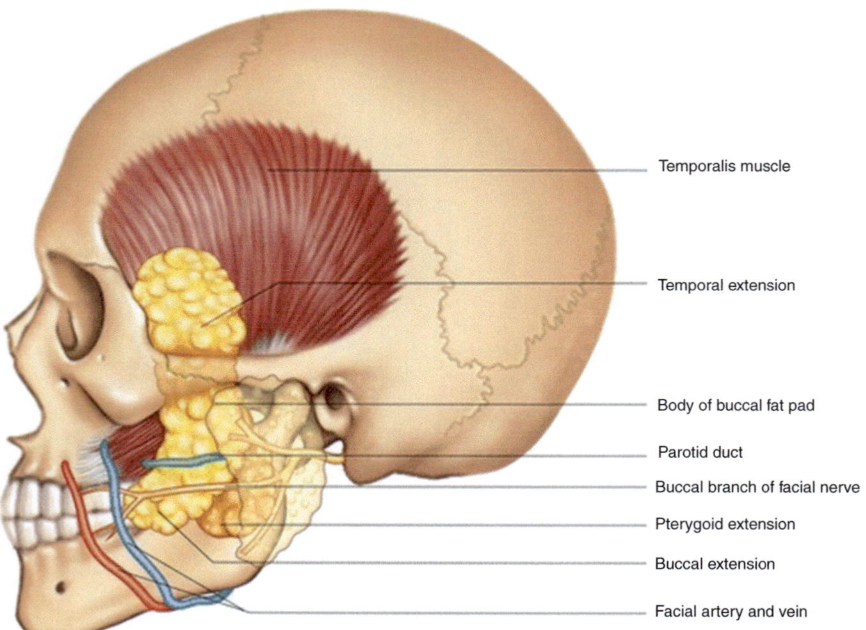

Fig. 2.11 Anatomical location of the buccal fat pad. The buccal fat pad is composed of a main body and four extensions (temporal, buccal, pterygoid, and pterygopalatine) [26]. Reproduced with permission from Kim, M.K., Han, W. and Kim, S.G. The use of the buccal fat pad flap for oral reconstruction. Maxillofacial Plastic and Reconstructive Surgery 2017; 39(1):1–9. Reproduced under a CC BY 4.0 licence

A more recent cadaveric study has shown that the buccal fat pad is divided into three lobes that are enclosed by separate membranes. This division is done according to the structure of the lobar envelopes, the formation of the ligaments, and the source of vessels [23, 25]:

- Anterior
  - Located below the zygoma
  - Extends anterior to the buccinator
- Intermediate
  - Located in the space around the lateral maxilla between the anterior and posterior lobes
- Posterior
  - Located in the masticatory space and its surrounding areas
  - Runs up to the infraorbital fissure and space around the temporalis muscle
  - Runs down towards the upper rim of the mandibular body
  - Has four extensions
    The buccal process (the most superficial process, under the parotid duct)

The pterygopalatine process (extends to the pterygopalatine fossa and encloses the pterygopalatine vessels)
The pterygoid process (remains in the pterygoid space)
The temporal process—this is subdivided into:
Superficial process
Profound process

Six ligaments anchor the various parts of the buccal fat pad, in addition to serving as entry points of vessels to the buccal fat pad. Each lobe is anchored by 2–4 ligaments to the surrounding structures.

The fat pad found between the superficial and the deep lamina of the deep temporal fascia, superiorly to the zygomatic arch, is another one of the deepest fat pads [10].

Ligaments

The superficial fascia is secured to the facial skeleton through a system of retaining ligaments, acting as anchor points binding the dermis to the skeleton with the components of this system passing through all facial layers [27]. There are three morphological forms of retaining ligaments of the face (Fig. 2.12):

- Ligaments
- Adhesions
- Septae

Interestingly, most facial ligaments are arranged into a single line lateral to the lateral orbital rim and extend from the temporal crest to the mandible [13]. This arrangement of ligaments is known as the line of ligaments. From superior to inferior, ligaments are [13] as follows:

- The temporal ligamentous adhesions
- Lateral orbital thickening
- Zygomatic ligament
- Mandibular ligament

The face is divided into two parts due to the presence of the line of ligament: medial to it is the medial midface, and lateral to it is the lateral midface. In the medial midface, a parallel arrangement of facial layers is not found because of the oblique course of mimetic muscles from bone to skin. On the other hand, fascial layers are arranged in a distinct parallel way in the lateral midface [13].

The facial retaining ligaments all have intrinsic viscoelastic properties, with some having more robust mechanical properties than others [25]. The zygomatic ligament is the strongest, followed by the orbital, mandibular, and maxillary

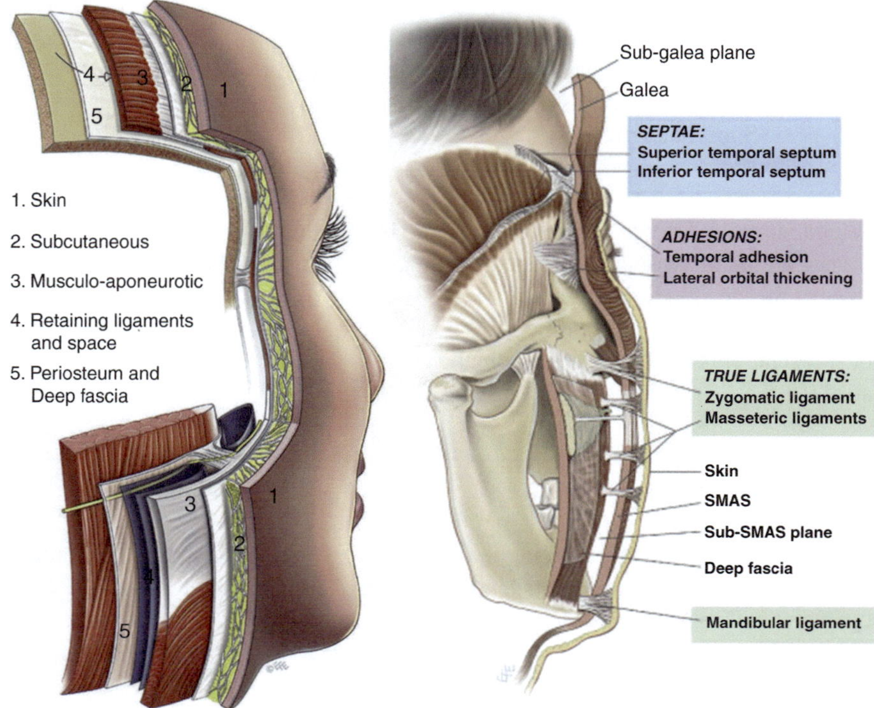

Fig. 2.12 The face is constructed of five basic layers; on the right-hand side, ligaments, septae, and adhesions can be seen. Reproduced with permission from Fitzgerald, R., Carqueville, J. and Yang, P.T., 2019. An approach to structural facial rejuvenation with fillers in women. International journal of women's dermatology, 5(1), pp. 52–67

ligaments. Regarding stiffness/rigidity, the zygomatic ligament is the most rigid, followed by the orbital, maxillary, and mandibular ligaments [28].

Musculature and SMAS

The facial musculature can be divided into two main groups:

- Muscles of mastication
- Mimetic muscles (muscles of facial expression)

Mimetic Muscles

The muscles of facial expression are employed to convey various emotions and feelings (Figs. 2.13 and 2.14) [29]. These muscles also provide a sphincteric function around the orifices. Lot [29] of these muscles lack bone attachments and are

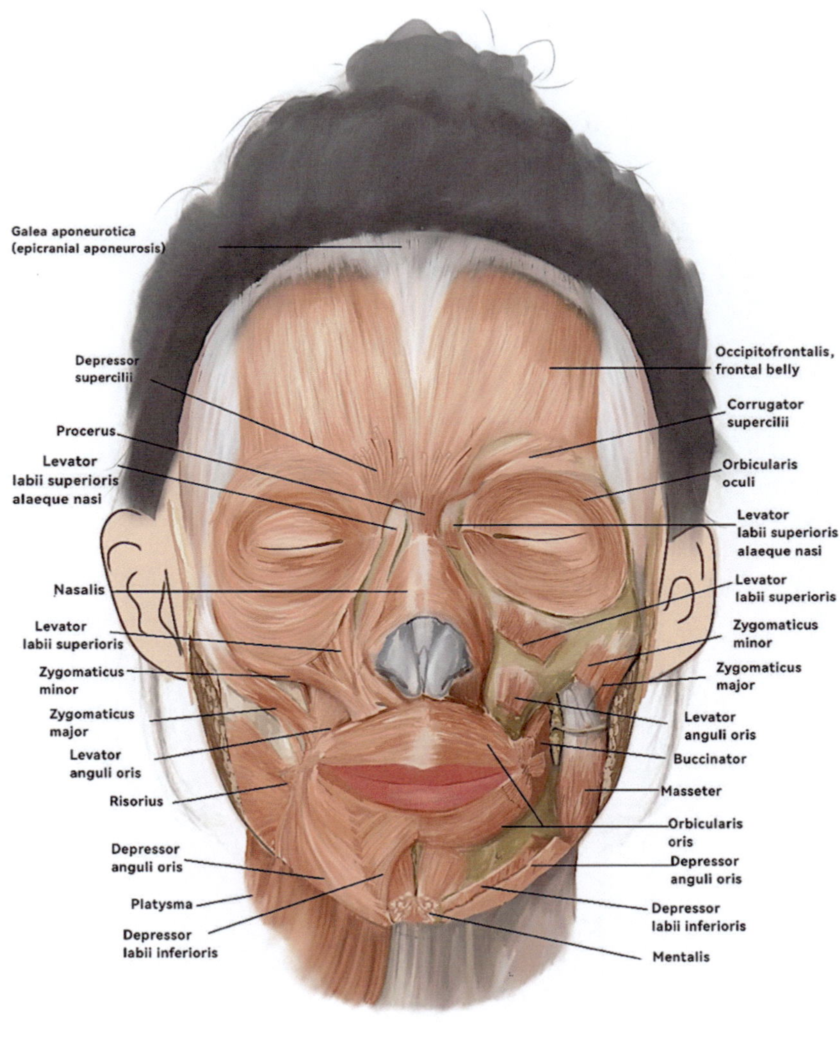

Fig. 2.13 Facial muscles

connected to the surrounding soft tissues and skin. They are arranged into four distinct layers [29]

- First layer
  - Orbicularis oculi
  - Risorius

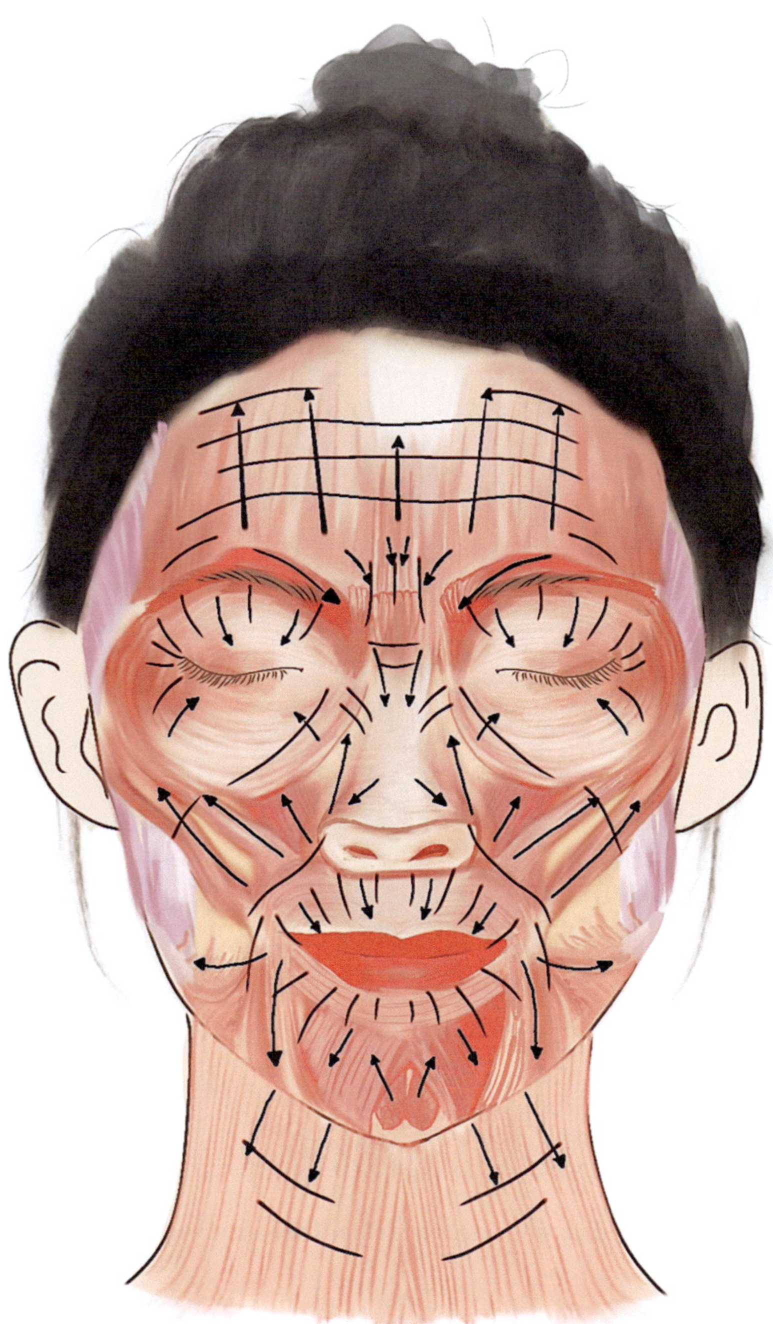

Fig. 2.14 Facial muscles and their actions

- – Zygomaticus minor
- – Depressor anguli oris
- Second layer
  - – Depressor labii inferior
  - – Zygomaticus major
  - – Levator labii superioris alaeque nasi
  - – Platysma
- Third layer
  - – Orbicularis oris
  - – Levator labii superioris
- Fourth layer
  - – Buccinator
  - – Mentalis
  - – Levator anguli oris

The top three layers are connected to the overlying dermis through an aponeurotic network of collagen and elastic fibres and fat cells. This superficial fascia is known as Superficial Musculoaponeurotic System (SMAS). This fascia is considerably distinctive in buccal, temporal, zygomatic, and platysma areas, serving as its anatomical borders [1]. It is regarded as the core tendon for the coordinated contraction of the face muscles and plays a functional role in displaying various facial emotions [30].

The following are prominent mimetic muscles (Figs. 2.13 and 2.14):

- **Frontalis:**
- It is the most significant muscle of the upper face and is the anterior belly of the occipitofrontalis muscle of the scalp with no bony attachment [29].
- Four types of frontalis muscle with four different patterns of horizontal parallel lines on the forehead skin have been reported [31]:
  - – Type I: Full form
  - – Type II: V-shaped
  - – Type III: Central
  - – Type IV: Lateral form
- Its function is to elevate the brows and create forehead furrows [29].
- **Orbicularis oculi:**
- It is a flat sphincter-like muscle lying directly under the skin of the eyelids, arranged in concentric bands around the upper and lower eyelid [29, 32].
- The orbicularis oculi muscle acts as a sphincter, causing the closing of the eyelids and aiding in the drainage of the eye's tears into the nasolacrimal duct system [32].
- The orbital portion of the orbicularis oculi is more engaged in voluntary eyelid closure, such as when winking or squeezing the eyelid. The preseptal piece is responsible for both voluntary and involuntary blink closing of the eye and maintaining the eyelids closed during sleep. The pretarsal region is more engaged in

the involuntary blinking of the eye and supporting closed eyelids during sleep [32].

- **Corrugator supercillii:**
- It is one muscle with two heads: a transverse head and an oblique head, arising from the superciliary arch/superomedial part of the orbital rim and inserting into the dermis of the middle of the eyebrow [29, 31, 33].
- Three types have been reported [31]:
  - Type I (fan-shaped): The muscle insertion in the deep layer of the medial half of the eyebrow
  - Type II: Insertion in the intermediate portion of the medial half of the eyebrow
  - Type III (narrow ribbon): A muscle strip inserted in the medial end of the eyebrow
- Its contraction results in brow depression and vertical wrinkles known as frown lines [29].
- **Procerus:**
- Two small pyramidal muscles arise from the nasal bone's lower part and insert into the skin between the eyebrows [31].
- Its contraction produces horizontal creases at the bridges of the nose [29].
- **Nasalis:**
- It consists of two parts: the upper part on the nasal dorsum, known as compressor naris, and the lower alar part, called dilator naris. The transverse part causes wrinkles over the dorsum of the nose, while the alar part causes dilation of the nasal apertures (flaring nostrils) [29].
- **Orbicularis oris:**
- A complex, multi-layered muscle that connects to the upper and lower lip dermis via a thin, superficial musculoaponeurotic system and acts as an attachment point for several other facial muscles in the perioral region [34].
- It is functionally composed of many components that work alone or with other facial muscles [35].
- The deeper fibres act as a sphincter of the mouth, originating from the angle of the mouth (modiolus) and are inserted in the lips' mucous membrane [29, 36].
- The superficial fibres are the retractor fibres associated with facial expressions and the precise lip motions required for speaking [36, 37].
- Other functions include protrusion of the lips, swallowing, mastication, and sucking, and contribution to the production of speech and sound and the position of dental arches/dentition [2, 36].
- **Buccinator:**
- It originates laterally from the alveolar processes of the mandible and maxillae and is inserted in the modiolus of the mouth [29].
- It plays a significant role in keeping the food within the vestibule [2]. It compresses the cheeks, expels air between the lips, and aids in mastication. It presses the cheeks during chewing and blowing against the molars.
- **Zygomaticus major:**
- Extending from the zygomatic bone, this muscle runs downwards to the angle of the mouth. During laughter, its contraction causes the mouth to elevate.

- **Zygomaticus minor:**
- This small muscle originates medially to the zygomaticus major muscle and inserts into the upper lip.
- It elevates the upper lip and also deepens the nasolabial sulcus [2].
- **Levator labii superioris:**
- It originates from the infraorbital margin and inserts into the upper lip, elevating the upper lip on contraction [2].
- **Risorius:**
- Its origin is from the parotid fascia and buccal skin, and its insertion is at the modiolus [29].
- It aids in laterally repositioning the oral commissures.
- **Levator anguli oris:**
- It originates from the canine fossa of the maxillae and is inserted into the angle of the mouth.
- Its contraction deepens the nasolabial sulcus [2].
- **Depressor anguli oris:**
- It originates from the anterolateral base of the mandible and extends up to the angle of the mouth [2].
- It draws the lateral borders of the mouth inferiorly [29].
- **Depressor labii inferioris:**
- It originates from the platysma and the anterolateral body of the mandible and is inserted in the lower lip.
- It helps in the retraction and eversion of the lips (pouting).
- **Mentalis:**
- Its origin is from the body of the mandible, and its insertion is into the skin of the chin.
- It causes elevation of the chin.
- **Platysma:**
- It is a sheet-like muscle originating from the subcutaneous tissue of the infraclavicular and supraclavicular regions. Its insertion is at the base of the mandible, the skin of the cheek & the lower lip, angle of the mouth (modiolus), and orbicularis oris. It has three parts (Fig. 2.15) [38]:
  - Pars labialis
  - Pars Modiolaris
  - Pars Mandibularis

It contributes to various facial expressions and the contraction of the soft tissues of the lower face and neck [29, 38].

Masticatory Muscles

Four muscles are involved in mastication (Fig. 2.16):

- Temporalis

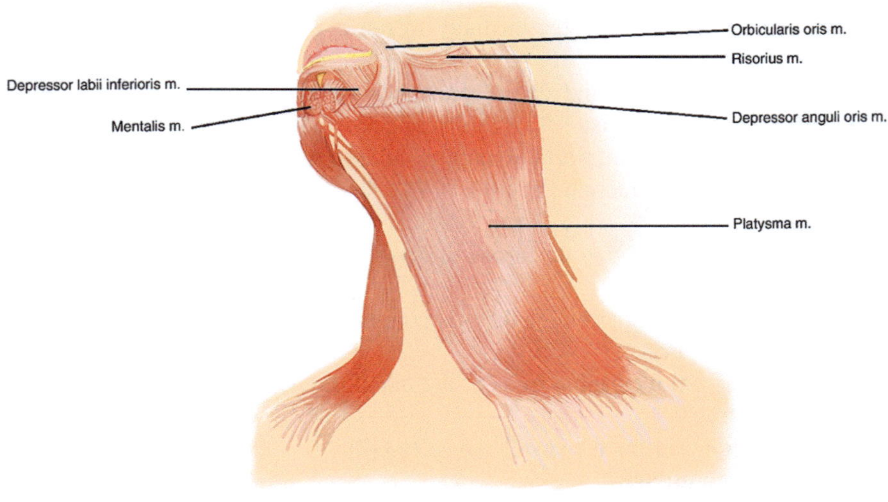

Fig. 2.15 Platysma muscles

- Masseter
- Lateral pterygoid
- Medial pterygoid

These muscles are located in the lateral portion of the face, deep to the deep fascia.

- **Temporalis:**
- It is a triangular muscle with a proximal attachment to the floor of the temporal fossa and the deep surface of the temporal fascia. Distally, it has a tip-shaped attachment to the coronoid process and the anterior border of the ramus of the mandible.
- It helps in the elevation and retraction of the mandible [29].
- **Masseter:**
- It is a quadrate muscle with a proximal attachment to the maxillary process of the zygomatic bone and zygomatic arch. Distally, it is attached to the angle and lateral border of the ramus of the mandible. It helps in the closing of the jaw by elevating the mandible [29].
- **Lateral pterygoid:**
- This muscle has two heads of origin. Its superior head originates from the infratemporal surface, while the inferior head arises from the lateral plate of the pterygoid process. The insertion of the muscle is into the neck of the mandible and the capsule of the temporomandibular joint. It helps in protrusion and side-to-side movement of the mandible [29].

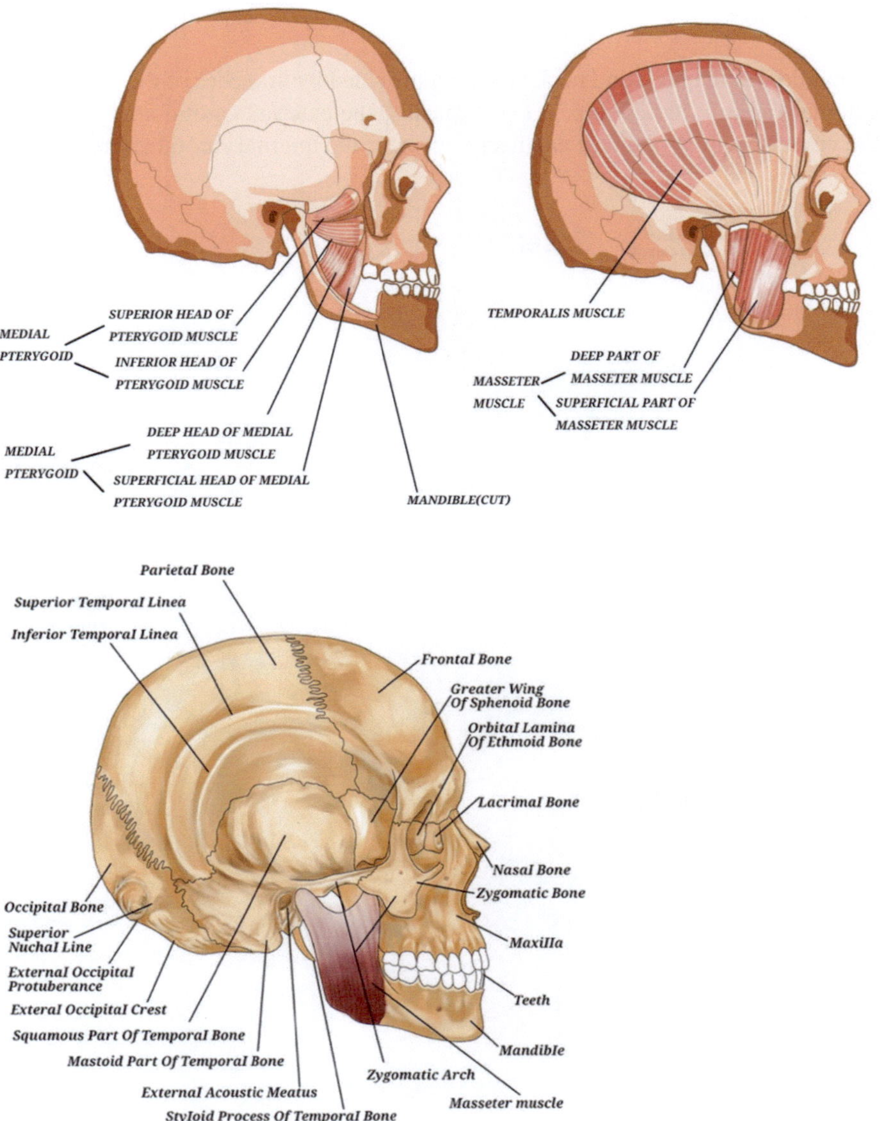

Fig. 2.16 Muscles of mastication: temporalis, masseter, medial, and lateral pterygoid. The Buccinator muscle is an accessory muscle of mastication. It compresses the cheeks inwards against molars and aids in chewing and swallowing

- **Medial pterygoid:**
- Its superficial head arises from the medial surface of the lateral pterygoid plate, while its deep head arises from the tuberosity of the maxillae. It is inserted into the medial surface of the ramus of the mandible. It acts synergistically with the masseter to elevate the mandible [29].

Vasculature

Blood flow to the head and neck is mainly provided by branches of the internal and external carotid arteries (Fig. 2.17). Typically, the external carotid artery provides the viscerocranium (the face and neck), whereas the internal carotid artery supplies

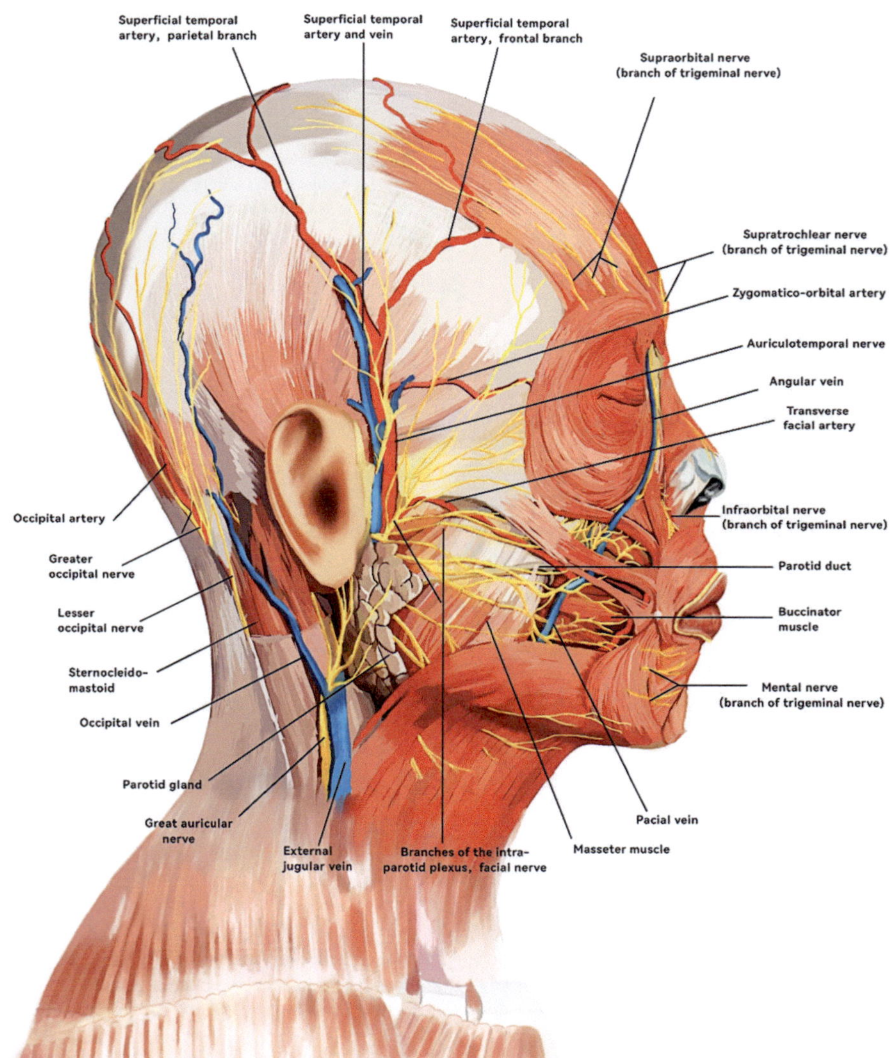

Fig. 2.17 Vasculature of the face

Table 2.3 Anastomoses between extracranial and intracranial arteries and their respective branches

Extracranial artery/branch	Intracranial artery/branch
Middle meningeal artery[a,b]	Orbital and anterior branch of OA[b]
Anterior deep temporal artery[a,b]	Lacrimal artery[b]
Infraorbital artery[a,b]	Medial and lateral muscular branches of the OA[b]
Infraorbital artery[a,b]	Dorsal nasal artery[b]
Sphenopalatine artery[b]	Anterior and posterior ethmoidal artery[b]
Superficial temporal artery anterior branch[b]	Supraorbital artery[b]
Superficial temporal artery anterior branch[b]	Supratrochlear artery[b]
Middle meningeal artery[a,b]	Superficial petrosal artery[b]
Accessory meningeal artery[a]	Inferolateral trunk
Middle meningeal artery[a]	Cavernous branch of the inferolateral trunk of ICA
Vidian artery[a]	Petrous/horizontal segment of ICA
Artery of foramen rotundum[a]	Inferolateral trunk
Transverse facial artery	Dorsal nasal artery
Facial artery	Dorsal nasal artery
Superior pharyngeal artery	Lateral clival artery
Occipital artery	Stylomastoid artery
Occipital artery	Vertebral artery segment 1–2
Ascending and deep cervical arteries	Vertebral artery segment 3–7

Reproduced with permission from Cotofana, Sebastian M.D., Ph.D.; Lachman, Nirusha Ph.D. Arteries of the Face and Their Relevance for Minimally Invasive Facial Procedures: An Anatomical Review, Plastic and Reconstructive Surgery: February 2019 - Volume 143 - Issue 2 - p 416–426 [39]
OA ophthalmic artery, *ICA* internal carotid artery
[a]Internal maxillary artery
[b]Branches of the ophthalmic artery

the neurocranium (i.e. the brain, orbit, and the bony cranial vault). Multiple connections between the external carotid artery and the internal carotid artery provide collateral blood flow, resulting in different vascular regions (Table 2.3, Figs. 2.18 and 2.19) [39]. Anastomotic pathways can compensate for decreased arterial blood flow in one zone. In contrast, these anastomotic pathways allow injectables that reach the arterial bloodstream to cross and enter the other vascular zone.

The primary supply of blood to the face is through the *external carotid artery*, but the internal carotid artery also contributes [40]. The ophthalmic artery, which originates from the internal carotid artery, is the primary arterial contributor to the forehead [41].

The arterial supply of the face is from different plexuses: deep plexus, subcutaneous plexus, and subdermal plexus [29]. These plexuses communicate through the perforating arteries. The deep facial plexus supplies the deeper parts lying under the

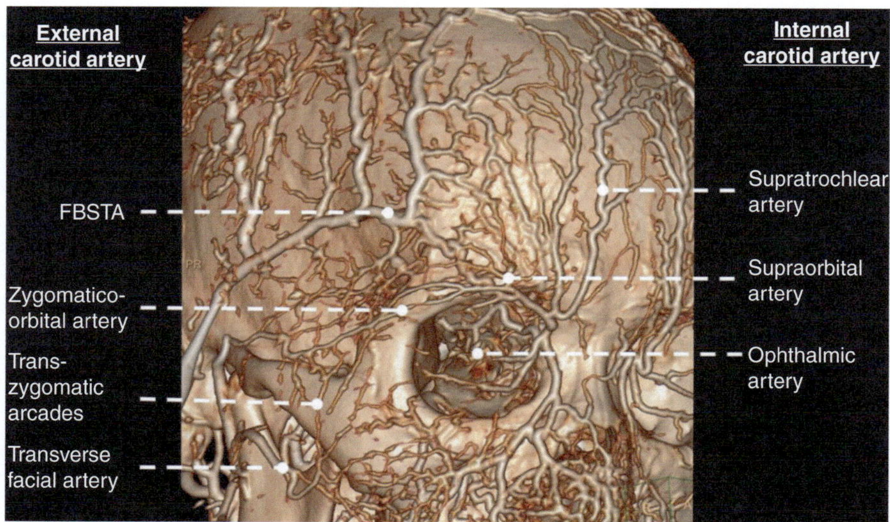

Fig. 2.18 Computed tomographic angiographic (CTA) scan of the right hemifacial side of a study participant. In this study, the relevant branches of the external carotid artery were the superficial temporal artery, the zygomatico-orbital artery, the transverse facial artery and the transzygomatic arcades. A strong vascular network around the forehead and orbit with multiple anastomotic connections can be seen in this CTA scan. FBSTA, frontal branch of the superficial temporal artery [46]. Reproduced with permission from Zhen-Hao Li, MD, Michael Alfertshofer, Wei-Jin Hong, MD, PhD, Xin-Rui Li, MD, You-Liang Zhang, MD, Nicholas Moellhoff, MD, Konstantin Frank, MD, Sheng-Kang Luo, MD, PhD, Sebastian Cotofana, MD, PhD, Upper Facial Anastomoses Between the External and Internal Carotid Vascular Territories – A 3D Computed Tomographic Investigation, Aesthetic Surgery Journal, 2022; sjac060

mimetic muscles. This plexus communicates with the subdermal plexus through musculocutaneous branches.

The main arteries of the face originate from either [41, 42]:

- Directly from the external carotid artery
  - Facial artery
  - Superficial temporal artery
- Branches of the external carotid artery
  - Transverse facial artery from the superficial temporal artery
  - Infraorbital artery from the maxillary artery

The main supply is through the main branch of the external carotid artery called the *facial artery* [29]. It starts at the lower border of the mandible, gives off different branches, and ultimately terminates by anastomosing with arteries of the internal carotid artery at the angle of the nose.

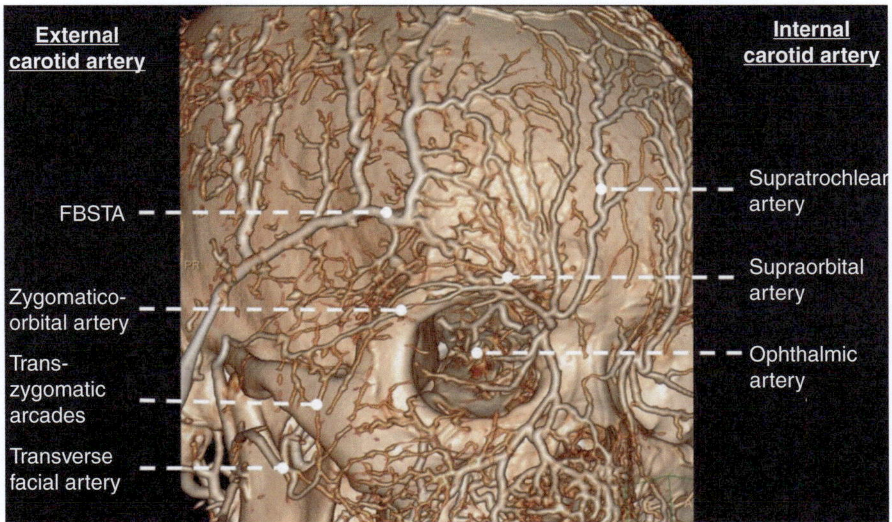

Fig. 2.19 Computed tomographic angiographic (CTA) scan of the right hemifacial side of a study participant. This CTA scan shows the most common type of location for the connection of communicating branches: both superficial and deep to the superficial fascia. The deep anastomosis can be identified due to the engulfed appearance, while the branches forming the superficial anastomosis appear to be more prominent. Reproduced with permission from Zhen-Hao Li, MD, Michael Alfertshofer, Wei-Jin Hong, MD, PhD, Xin-Rui Li, MD, You-Liang Zhang, MD, Nicholas Moellhoff, MD, Konstantin Frank, MD, Sheng-Kang Luo, MD, PhD, Sebastian Cotofana, MD, PhD, Upper Facial Anastomoses Between the External and Internal Carotid Vascular Territories – A 3D Computed Tomographic Investigation, Aesthetic Surgery Journal, 2022; sjac060

The facial artery originates from the carotid triangle (the superior belly of the omohyoid muscle, the sternocleidomastoid, and the posterior belly of the digastric) and supplies the anatomical structures of the superficial face. It has a tortuous course that enables stretching during facial actions, e.g. mastication [43].

The facial artery originates deep within the platysma muscle and becomes superficial soon after. The vessel courses deep to the posterior belly of the digastric and stylohyoid muscles, continuing along the posterior surface of the submandibular gland [44]. The artery moves upward over the body of the mandible, passing alongside the anteroinferior border of the masseter muscle. The pulse of the facial artery can easily be palpated in this region. The artery continues superiorly at an oblique angle towards the oral commissure. Following this, the artery ascends along the side of the nose, terminating at the medial canthus of the eye as the angular artery [45]. The table below summarises the arteries of the face.

Venous Drainage

The internal jugular vein is a paired vein that gathers blood from the brain, superficial facial areas, and neck, sending it to the right atrium (Fig. 2.20) [47].

Many veins accompany the eponymous arteries in the face. Exceptions include the inferior ophthalmic vein and retromandibular vein [41]. The facial vein and artery follow distinct paths in the face and are spaced apart by a specific distance. While the facial vein and artery are located adjacent to one another at the mandible's lower border, the artery follows a convoluted journey via the midface muscles of facial expression, whilst the vein follows a straight path from the medial canthus to the lower mandible [41]. There are many communications between facial and intra-cerebral veins. Valves are reported to be present in many of the veins in the facial region.

Superficial veins of the face are of clinical importance because they also communicate with the cavernous sinus. Thus, especially in the area around the nose, the medial part of the lips and medial canthus is known as the "danger area" because it is drained by the facial vein, and the facial vein communicates with the cavernous sinus [29]. Infection can spread from the external face to the cavernous sinus through this communication.

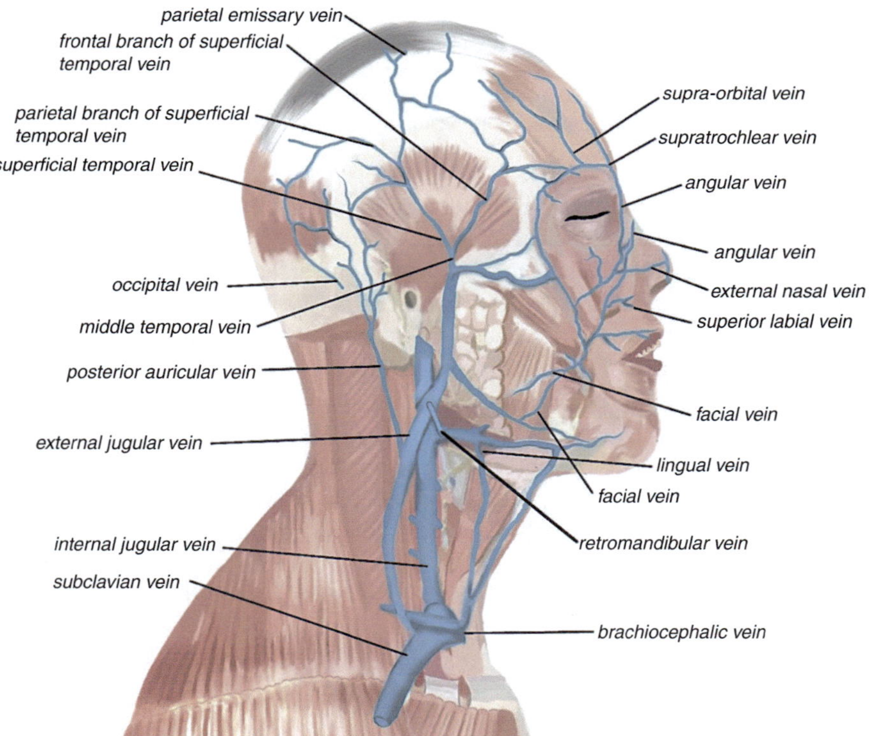

Fig. 2.20 Venous drainage of the face

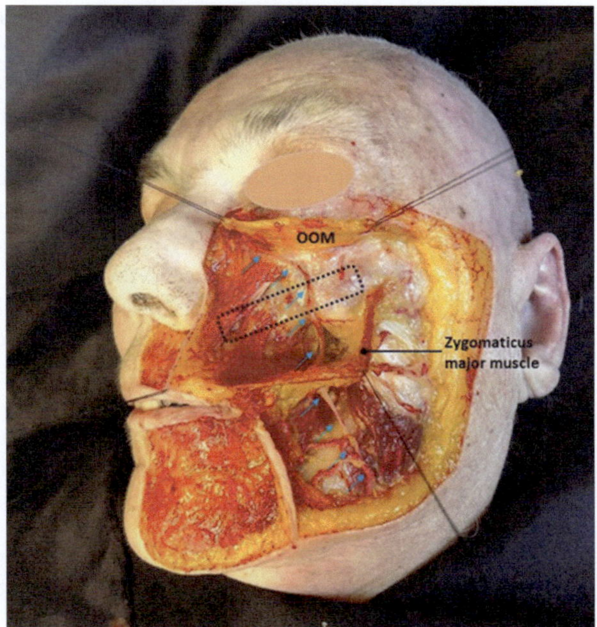

Fig. 2.21 Cadaveric dissection of the left side of the face of a fresh male cadaveric specimen. The facial/angular vein is indicated by the blue arrows. The ultrasound transducer was positioned cranial to the zygomaticus major muscle and inferior to the attachment of the orbicularis oculi muscle (OOM), as indicated by the dotted square [48]. Reproduced with permission from Cotofana, S, Lowry, N, Devineni, A, et al. Can smiling influence the blood flow in the facial vein? An experimental study. J Cosmet Dermatol. 2019

Minimally invasive and surgical interventions that modify the SMAS, the periocular musculature or the deep midfacial fat compartments could impact angular/facial venous flow (Fig. 2.21) [48].

Lymphatics

The lymphatic system is comprised of a capillary network made up of pre-collecting and collecting lymph capillaries, lymphatic trunks and ducts, and lymph nodes [41, 49]. Lymph vessels are part of the circulatory system. They are small and transparent channels. Lymph vessels, through the lymphatic ducts, offer alternative routes for returning interstitial fluid (lymph) to the subclavian veins. Lymphatic channels develop a muscular wall and subsequently an adventitia as they grow in size on their route to collecting lymph nodes. These extra layers contribute to the reduction of trans-mural absorption. As a result, lymphatic absorption occurs at a lower rate in the deeper subcutaneous and muscular layers [50]. It is believed that lymphatics drain inwardly from superficial to deep as they progress toward the larger lymphatic vessels and nodes preceding moving into the systemic circulation [50].

Lymph-collecting vessels are found in three regions of the superficial tissue of the head and neck [49]:

- The scalp
- The face
- The cervical region

These vessels are dense in the scalp and lateral neck area and sparse in the facial, anterior, and posterior neck (Fig. 2.22) [49]. Lymphatic drainage of the face is limited to certain areas. The lymphatic vessels of the face travel radially from medial to lateral toward their first-tier lymph nodes found in the deep aspect of the subcutaneous tissue between the eyebrow and the inferior border of the mandible [49].

Superficial lymphatic vessels accompany facial veins, while, on the other hand, deep lymphatics run parallel to arteries, and all these drain into deep cervical lymph nodes [2], which is a whole chain of lymph nodes along the internal jugular vein. Lymph from these lymph nodes passes to the jugular lymphatic trunk, which ultimately drains into the thoracic duct on the left side and brachiocephalic vein on the right side. Following is a summary of lymphatic drainage of different face regions [2]:

- *Superficial parotid lymph nodes*: lateral part of face and scalp, and eyelids
- *Deep cervical lymph nodes*: lymph from deep parotid nodes

Peripheral lymph nodes and associated anatomic sites	
Lymph Node Group	**Sites**
Preauricular	Conjunctiva, anterior and temporal scalp, anterior ear canal
Posterior auricular	Parietal and temporal scalp
Parotid	Forehead, midface, temporal scalp, external ear canal, middle ear, parotid glands, gums
Cervical-superficial	Parotid gland, lower larynx, lower ear canal
Cervical	Larynx, thyroid, palate, esophagus, paranasal sinuses, tonsils, adenoids, posterior scalp and neck, nose
Occipital	Posterior scalp
Submandibular	Nose, lips, tongue, cheek, submandibular gland, buccal mucosa
Submental	Floor of mouth, lower lip
Supraclavicular	Chest and abdomen (left supraclavicular, abdomen; right supraclavicular, mediastinum and lungs)
Axillary	Lower neck, upper extremity, lateral breast, chest wall
Deltopectoral	Upper extremity
Epitrochlear	Upper extremity below the elbow
Inguinal	Lower extremity, genital region, buttock, abdominal wall below the umbilicus
Popliteal	Lower extremity below the knee

Adapted from Henry M, Kamat D. Integrating basic science into clinical teaching initiative series: approach to lymphadenopathy. Clin Pediatr (Phila) 2011;50(8):685, with permission; and Friedmann AM. Evaluation and management of lymphadenopathy in children. Pediatr Rev 2008;29(2):54, with permission.

Fig. 2.22 Lymph-collecting vessels are found in three regions of the superficial tissue of the head and neck. Peripheral lymph nodes and associated anatomic sites. Reproduced with permission from Motyckova, Gabriela, and David P. Steensma. "Why does my patient have lymphadenopathy or splenomegaly?" Hematology/Oncology Clinics 26.2 (2012): 395–408 [51]

- *Submandibular lymph nodes*: upper lip and lateral parts of the lower lip
- *Submental lymph nodes*: chin and central part of the lower lip

According to facial areas [41, 49]:
The forehead
An average of four lymph vessels (range of three to five) drained to:

- The pre-auricular lymph nodes
- Deep parotid lymph nodes
- Retroauricular, nasolabial, or buccinator lymph nodes (occasional).

The eyelids
Distinct lymph vessels originating from the medial and lateral eyelid commissures drain to:

- Pre-auricular lymph nodes (mainly)
- The parotid lymph nodes (mainly)
- Submandibular lymph nodes
- Buccinator lymph nodes (rarely)

The nose
Drain into:

- The buccinator lymph nodes
- Submandibular lymph nodes
- Nasolabial lymph nodes (rarely)

Perioral region
Labial lymph vessels arise adjacent to the lip commissures and drain to:

- The buccinator lymph nodes
- Submandibular lymph nodes
- Submental lymph nodes (rarely)

The chin
Drain into:

- The submental lymph nodesBoth submental and submandibular lymph nodes

Nerve Supply of Face

The nerve supply of the face consists of two types: cutaneous nerve supply and motor nerve supply. The main and primary cutaneous nerve supply of the face is through the trigeminal nerve (cranial nerve V) [40]. The motor supply of the muscles of the face is through the facial nerve (cranial nerve VII) and the mandibular branch (V3) of the trigeminal nerve.

- **Cutaneous Nerve Supply**
- The cutaneous nerve supply of the face is primarily supplied by the three branches of the trigeminal nerve, which further give off branches to different parts of the face. The three main branches of the trigeminal nerve are [2] as follows:
  - Ophthalmic nerve (V1)
  - Maxillary nerve (V2)
  - Mandibular nerve (V3)
- These three branches further give off branches to supply different regions of the face (Figs. 2.23 and 2.24) [2].
- **Motor nerve supply:**
- The nerve supply of mimetic muscles is through branches of the facial nerve, while that of the masticatory muscles is through the mandibular nerve.
  - **Mimetic muscles:**
  - The facial nerve's motor root supplies the muscles of expression (Figs. 2.25 and 2.26). It exits the cranial cavity through *stylomastoid foramen* and then enters the parotid gland, where it gives off five terminal branches, which, along with their distribution, are as follows [2]:

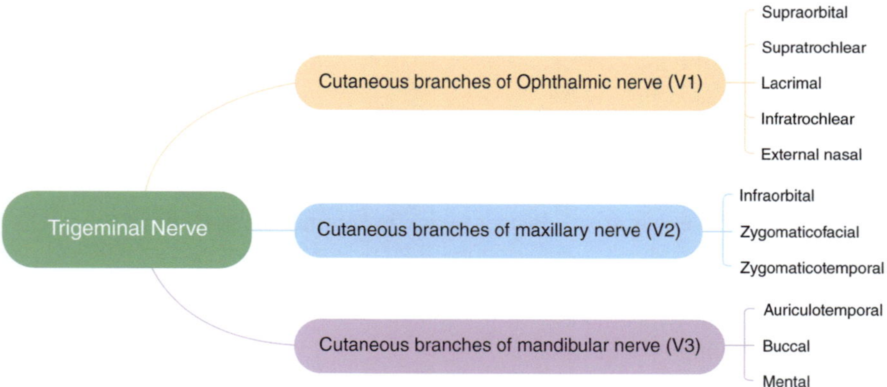

Fig. 2.23 Cutaneous nerve supply of the face is primarily supplied by the three branches of the trigeminal nerve, which further give off branches to different parts of the face

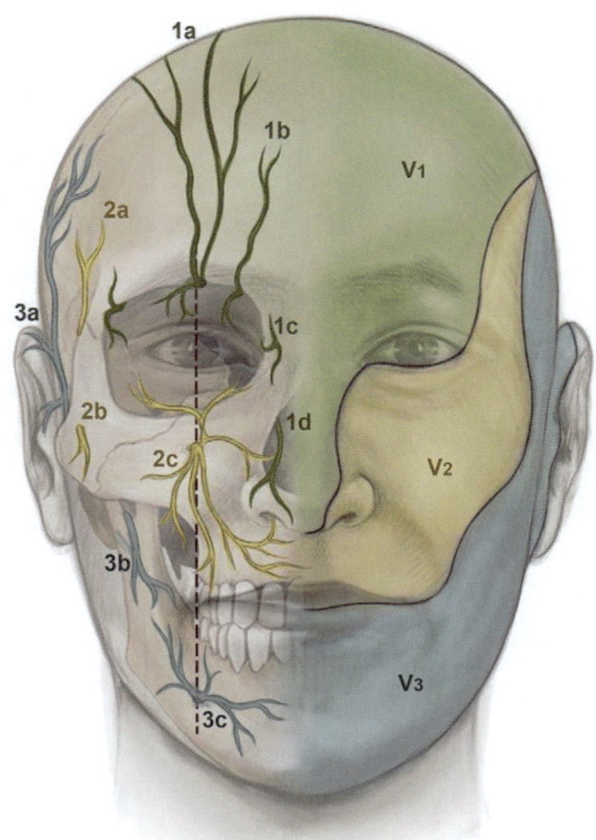

Fig. 2.24 Cutaneous innervation of the face. Ophthalmic nerve (V1), (1a) supraorbital nerve, (1b) supratrochlear nerve, (1c) infratrochlear nerve, (1d) external nasal nerve; Maxillary nerve (V2), (2a) zygomaticotemporal nerve, (2b) zygomaticofacial nerve, (2c) infraorbital nerve; Mandibular nerve (V3), (3a) auriculotemporal nerve, (3b) buccal nerve, (3c) mental nerve. Reproduced with permission from Marur, T., Y. Tuna, and S. Demirci, Facial anatomy. Clinics in Dermatology, 2014. 32(1): p. 14–23 [29]

- **Masticatory muscles:**
- When the mandibular nerve emerges from the trigeminal ganglion, it immediately receives the motor root of the trigeminal nerve and enters the infratemporal fossa through the foramen ovale. It gives off the following four branches, which supply the muscles of mastication [2]:

  Deep temporal nerve: supplies the temporalis

  Masseteric nerve: supplies the masseter muscle

  The medial pterygoid nerve: supplies the medial pterygoid muscle

  Lateral pterygoid nerve: supplies the lateral pterygoid muscle

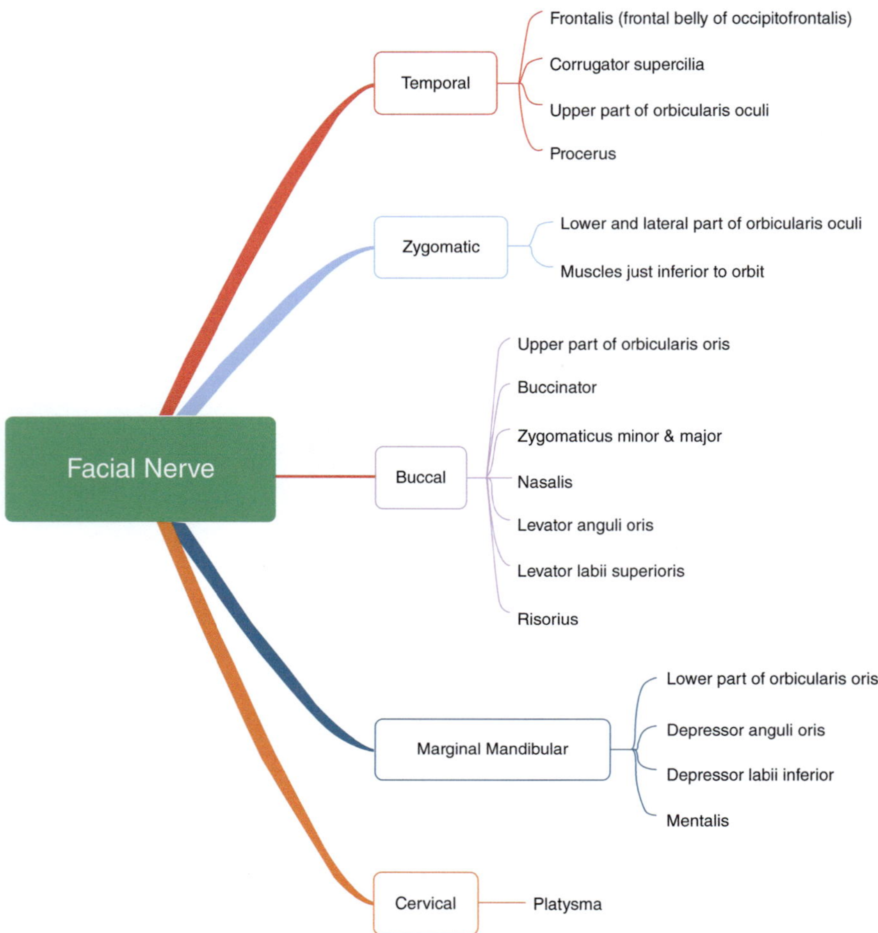

Fig. 2.25 Branches of the facial nerve: muscles of facial expression and innervation by the facial nerve (cranial nerve II)

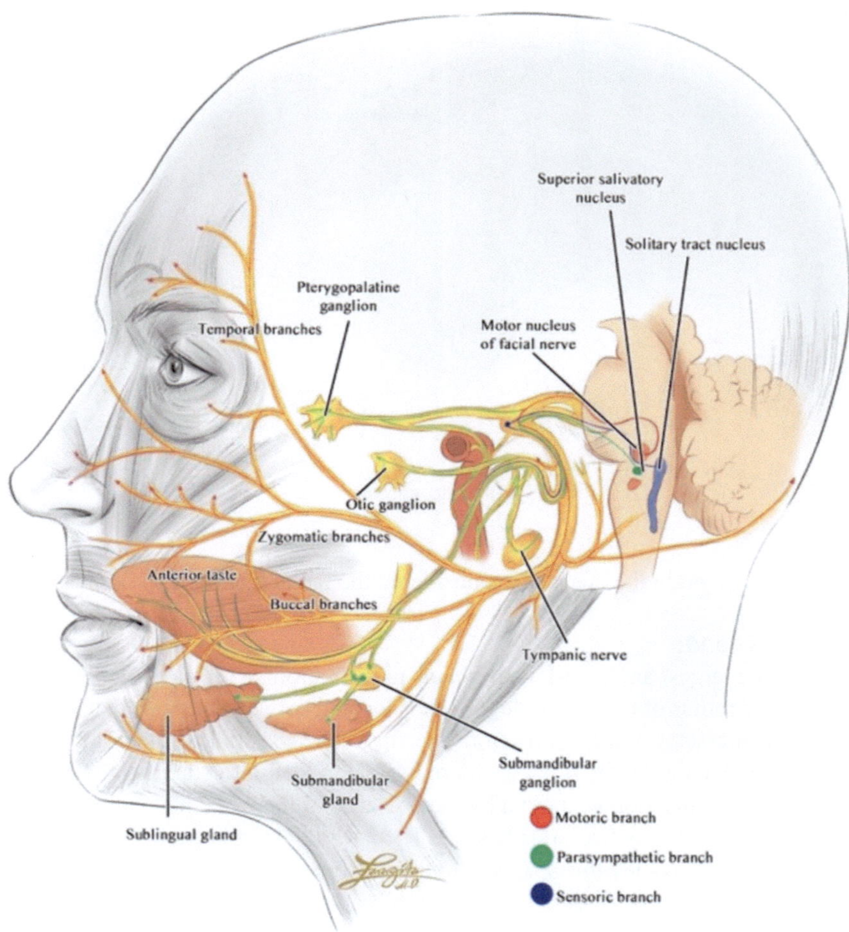

Fig. 2.26 Facial nerve course of motor, sensory, and parasympathetic innervation. Reproduced with permission from Nugroho, S.W., et al., Predicting outcome of hemifacial spasm after microvascular decompression with intraoperative monitoring: A systematic review. Heliyon, 2021. 7(2): p. e06115 [52]

Glands of Face

There are three major salivary glands in the face (Fig. 2.27) [2].

Parotid gland
Submandibular gland
Sublingual gland

Fig. 2.27 Salivary glands

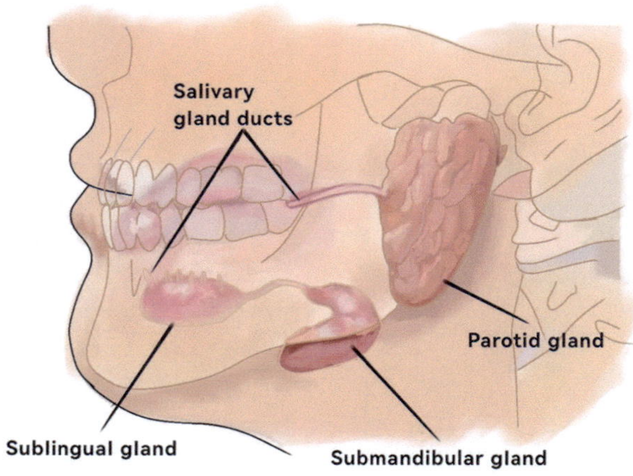

The lacrimal gland in the eye is also considered the facial gland that produces tears.

- **Parotid Gland:**

  It is the largest among all other glands in the region and is palpable because it lies on the ramus of the mandible [53]. It is located between the sternocleidomastoid and masseter and extends from the tip of the mastoid to the angle of the mandible. Anatomically, it is considered to be divided into superficial and deep portions. This division is marked by the presence of the facial nerve that enters it and divides it into its five branches [2]. The parotid gland is enclosed in a tough capsule known as the *parotid sheath*, derived from investing layer of deep cervical fascia [2]. Stensen's duct emerges from its anterior portion. It runs over the masseter muscle and buccal fat pad, then turns medially, and opens into the vestibule of the mouth after piercing the buccinator [53]. Its lymphatic drainage is into *parotid lymph nodes*, which drain into the internal jugular chain lymph nodes. The sympathetic supply is from the *external carotid nerve plexus*, and secretory fibres come from the *otic ganglion* through the auriculotemporal nerve [2].

  It is an area of importance for both surgical and non-surgical procedures due to the presence of important facial structures, including the facial nerve.

  Submandibular Gland:

  It is the second-largest salivary gland, having half the weight of the parotid gland [53]. It lies on the body of the mandible, partially superficial and partially deep to the mylohyoid muscle. Its main excretory duct, Wharton's duct, arises from the portion that lies between the mylohyoid and hyoglossus muscles [53]. Along its course, the lingual nerve loops under the duct. It opens by one to three small orifices on a small lingual papilla [2]. Deep to the gland is the hypoglossal nerve, which accompanies the vein. *Submental arteries* are the main arterial supply of the gland, and veins accompany these arteries. Its lymphatic drainage is into the *deep cervical lymph nodes*, especially the *jugulo-omohyoid nodes* [2].

Secretory parasympathetic supply is from the *submandibular ganglion*, which receives fibres from the *chorda tympani* branch of the facial nerve. The sympathetic supply is from the *superior cervical ganglion* [2].

- **Sublingual Gland:**

It is an almond-shaped gland and is the smallest of all the salivary glands. It is located deep in the floor of the mouth between the mandible and genioglossus muscle [54]. About 20 small ducts, known as the ducts of Rivinus, arise from this and open into the floor of the mouth near the lingual papilla area[53]. Its arterial supply is provided by the *sublingual* and *submental arteries*. Lymphatic drainage is into the *submental nodes* and *submandibular nodes* [2]. The nerve supply of the gland is the same as that of the submandibular gland.

Fascial Spaces

There are two types of fascial spaces [55]:

- The soft tissue spaces
- The spaces within bony cavities

The fascial spaces are gliding planes that become increasingly visible as laxity decreases with age [55]. These are important, as infection can spread through these spaces and can become life-threatening. Therefore, dentists, ENT, and maxillofacial surgeons are very familiar with the location and boundaries of these spaces.

Following are the important fascial spaces of the face and neck (Figs. 2.28 and 2.29) [55, 56].

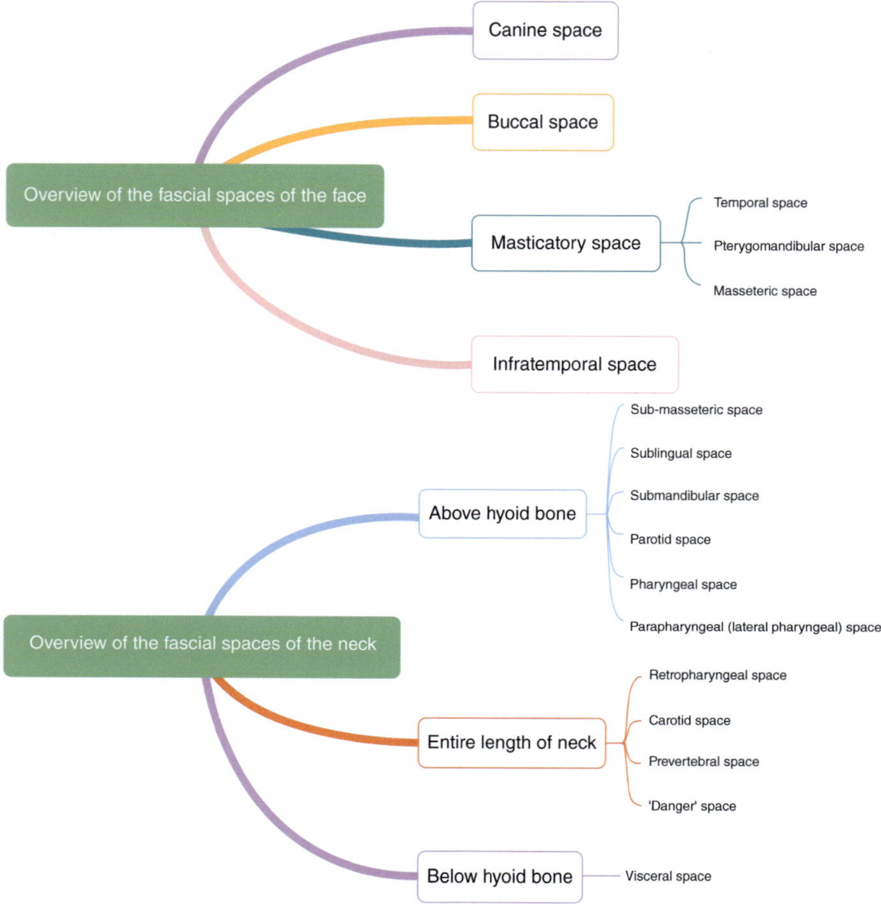

Fig. 2.28 Important fascial spaces of the face and neck

Fig. 2.29 Spatial anatomy of the midcheek showing the following spaces: preseptal, prezygomatic, masticator, and oral cavity. The orbicularis retaining ligament (above) separates the preseptal space of the lower lid from the prezygomatic space. The zygomaticocutaneous ligaments (below) separate the prezygomatic space from the masticator space [55]. Reproduced with permission from Mendelson, B.C. and Jacobson, S.R., 2008. Surgical anatomy of the midcheek: facial layers, spaces, and the midcheek segments. Clinics in plastic surgery, 35(3), pp. 395–404

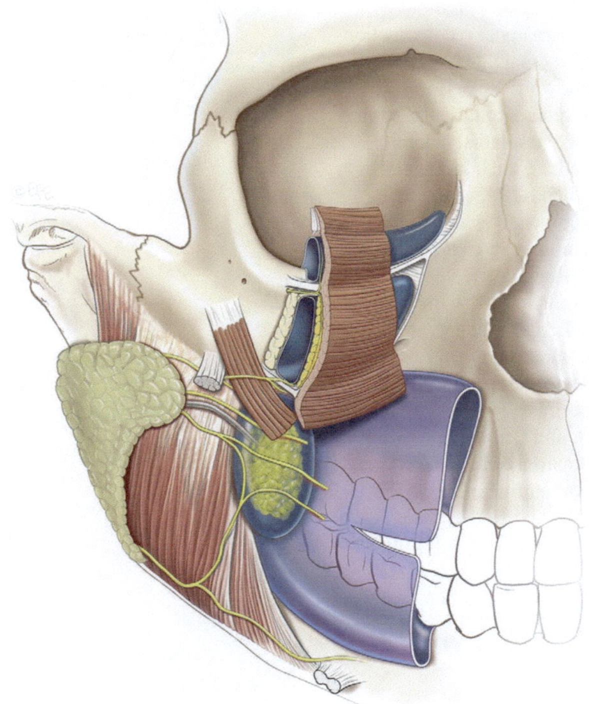

Thread Lifting Procedures

Thread lifting is a minimally invasive treatment that aims to lift and reposition ptotic soft tissue. This technique has grown in popularity. This is accomplished by manually elevating the ptotic soft tissue following thread insertion, followed by the biostimulatory effect of threads. In-depth knowledge of anatomy, thread materials, patient selection, and the procedure are critical for a successful outcome.

Too superficial placement of the threads in the dermal plane is ineffective, palpable to the patients, and possibly visible. Too deeply placed threads result in damage and injury to the deep anatomical structures such as the arteries, veins, and nerves of the face. Therefore, it is critical to identify the correct tissue layers of the face to place the threads according to the treatment aims and objectives.

The primary target layer for thread insertion is the subcutaneous layer (Fig. 2.30). It comprises subcutaneous fat, which gives the skin its volume and movement, and the fibrous retinacula cutis, which links the dermis to the underlying SMAS. The subcutaneous layer is superficially lined with tiny retinacula cutis fibres. The fibrotic network becomes sparser, and thicker fibrotic branches develop as it becomes deeper into the retinacula cutis. This particular arrangement of the retinacula cutis affects the interaction of the barbs with the fibrotic network of the subcutaneous fat [57].

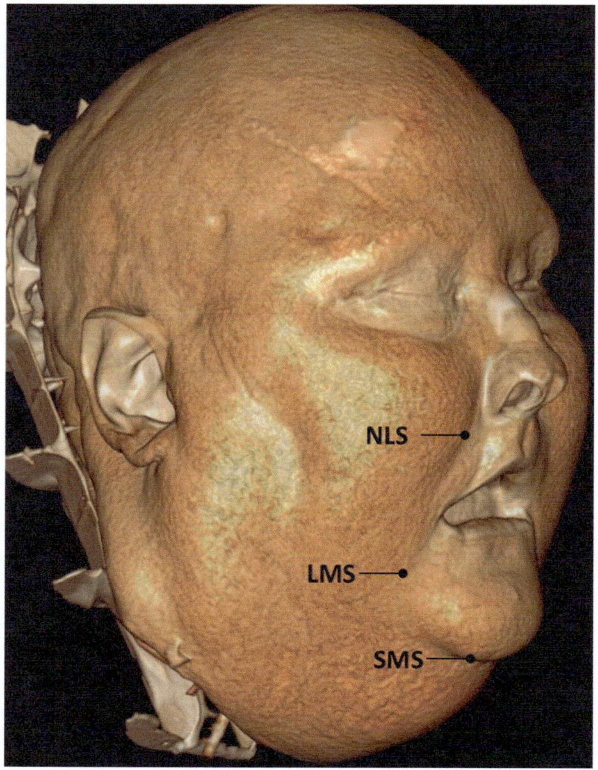

Fig. 2.30 Three-dimensional reconstruction of a cranial CT scan showing the perioral region, including the chin. The nasolabial sulcus (NLS), the labiomental sulcus (LMS), and the submental sulcus (SMS) are indicated. There are no distinct layered arrangements with subcutaneous fat compartments in this region. Reproduced with permission from Cotofana, S. and Lachman, N., 2019. Anatomy of the facial fat compartments and their relevance in aesthetic surgery. JDDG: Journal der Deutschen Dermatologischen Gesellschaft, 17(4), pp. 399–413 [13]

Injury to facial structures should be avoided during thread lifting procedures. Damage to the blood vessels, nerves, and parotid duct can occur via needles, cannula, or cogs.

Areas that require significant attention include:

1. The temporal area

    Threads are commonly used for the vertical repositioning of soft tissues. Hence, the temporal region is a common insertion point. Furthermore, the temporal fascia creates a stronger fixing point than the subcutaneous fat layer [7]. Damage to the superficial temporal artery/vein, the zygomatico-orbital artery, and temporal branches of the facial nerve should be prevented.

2. Zygomatic arch

    Care is to be taken due to the curvature of the zygomatic arch and changes in tissue thickness in this region. Therefore, remaining in the intended facial layer is important.

3. The parotid region

    This area houses important structures, including the parotid gland and duct, facial nerve branches, and transverse facial artery. The threads must strictly be placed in the subcutaneous layer. Incorrect insertion of threads in this region can have devastating effects.

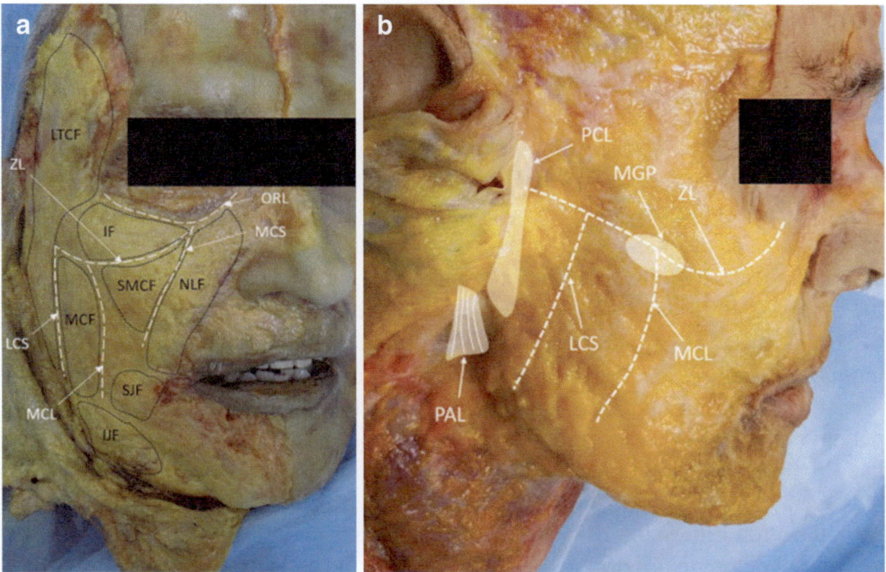

Fig. 2.31 (**a**) Superficial fat compartments (**b**) Main ligaments used as anchoring points. *IF* infraorbital fat; *SMCF* superficial medial cheek fat; *NLF* nasolabial fat; *MCF* middle cheek fat; *LTCF* lateral temporal-cheek fat; *SJF, IJF* superior, inferior jowl fat; *ORL* orbicularis retaining ligament; *ZL* zygomatic ligament; *MCS* medial cheek septum; *MCL* masseteric cutaneous ligament; *LCS* lateral cheek septum; *ZL* zygomatic ligament; *MGP* Mc Gregor patch; *PCL* parotid cutaneous ligament; *PAL* platysma auricular ligament. Reproduced with permission from Fundaro, S.P., Goh, C.L., Hau, K.C., Moon, H., Lao, P.P. and Salti, G., 2021. Expert consensus on soft-tissue repositioning using absorbable barbed suspension double-needle threads in Asian and Caucasian patients. Journal of Cutaneous and Aesthetic Surgery, 14(1), p. 1

4. Ligaments

Facial ligaments act as anchors for the barbed threads [11, 57]:

- Osteocutaneous ligaments:
  - Connect the periosteum to the dermis
  - Pass through all anatomical layers of the face
- Fasciocutaneous ligaments:
  - Coalesce between the superficial and deep fasciae of the face

The ligaments in the upper and lateral cheek provide a firm anchoring point (Fig. 2.31). Therefore, these enhance the repositioning capacity of the threads. The main retaining structures used as anchoring points are [11, 18, 57–60]:

- The Mc Gregor patch
- The platysma auricular ligament
- The parotid cutaneous ligament
- The zygomatic ligament

Conclusion

The intricacy of facial anatomy cannot be overstated, with its myriad layers exhibiting a complex structural interplay and variable thicknesses across different facial regions. A holistic understanding of this anatomy is pivotal for aesthetic practitioners, forming the foundation upon which all successful interventions are built. However, anatomical knowledge alone is insufficient. A deep comprehension of the materials used, specifically the characteristics and suitability of different threads, is equally crucial. It is this intersection of anatomy and material science that informs the approach to thread lifting procedures. Patient selection is another critical facet of successful aesthetic interventions. The practitioner must consider the patient's unique anatomical features, aesthetic goals, overall health, and suitability for the procedure. This individualised approach ensures the treatment plan is tailored to the patient's needs, optimising the potential for a successful outcome. The procedure itself requires skill and precision, with the practitioner needing to navigate the complex facial anatomy while applying the appropriate thread material. Mastery of the procedure minimises the risk of complications and maximises the likelihood of a successful outcome. Therefore, the success of thread lifting procedures hinges on a multifaceted understanding encompassing facial anatomy, thread material properties, patient selection, and procedural expertise. By embracing this comprehensive approach, practitioners can enhance their ability to deliver safe and effective aesthetic outcomes.

References

1. Prendergast PM. Anatomy of the face and neck. In: Cosmetic surgery. Springer; 2013. p. 29–45.
2. Moore KL, Dalley AF. Clinically oriented anatomy. Wolters Kluwer India Pvt Ltd.; 2018.
3. Prendergast PM. Facial anatomy. In: Advanced surgical facial rejuvenation. Springer; 2012. p. 3–14.
4. Fitzgerald R, Carqueville J, Yang P. An approach to structural facial rejuvenation with fillers in women. Int J Women's Dermatol. 2019;5(1):52–67.
5. Ingallina F, et al. Reevaluation of the layered anatomy of the forehead: introducing the subfrontalis fascia and the retrofrontalis fat compartments. Plast Reconstr Surg. 2022;149(3):587–95.
6. Kim H-J, et al. General anatomy of the face and neck. In: Clinical anatomy of the face for filler and botulinum toxin injection. Singapore: Springer Singapore; 2016. p. 1–53.
7. Kim B, Oh S, Jung W. Anatomy for absorbable thread lifting. In: The art and science of thread lifting. Springer; 2019. p. 13–29.
8. Kim YS, et al. Regional thickness of facial skin and superficial fat: application to the minimally invasive procedures. Clin Anat. 2019;32(8):1008–18.
9. Rohrich RJ, Pessa JE. The fat compartments of the face: anatomy and clinical implications for cosmetic surgery. Plast Reconstr Surg. 2007;119(7):2219–27.
10. Kruglikov I, et al. The facial adipose tissue: a revision. Facial Plast Surg. 2016;32(6):671–82.
11. Stuzin JM, Baker TJ, Gordon HL. The relationship of the superficial and deep facial fascias: relevance to rhytidectomy and aging. Plast Reconstr Surg. 1992;89(3):441–9. discussion 450
12. Bertossi D, et al. Classification of fat pad of the third medium of the face. Union of Aesthetic Medicine–UIME; 2015. p. 103.

13. Cotofana S, Lachman N. Anatomy of the facial fat compartments and their relevance in aesthetic surgery. J Dtsch Dermatol Ges. 2019;17(4):399–413.
14. Saban Y, et al. Facial layers and facial fat compartments: focus on midcheek area. Facial Plast Surg. 2017;33(05):470–82.
15. Sandoval SE, et al. Facial fat compartments: a guide to filler placement. In: Seminars in plastic surgery. Thieme Medical Publishers; 2009.
16. Stuzin JM, Rohrich RJ, Dayan E. The facial fat compartments revisited: clinical relevance to subcutaneous dissection and facial deflation in face lifting. Plast Reconstr Surg. 2019;144(5):1070–8.
17. Cohen SR, Womack H. Injectable tissue replacement and regeneration: anatomic fat grafting to restore decayed facial tissues. Plast Reconstr Surg Glob Open. 2019;7(8).
18. Mendelson BC, et al. Surgical anatomy of the lower face: the premasseter space, the jowl, and the labiomandibular fold. Aesthet Plast Surg. 2008;32(2):185–95.
19. Mendelson BC, Wong C-H. Surgical anatomy of the middle premasseter space and its application in sub–SMAS face lift surgery. Plast Reconstr Surg. 2013;132(1):57–64.
20. Wong C-H, Mendelson B. Facial soft-tissue spaces and retaining ligaments of the midcheek: defining the premaxillary space. Plast Reconstr Surg. 2013;132(1):49–56.
21. Cotofana S, et al. Midface: clinical anatomy and regional approaches with injectable fillers. Plast Reconstr Surg. 2015;136(5):219S–34S.
22. Zenker W. New findings in temporal muscle in man. Zeitschrift fur Anatomie und Entwicklungsgeschichte. 1955;118(4):355–68.
23. Yousuf S, et al. A review of the gross anatomy, functions, pathology, and clinical uses of the buccal fat pad. Surg Radiol Anat. 2010;32(5):427–36.
24. Kahn J, Wolfram-Gabel R, Bourjat P. Anatomy and imaging of the deep fat of the face. Clin Anat. 2000;13(5):373–82.
25. Zhang H-M, et al. Anatomical structure of the buccal fat pad and its clinical adaptations. Plast Reconstr Surg. 2002;109(7):2509–18; discussion 2519.
26. Kim M-K, Han W, Kim S-G. The use of the buccal fat pad flap for oral reconstruction. Maxillofac Plast Reconstr Surg. 2017;39(1):1–9.
27. Alghoul M, Codner MA. Retaining ligaments of the face: review of anatomy and clinical applications. Aesthet Surg J. 2013;33(6):769–82.
28. Brandt MG, et al. Biomechanical properties of the facial retaining ligaments. Arch Facial Plast Surg. 2012;14(4):289–94.
29. Marur T, Tuna Y, Demirci S. Facial anatomy. Clin Dermatol. 2014;32(1):14–23.
30. Broughton M, Fyfe GM. The superficial musculoaponeurotic system of the face: a model explored. Anat Res Int. 2013;2013:794682.
31. Abramo AC, et al. Anatomy of forehead, glabellar, nasal and orbital muscles, and their correlation with distinctive patterns of skin lines on the upper third of the face: reviewing concepts. Aesthet Plast Surg. 2016;40(6):962–71.
32. Tong J, Lopez MJ, Patel BC. Anatomy, head and neck, eye orbicularis oculi muscle. StatPearls; 2020.
33. Yu M, Wang S-M. Anatomy, head and neck, eye corrugator muscle. StatPearls; 2020.
34. Ghassemi A, et al. Anatomy of the SMAS revisited. Aesthet Plast Surg. 2003;27(4):258–64.
35. Vinkka-Puhakka H, Kean MR, Heap S. Ultrasonic investigation of the circumoral musculature. J Anat. 1989;166:121–33.
36. Jain P, Rathee M. Anatomy, head and neck, orbicularis oris muscle. StatPearls; 2020.
37. Nicolau PJ. The orbicularis oris muscle: a functional approach to its repair in the cleft lip. Br J Plast Surg. 1983;36(2):141–53.
38. de Almeida AR, Romiti A, Carruthers JD. The facial platysma and its underappreciated role in lower face dynamics and contour. Dermatol Surg. 2017;43(8):1042–9.
39. Cotofana S, Lachman N. Arteries of the face and their relevance for minimally invasive facial procedures: an anatomical review. Plast Reconstr Surg. 2019;143(2):416–26.
40. Bentsianov B, Blitzer A. Facial anatomy. Clin Dermatol. 2004;22(1):3–13.

41. von Arx T, et al. The face–a vascular perspective. A literature review. Swiss Dental J. 2018;128(5):382.
42. von Arx T, Abdelkarim AZ, Lozanoff S. The face—a neurosensory perspective. A literature review. Swiss Dental J SSO. 2017;127(5):1066–75.
43. Meegalla N, et al. Anatomy, head and neck, facial arteries. 2019.
44. Vadgaonkar R, et al. Variant facial artery in the submandibular region. J Craniofac Surg. 2012;23(4):e355–7.
45. Niranjan NS. An anatomical study of the facial artery. Ann Plast Surg. 1988;21(1):14–22.
46. Li Z-H, et al. Upper facial anastomoses between the external and internal carotid vascular territories—a 3D computed tomographic investigation. Aesthet Surg J. 2022;42:1145–51.
47. Rivard AB, Burns B. Anatomy, head and neck, internal jugular vein. 2018.
48. Cotofana S, et al. Can smiling influence the blood flow in the facial vein? An experimental study. J Cosmet Dermatol. 2020;19(2):321–7.
49. Pan W-R, Le Roux CM, Briggs CA. Variations in the lymphatic drainage pattern of the head and neck: further anatomic studies and clinical implications. Plast Reconstr Surg. 2011;127(2):611–20.
50. Meade RA, et al. Facelift and patterns of lymphatic drainage. Aesthet Surg J. 2012;32(1):39–45.
51. Motyckova G, Steensma DP. Why does my patient have lymphadenopathy or splenomegaly? Hematol/Oncol Clin. 2012;26(2):395–408.
52. Nugroho SW, et al. Predicting outcome of hemifacial spasm after microvascular decompression with intraoperative monitoring: a systematic review. Heliyon. 2021;7(2):e06115.
53. Silvers AR, Som PM. Salivary glands. Radiol Clin N Am. 1998;36(5):941–66.
54. Ghannam MG, Singh P. Anatomy, head and neck, salivary glands. 2019.
55. Mendelson BC, Jacobson SR. Surgical anatomy of the midcheek: facial layers, spaces, and the midcheek segments. Clin Plast Surg. 2008;35(3):395–404.
56. Kwon PH, Laskin DM. Clinician's manual of oral and maxillofacial surgery. Quintessence Publishing Company; 2001.
57. Fundaro SP, et al. Expert consensus on soft-tissue repositioning using absorbable barbed suspension double-needle threads in Asian and Caucasian patients. J Cutan Aesthet Surg. 2021;14(1):1–13.
58. Furnas DW. The retaining ligaments of the cheek. Plast Reconstr Surg. 1989;83(1):11–6.
59. Ozdemir R, et al. Anatomicohistologic study of the retaining ligaments of the face and use in face lift: retaining ligament correction and SMAS plication. Plast Reconstr Surg. 2002;110(4):1134–47; discussion 1148–9.
60. Mendelson BC. SMAS fixation to the facial skeleton: rationale and results. Plast Reconstr Surg. 1997;100(7):1834–42; discussion 1843–5.

Anatomy and Pathophysiology of Facial Ageing

3

Souphiyeh Samizadeh

Abstract

Ageing represents a constellation of interconnected and intertwined internal and external processes resulting in the manifestation of distinct phenotypes. These encompass changes in body composition, metabolic processes, variations in energy consumption and production, along with dysregulation of homeostasis, culminating in an accumulation of unrepaired damage. Facial ageing mirrors this multilayered and multilevel pattern of physiological changes, manifesting as alterations in skin, subcutaneous fat distribution, muscular tone, and bone structure. This interplay is mediated through the same array of processes and mechanisms implicated in systemic ageing, revealing facial ageing as a visible and complex sub-phenotype of the ageing process. In-depth understanding of the network governing ageing, and more specifically facial ageing, can illuminate the pathways to develop strategies mitigating the impact of ageing and improving overall health span. This chapter thus delves into a detailed discussion on facial ageing, aiming to provide an encompassing perspective on the complexities inherent to this fascinating sub-phenotype of the ageing process.

Keywords

Ageing · Facial ageing · Facial rejuvenation · Ligaments · Musculature · Skin ageing

S. Samizadeh (✉)
King's College London, London, UK

University College London, London, UK

Great British Academy of Aesthetic Medicine, London, UK
e-mail: info@baamed.co.uk

© Springer Nature Switzerland AG 2024
S. Samizadeh (ed.), *Thread Lifting Techniques for Facial Rejuvenation and Recontouring*, https://doi.org/10.1007/978-3-031-47954-0_3

Ageing

The ageing process is governed by a network of interconnected and intertwined internal and external processes that result in the development of distinctive phenotypes, including changes and alterations in body composition, metabolic processes, energy consumption and imbalances in energy production and consumption, dysregulation of homeostasis, loss of neuroplasticity and neurodegeneration, and the resultant accumulation of unrepaired damage (Fig. 3.1) [1]. The proinflammatory state of ageing is a crucial concept, and many environmental factors contribute to this state. These sum up to genetic, chemical, and biochemical changes. Such changes result in enhanced susceptibility to disease, reduction in functional reserves, reduction of the healing capacity and stress resistance, and therefore, unstable health and, lastly, failure to thrive [1].

The facial ageing process is multifactorial, mediated by both intrinsic and extrinsic factors (refer to Fig. 3.2). Intrinsic ageing, largely dictated by genetic predispositions, is characterised by predetermined cellular and physiological changes. However, the extent of their manifestation is modulated by extrinsic factors,

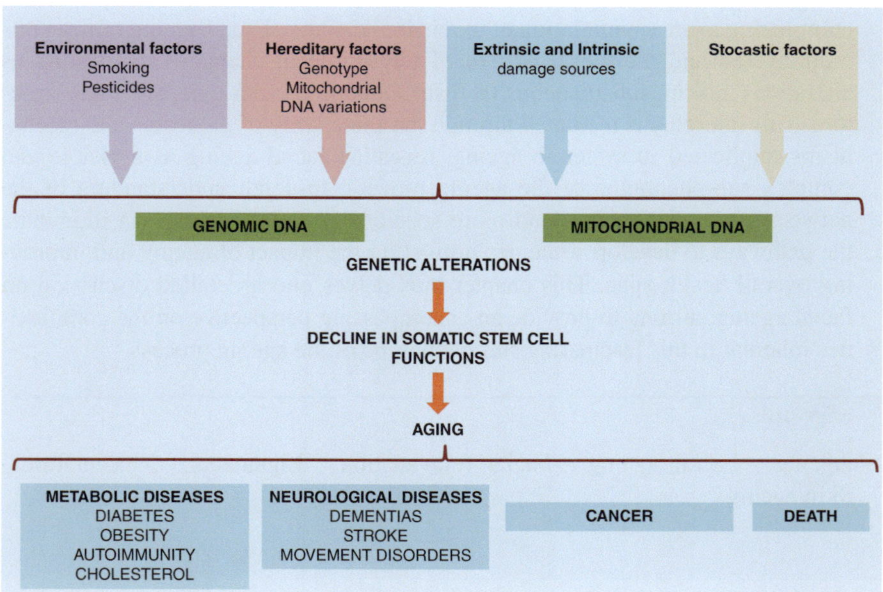

Fig. 3.1 Representation of genetic factors' that influence ageing and lifespan. The environmental conditions (stress, pesticides), individual genotype (genomic and mitochondrial DNA), and stochastic factors can induce genetic and epigenetic alterations that cause a decline in somatic stem cell function, which can be the origin of metabolic, degenerative diseases, cancer, and ageing in individuals. Reproduced with permission from Rodríguez-Rodero S, Fernández-Morera JL, Menéndez-Torre E, Calvanese V, Fernández AF, Fraga MF. Aging genetics and aging. Aging Dis. 2011;2(3):186–95 [2]

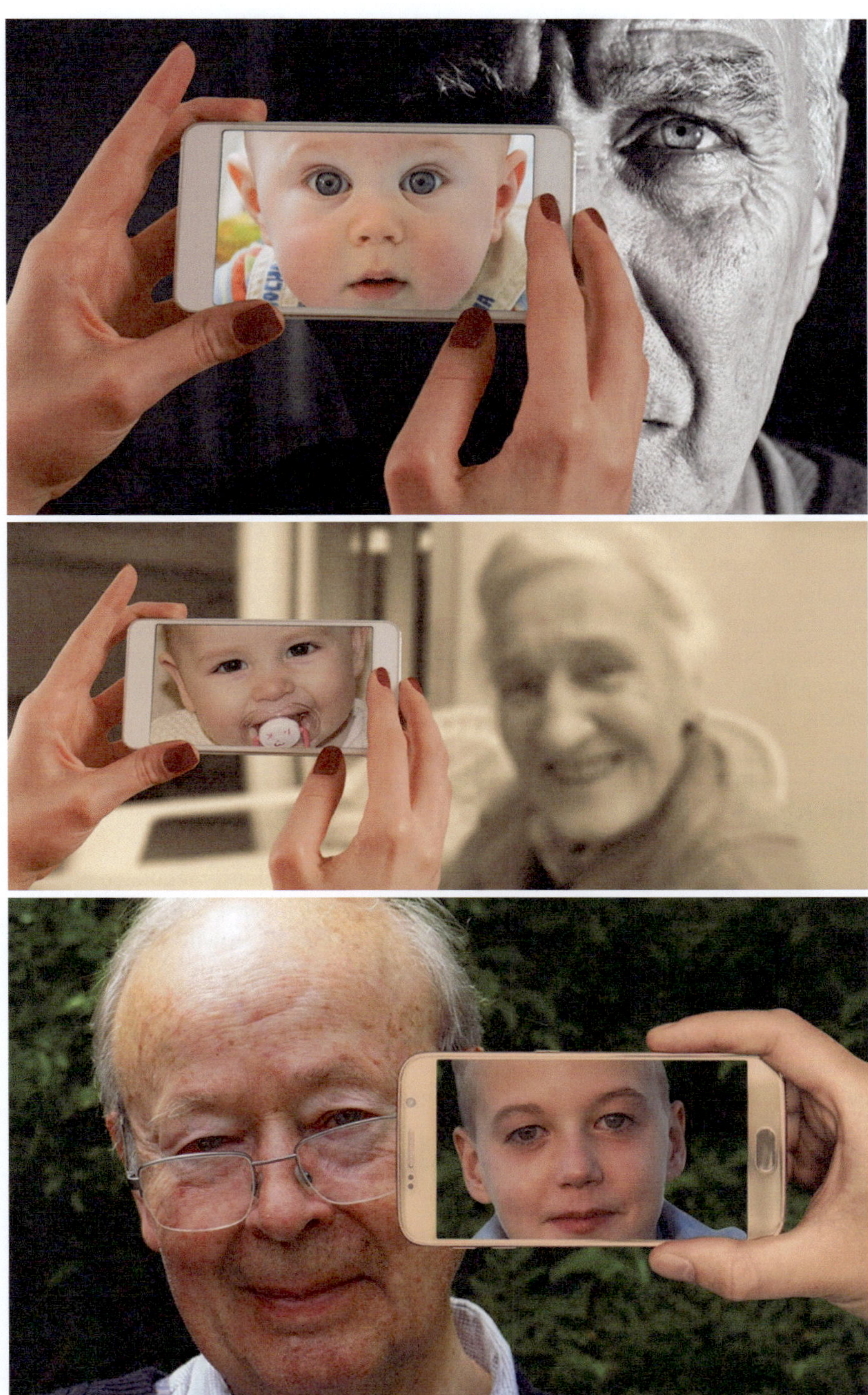

Fig. 3.2 The face goes through ageing changes that are not only skin deep, with internal and external influencing factors. Image credit: Pixabay

influencing the expression and activation of various genes associated with ageing. Throughout an individual's lifetime, cells are perpetually exposed to a myriad of environmental factors, encompassing dietary elements, pharmacological agents, chemical compounds, fluctuations in temperature, varying oxygen levels, differential light exposure, and the presence of mutagenic agents. These external variables play a crucial role in modulating gene expression patterns, consequently influencing the ageing phenotype. This underscores the interplay between genetics and environment in the context of facial ageing, where the underlying genetic code provides the potential landscape for ageing, and environmental influences shape its realisation. This complex interaction necessitates further investigation to elucidate the nuances of the facial ageing process.

Emerging research has indicated that perceived advanced ageing—often encapsulated in the notion of "looking old for your age"—is associated with an increased mortality risk [3]. This association implies a potential link between physical appearance, ageing biology, and overall health outcomes. Therefore, a comprehensive exploration of this correlation is merited, as it could elucidate the intricacies of ageing and longevity. Concurrently, the societal trend towards rejuvenation interventions to counteract visible signs of ageing introduces a novel angle to this investigation. The interplay between the increasing popularity of rejuvenation procedures and the pursuit of longevity presents a compelling research avenue. Analysing the potential impacts of rejuvenation therapies on biological ageing, and consequently on longevity, might yield valuable insights into the multidimensional aspects of ageing and provide pathways for novel antiageing strategies.

The Ageing Face

The ontogenesis of facial bones and soft tissues is a meticulously regulated process, with the key structural elements of the face being established before the onset of puberty. By the age of 6, approximately 90% of the overall growth is achieved, signifying the considerable extent of facial development during early childhood [4].

The ageing of the face, however, continues throughout life, being subjected to a confluence of intrinsic and extrinsic factors. These processes induce alterations across multiple facial layers, affecting the skeletal framework, musculature, and cutaneous structures [5] The skeletal changes comprise modifications in bone density and structure, while muscular adaptations involve alterations in the function and structure of both mimetic and masticatory muscles. In the cutaneous layer, changes include reduced elasticity, collagen degradation, and the alteration of skin appendages. Ageing further results in ligamentous attenuation and variances in the size and position of facial fat pads, including both atrophy and hypertrophy. These transformations, coupled with the gravitational descent of fat, contribute to the typical features of an aged face and ageing of its appendages. To fully comprehend these changes, an understanding of the alterations across various facial layers is essential (Fig. 3.3). It is crucial to maintain an integrated perspective on the three-dimensional (3D) structure of the face, recognising the interdependence of each facial structure

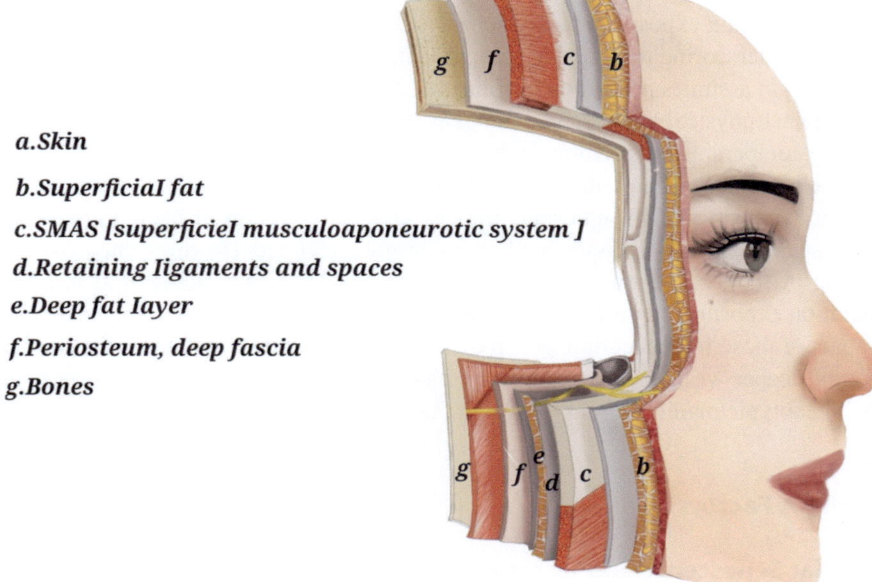

Fig. 3.3 Facial layers

and its relationship with surrounding structures. Paramount among these modifications are changes in soft tissues (in terms of quality, quantity, and dynamics), and hard tissues, including bones, dentition, and cartilaginous structures [6]. This holistic understanding of facial ageing can lead to more comprehensive and effective strategies for managing the aesthetic and functional impacts of this complex process.

A multitude of extrinsic factors exert direct and deleterious effects on facial ageing. Known accelerants of premature ageing encompass ultraviolet radiation exposure, tobacco consumption, habitual alcohol intake, and a low body mass index (BMI) [3, 7–10]. A pivotal study exploring the influence of environmental determinants on facial ageing, as gauged by perceived age, reported a nuanced landscape of influencers. Extrinsic damage-driven factors, such as sun exposure, smoking, and low BMI, were identified as negative influencers, exacerbating perceived ageing. Conversely, high social status, low scores on depression scales, and marital status were associated with a perceived younger age. However, the study noted an interesting divergence in this association across different genders [7].

Skin

The skin, representing the body's most expansive organ, is particularly susceptible to an array of intrinsic and extrinsic factors. Extrinsic factors such as free radicals, ultraviolet radiation, tobacco use (nicotine), habitual sleep position, suboptimal nutrition, and environmental pollutants can instigate cumulative harm to the skin. Historically, sun exposure was posited to account for approximately 80% of facial ageing, underscoring the considerable influence of environmental variables [11].

The skin assumes numerous fundamental functions, serving as a protective barrier against physical insults and pathogens, mediating immune surveillance, maintaining temperature regulation, upholding homeostasis, preventing percutaneous fluid, electrolyte and protein loss, and facilitating sensory perception [12].

Intrinsic skin ageing represents the "natural" progression of ageing across all tissues and is intimately associated with chronological age. However, the extrinsic ageing of the skin is primarily driven by factors such as ultraviolet and infrared radiation exposure, environmental pollutants, and tobacco smoking. The collective impact of these factors culminates in marked skin alterations, including the formation of deeper wrinkles and pigmentary changes, thus contributing significantly to the phenotypic manifestations of ageing [13].

Intrinsic Factors

Cellular Senescence and Telomeres

Diploid cells, including fibroblasts, exhibit a finite lifespan due to their limited proliferative capacity, a phenomenon termed replicative senescence. This is most conspicuously evidenced by the progressive shortening of telomeres, the repetitive DNA sequences located at the termini of chromosomal DNA. With each cellular division, telomeres undergo attrition, eventually reaching a critically short length that triggers cellular senescence, inhibiting further cell division [14]. Importantly, senescent cells are not simply non-proliferative; they also undergo substantial alterations in their functional phenotype. These changes include the upregulation of growth factors, proteins responsible for degrading the extracellular matrix (ECM), and pro-inflammatory cytokines. The resultant shift in the cellular milieu significantly contributes to the ageing process, implicating cellular senescence as a fundamental mechanism underpinning ageing [15]. Consequently, a comprehensive understanding of the process of replicative senescence, its underlying molecular mechanisms, and its wider physiological implications could be pivotal in developing novel strategies to manage ageing. The concept of modulating replicative senescence refers to the potential for manipulating the cellular and molecular processes that lead to this state. This could be achieved by interventions that either delay the onset of senescence, enhance the removal of senescent cells, or even rejuvenate senescent cells, thereby restoring their normal cellular function.

Modulating replicative senescence holds significant promise as an approach to mitigate the impacts of ageing. By delaying or reversing senescence, we might be able to prevent or mitigate many age-associated changes and conditions, including skin ageing, chronic diseases, and possibly extend healthy lifespan. In this context, research into the triggers and controllers of replicative senescence is a critical area of study in ageing research. This could lead to the development of pharmacological agents, lifestyle modifications, or other interventions capable of modulating this process, potentially altering our ability to manage ageing and its related pathologies.

Free Radicals

Oxidative stress, resulting from an imbalance between the production of free radicals—predominantly reactive oxygen species (ROS)—and the capability of antioxidant defence systems, is a pivotal factor in the ageing process. According to the free radical theory of ageing, ROS are instrumental in both intrinsic and extrinsic skin ageing. A major cellular source of oxidative stress is the mitochondria, the organelles primarily responsible for energy production within cells [15].

Despite the skin's energy requirements being less pronounced compared to metabolically active organs such as skeletal muscle, mitochondria maintain a critical role within the skin's cellular physiology. Their functions extend beyond energy production, contributing significantly to cell signalling, wound healing, pigmentation, homeostatic vasculature regulation, and hair development. Moreover, mitochondria are integral to the skin's defensive capacity against microbial infections. For instance, in response to hypoxia-induced metabolic stress during Staphylococcus aureus skin infection, the skin's cells have been demonstrated to rapidly increase glycolytic activity and ATP production, leading to the activation of hypoxia-inducible factor 1-alpha (HIF1α) and recruiting immune cells to bolster the skin's defences.

Additionally, mitochondrial activity and ROS generation contribute to the regulation of stem cell differentiation, which is closely linked with epidermal homeostasis and hair follicle growth. Consequently, ROS signalling mediated by mitochondria plays a significant role in skin development and function. Nonetheless, mitochondrial dysfunction, such as mtDNA mutations and associated functional declines, has been linked with skin ageing manifestations, including stress-induced wrinkle formation, pigmentation changes, hair greying, and hair loss.

While our understanding of the intricate mechanisms underpinning skin ageing has significantly advanced, many aspects remain elusive. Mitochondrial function is likely intertwined in a complex cascade of events leading to functional tissue decline and the overall ageing process. From a scientific perspective, dissecting the processes driving skin ageing is crucial. This knowledge not only holds the potential to inform the development of preventive clinical interventions but could also guide the formulation of enhanced antiageing products, specifically tailored to the needs of aged skin [16].

Hormonal Factors

As ageing progresses, the production of sex hormones in gonadal and adrenal glands undergoes a substantial decrease. The reduction in the levels of oestrogens and androgens culminates in a series of dermatological alterations, including skin dryness, wrinkle formation, epidermal thinning, collagen degradation, and augmented skin laxity.

Particularly during menopause, a period marked by a substantial reduction in the levels of oestrogen and progesterone, severe cutaneous consequences ensue. These hormonal shifts trigger a decrease in skin suppleness, an increase in the development of wrinkles, pronounced skin dryness, and reduced vascularity. Consequently, the skin becomes more brittle, impairing its protective capabilities and retarding the wound healing process [17].

These changes underscore the significant role that sex hormones play in skin physiology and homeostasis, and how their decline with ageing contributes to the dermatological manifestations of ageing. Therefore, understanding these hormonal changes and their effects on skin biology can inform interventions aimed at mitigating these changes, enhancing skin health, and potentially decelerating the visible signs of ageing.

Extrinsic Factors

Extrinsic determinants exert a considerable influence on facial ageing. Given the critical role of environmental elements in skin ageing, particularly their direct impact on the epidermis, extrinsic skin ageing has traditionally been conceptualised as an external mechanism. Specifically, this suggests that damage sustained by the epidermal compartment—instigated by factors such as ultraviolet radiation, pollution, and lifestyle choices—not only incites observable epidermal ageing but also instigates a cascading effect that drives ageing in the dermal compartment. This conceptualisation underscores the interconnectedness of the various skin layers and the notion that perturbations at one level can induce changes throughout the entire skin structure [18].

Understanding this cascade of events is key to formulating comprehensive strategies for preventing or mitigating the impacts of extrinsic skin ageing. Thus, interventions aimed at protecting the skin from environmental damage could potentially attenuate both epidermal and dermal ageing, consequently preserving overall skin health and aesthetics.

Photoageing

Exposure to ultraviolet sunlight (UVR) is a recognised primary instigator of skin ageing. Both UVB (290–315 nm) and UVA (315–400 nm) rays contribute significantly to extrinsic skin ageing, with the longer wavelength segment of UVA, namely UVA1 (340–400 nm), bearing particular relevance. This is due to its ability to deeply penetrate human skin and directly influence dermal fibroblasts, cells integral to the skin's structure and function [19].

Photodamage, often referred to as photoageing, refers to the cumulative and persistent structural and physiological alterations in the skin due to chronic UVR exposure. It represents a distinct subclass of extrinsic ageing and is characterised by a combination of clinical, histological, and functional changes that differentiate it from intrinsic or chronological ageing.

Clinically, photoaged skin exhibits coarse wrinkles, uneven pigmentation, loss of elasticity, and a leathery texture. At the microscopic level, photodamage manifests as alterations in the skin's collagenous framework, with increased elastosis and a disorganised distribution of collagen fibres, along with an increased deposition of abnormal elastin-containing material.

The underlying mechanism of photoageing primarily involves UVR-induced DNA damage and the generation of ROS, which instigate a cascade of biochemical reactions leading to the activation of transcription factors such as nuclear factor-kappa B (NF-κB) and activator protein-1 (AP-1). This activation results in the upregulation of matrix metalloproteinases (MMPs), enzymes that degrade the extracellular matrix, especially collagen, a crucial structural component of the dermis.

Moreover, UVR exposure can also suppress the skin's immune response, further contributing to the deterioration of skin structure and function over time. It's important to note that the degree of photodamage is not merely dependent on UVR intensity but also on individual characteristics like skin type and pigmentation, which influence the skin's susceptibility to UVR.

Emerging evidence also suggests a role for blue light-induced skin pigmentation in the ageing process. Clinical trials have indicated that sunscreens capable of protecting against blue light can aid in reducing the recurrence of skin lesions in patients with melasma. The blue light spectrum, largely emitted by digital screens, may induce exposure to reactive oxygen species (ROS) in human skin, leading to morphological alterations in fibroblasts [18].

These findings underline the wide-ranging impact of various components of the light spectrum on skin health and ageing, from ultraviolet to visible light. Given the ubiquity of these exposures in daily life, understanding their precise effects on skin biology is critical for developing effective strategies to protect the skin and counteract the signs of ageing.

Air Pollution

The association between traffic-related air pollution and skin ageing has been well-established. Traffic-related air pollutants, for which skin ageing is well-established, are high in polycyclic aromatic hydrocarbons (PAHs). They are produced by incomplete combustion of organic material like coal or oil. PAHs are lipophilic and may permeate the epidermal barrier. It is also known that aryl hydrocarbon receptor ligands, such as PAHs and dioxin, promote melanocyte growth and hence skin pigmentation [20].

There is a possible relationship between air pollutants (PAHs) and skin ageing. Deposition of these particles on the skin and follicular structure can harm the living cells and result in pigmentation in that specific region (pigmented spot), influencing the gene expression patterns of those cells. Indoor air pollution has also been recognised as a risk factor for premature skin ageing. Indoor air pollution is associated with domestic activities like cooking, heating, and lighting, particularly in underdeveloped countries [21].

Ozone (O3) quickly oxidises skin macromolecules such as lipids and proteins, producing radical species such as radical hydroxyl and causing oxidative stress.

Higher ground ozone levels are directly related to higher temperatures and lead to wrinkling of facial skin. Furthermore, particulate matter from traffic pollution and ultraviolet radiation from sunlight have been reported to have synergistic effects on the ageing of the skin [18].

Tobacco Smoking and Alcohol Use

The detrimental effects of tobacco and alcohol consumption on skin health and the ageing process are well-documented, largely owing to their impact on oxidative stress mechanisms and the body's natural antioxidative defences.

Tobacco smoke contains a plethora of harmful substances, including free radicals and reactive oxygen species (ROS), which are known to instigate ageing changes across multiple skin layers, including the epidermis, dermis, and lipid-rich layers. With the degradation of these structural components of the skin, signs of ageing, such as diminished facial volume, become more prominent. Specific facial characteristics like tear troughs (depressions beneath the lower eyelid) and fat pads (areas of puffiness) are more apparent as a result of these changes [22].

The role of alcohol consumption in influencing skin health is multifaceted and complex. Alcohol consumption has been found to affect the skin's antioxidant defence mechanisms, thus augmenting the skin's susceptibility to ultraviolet (UV) light-induced damage. It can lead to dehydration, compromising the skin's barrier function and leading to dryness, which may exacerbate the visibility of wrinkles and fine lines. Alcohol has also been implicated in disrupting various physiological processes, leading to nutritional deficiencies and affecting skin health over time. Furthermore, alcohol's vasodilatory effect can result in persistent skin redness and the formation of telangiectasias, contributing to an aged appearance. It is also worth noting that heavy alcohol consumption can interfere with the absorption and utilisation of vital skin-healthy nutrients, like vitamins A and C, hastening the ageing process [23].

The synergistic effects of alcohol consumption and tobacco smoking present a potent challenge to skin health and ageing, implicating multiple physiological pathways and exacerbating skin damage. Cigarette smoke is a potent source of free radicals and reactive oxygen species (ROS), which induce oxidative stress and damage in the skin layers, thereby promoting ageing changes. Concurrently, alcohol intake further weakens the skin's antioxidative defence mechanisms, making the skin more vulnerable to the harmful effects of these free radicals and ROS. Moreover, both alcohol and tobacco have profound effects on cutaneous blood flow. Smoking results in vasoconstriction, reducing blood supply to the skin, which, over time, can lead to skin pallor and an unhealthy, aged appearance. Conversely, alcohol causes vasodilation, which can result in skin redness and the formation of telangiectasias, further contributing to an aged skin appearance. Furthermore, chronic alcohol consumption can lead to dehydration and nutritional deficiencies, notably in vitamins A and C, which are essential for skin health and resilience. These deficiencies, coupled with the reduced blood supply to the skin due to smoking, significantly compromise the skin's regenerative capabilities and accelerate the ageing process. Taken together, the combined effects of alcohol and tobacco present a potent threat to skin health, leading to accelerated ageing. Understanding these interactions underscores the importance of a holistic approach to skin health, encompassing both skincare strategies and lifestyle modifications, including the cessation of smoking and moderated alcohol consumption.

Ageing and the Skin

The age-associated alterations in gene expression within the human epidermis were explored in a 2013 study. Findings suggested the maintenance of the core skin developmental program throughout ageing, with concurrent ageing-associated subtle destabilisation occurring at the level of the epigenome in gene regulatory elements [24].

The functional capacity and structural stability of the skin are inevitably compromised as a result of ageing, leading to a loss of skin integrity [25]. This deterioration of the skin, a vital organ, gives rise to compromised barrier function, attributing to considerable morbidity [12]. Additionally, ageing brings about a transformation in neurosensory perception [26]. Age-associated skin becomes increasingly susceptible to widespread dryness, itching, infection, vascular complications, autoimmune disorders, and a heightened risk of cutaneous malignancies [12]. Photodamaged skin, in particular, presents a leathery and dry appearance [27]. Oxidative stress is widely considered a principal contributor to the ageing process [28]. Altered protein structure can be seen in aged skin and more so in photoaged skin [27]. Among the various mechanisms implicated in skin ageing, reactive oxygen species, mitochondrial DNA mutations, hormonal shifts, and telomere shortening are prominent [29].

Ageing induces visible transformations at the surface of the skin, reflecting changes within the multiple layers of the skin, including the epidermis, dermis, hypodermis, and subcutaneous tissues (Fig. 3.4). Epidermal ageing is characterised by thinning of the epidermis and pigmentary changes, such as the emergence of "age spots" or skin unevenness. Dermal ageing involves dermal thinning, resulting from the diminution of fibroblasts, a decrease in collagen synthesis, and augmented UV-induced collagen degradation. The dermal elastin network is progressively demolished, leading to loss of skin elasticity due to curtailed elastin synthesis and

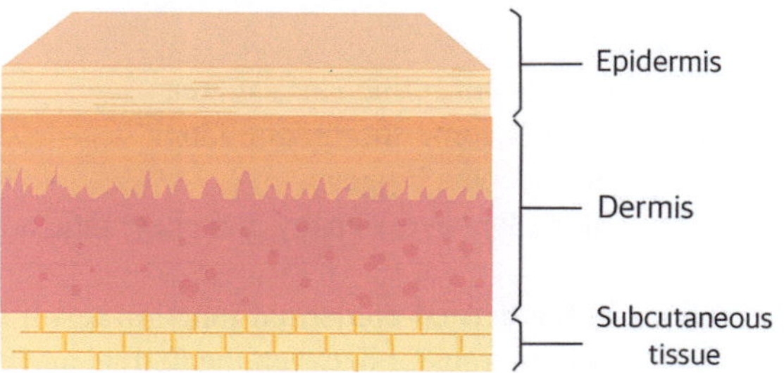

Fig. 3.4 Ageing changes occur within the epidermis, dermis, and subcutaneous tissue

intensified degradation or de-structuring of elastic fibres. Sebum production, water and lipid content, water and fat emulsion, water-binding capacity, and barrier integrity are all compromised, resulting in diminished moisture retention and a weakened skin barrier [26, 30]. These alterations contribute to skin sagging, an increased predisposition to the development of wrinkles and cellulite [31–33]. Aged skin has the following clinical characteristics [2, 34–36]:

- Loss of hydration
- Rough texture
- Irregular pigmentation
- Yellowish colour
- Telangiectasia
- Deep rhytids or furrows and fine lines
- Dermal thinning

Progressive reduction in cutaneous thickness starts in the 20 s, principally in cheeks, temples, and orbit, and the first signs of ageing become apparent in the 30 s [37–39]. The skin is furthermore affected by soft tissues and the skeletal structure changes.

The following section offers a brief overview of some age-related skin changes; however, an exhaustive examination of skin ageing far exceeds the scope of the present chapter.

Epidermis

Epidermal ageing is illustrated by morphologic changes involving the dermal-epidermal junction flattening and reduced thickness [40]. The changes include [26, 27, 30, 40–42]:

- The epidermis becomes thinner
  - F > M
  - Face, neck, the upper part of the chest, and the extensor surface of the hands and forearms
- Decrease in cell turnover
- No changes in stratum corneum
- Alteration in the dermal-epidermal junction
  - Flattening
  - Diminished connecting surface area
- Keratinocytes become shorter and fatter
- Corneocytes become bigger
- Decrease in melanocyte density and enzymatic activity—uneven pigmentation

Alterations in the dermal-epidermal junction result in the fragility of the skin and reduced nutritional transfer between the dermal and epidermal layers. Furthermore, this means diminished resistance to shearing forces and enhanced susceptibility to insult [26]. Reduced cell turnover inevitably means mounds of corneocytes that change the skin's surface characteristics, making it feel and look older, rough, and dull in appearance [43]. Changes in the dermo-epidermal junction and the resultant reduction in nutrient and oxygen supply cause an amplified risk of dermo-epidermal separation. A possible mechanism by which rhytids form [26, 44, 45].

Dermis

Ageing impinges upon all three principal constituents of the dermis: collagen, elastin, and glycosaminoglycans, thereby altering the structural and functional integrity of the skin [43]. Changes include [27, 46]:

- Reduction in thickness
- Reduction in the number of mast cells and fibroblasts
- Reduction in the number of blood vessels
- Collagen
  - Reduced production
  - Changes in arrangement/disorganised collagen fibrils/thickened fibrils
  - Greater degradation
  - The buildup of abnormal elastin-containing material
  - Changes in the ratio of Type III to Type I collagen
      Loss of collagen I
      Loss of collagen IV—loss of structural integrity and wrinkle formation

Reduced blood vessels with ageing cause a diminishing blood supply to the dermis [47]. The changes in the dermis and the loss of molecular integrity result in [26, 44, 48].

- Reduced and declined elasticity
- Increase in the rigidity of the skin
- Reduced torsion extensibility
- Increased susceptibility to tear
- Altered recovery from mechanical depression
- Fast erosion in women

Collagen

Collagen comprises up to 80% of the dry weight of the dermis. It is mainly responsible for the tensile strength of the skin. With ageing [27, 49–52]:

- Decreased collagen content
- Rate of collagen synthesis decreases
- The activity of enzymes for post-translational modification decreases

- Collagen solubility decreases
- The density of the collagen—reduction in ground substance
- Collagen fibres:
  - The thickness of bundles decreases and becomes disorganised
  - Aggregates of loosely woven, mainly straight fibres
  - Increased straight fibres mean increased tensile strength and less the skin can stretch
- The ratio of type III to type I collagen increases
- Photoaged: Fibres are fragmented, thickened, and more soluble

The reduction in collagen deposition with ageing could be due to dermal atrophy and may be related to poor wound healing [27, 50].

Elastin [43, 53]

Elastin is a protein, part of the molecular components of the extracellular matrix, and provides support to the blood vessels, lungs, and the skin [54]. Elastin has short repeated 3–9 amino acid sequences. These form flexible and dynamic structures and are essential functions for cutaneous homeostasis.

- Reduction of elastin content
- Thickening and coiling of fibres in the papillary dermis due to sun exposure
- Reduction in the number of microfibrils
- Increased interfibrillar areas
- Fragmentation of elastic fibres (decreased number and diameter)

The flexible fibre network shows age-related changes after the age of 30. In sun exposure, excessive accumulation of elastic material occurs and accumulates (Fig. 3.5) [27].

Glycosaminoglycans (GAGs)

Glycosaminoglycans (GAGs) are polysaccharide chains containing long repetitions of specific disaccharide units [1]. Hyaluronic acid is made by HA synthase in the plasma membrane. It is then secreted to extracellular spaces in GAG form alone [55]. Hyaluronic acid has many functions, including space-filling, regulating many physiological functions such as cell proliferation, adhesion, migration, differentiation, inflammatory response, and wound healing [55, 56]. Skin hydration is strongly and directly linked to the content and distribution of dermal GAGs, particularly hyaluronic acid [27].

- Decrease in total GAG contents.
- Chronic sun exposure alters both the content and distribution of dermal glycosaminoglycans [57].

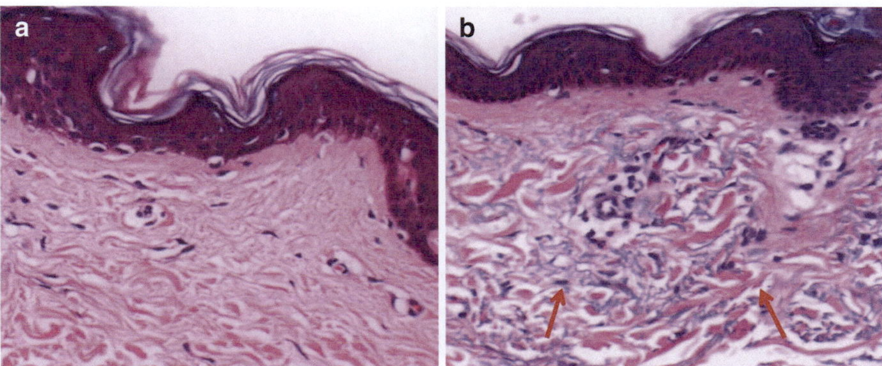

Fig. 3.5 Changes in elastic fibre organisation with skin photoageing. (**a**) Skin from a region that has not been exposed to solar radiation. (**b**) Skin from a region exposed to solar radiation. The skin fragments were obtained from participants in the same age group (45–50 years). The disorganisation of the elastic fibres (arrows) with fragmented material and accumulation characteristic of solar elastosis is observed in the skin exposed to solar radiation. Haematoxylin–eosin staining. Magnification 20× [54]. Reproduced with permission from Weihermann AC, Lorencini M, Brohem CA, de Carvalho CM. Elastin structure and its involvement in skin photoageing. International Journal of Cosmetic Science. 2017;39(3):241–7

- Impairment of glycosaminoglycans and small leucine-rich proteoglycans synthesis [58].
- GAGs increase in photoaged skin. However, abnormally deposited on elastic material interferes with water-binding by GAGs [27].

With ageing, there is a decrease in the number of monocytes and vascular network (most noticeable in the papillary dermis). Decreased vascular network and blood flow result in [43]:

- Diminished nutrient exchange
- Repressed thermoregulation
- Decreased skin surface temperature
- Skin pallor

While the primary target audience for this chapter comprises aesthetic practitioners, acquiring a comprehensive understanding of skin ageing is essential for all healthcare professionals. Ageing introduces disruptions to the structural and functional integrity of the skin, potentially influencing quality of life and contributing to morbidity. Hence, all healthcare professionals are in a unique position to assist patients within our ageing population, imparting knowledge regarding skincare that can help preserve skin function, maintain stability, and avert disease. It's worth highlighting that the skin exhibits a significant capacity for regeneration, which underscores the value of a well-informed approach to skin health and ageing.

Subcutaneous Tissue

The subcutaneous tissue comprises adipose cells, which underpin the connective tissue framework in conjunction with capillary plexuses, dermal papillae, and eccrine ducts [28, 37]. Ageing induces a state of atrophy within subcutaneous fat layers, which is markedly evident in areas such as the hands, shins, and particularly, the face. Indeed, the ageing-related changes observed in the facial region are primarily attributable to the reduction of subcutaneous fat in the head and neck [4, 43, 59]. The resulting loss of facial fat, including the temporal and buccal fat pads, manifests in visible changes such as the deepening of nasolabial folds, the concavity of cheeks, hollowing in the periorbital region, and increased visibility of facial musculature, all of which contribute to the phenomenon of facial skeletonisation (Fig. 3.6).

The superficial adipose layer houses an array of structures, including eccrine glands, hair bulbs, blood vessels, lymphatic channels, and nerves. Importantly, this layer acts as an interface between the skin and the underlying muscles of facial expression. However, with ageing-induced fat atrophy in this layer and skin thinning, the underlying muscles become more prominent, with repeated contractions resulting in overstated expressions. This deflation and volume loss further result in skin laxity and diminished tissue elasticity [37].

Within this subcutaneous layer, additional adipose tissue is compartmentalised into discrete pockets present in both superficial and deep layers, commonly referred to as "fat pads". Notably, the medial midface region holds a more substantial amount of dispersed subcutaneous fat compared to other facial regions [37].

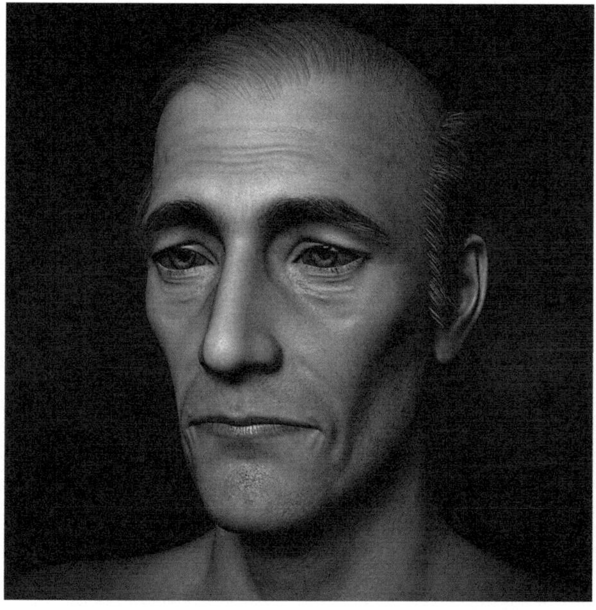

Fig. 3.6 Loss of facial fat, including the temporal and buccal fat pads, deepening of nasolabial folds, cheeks becoming concave, hollowing of the periorbital region, and visibility of facial musculature result in facial skeletonisation. Image credit: Pixabay

Subcutaneous Tissue, Fat Pads, Ligaments, and Facial Spaces

Age-associated transformations in the subcutaneous white adipose tissue (sWAT) of the facial region, encompassing alterations in volume, modifications in collagen content, and changes in the adhesion between dermal and adipose layers, can significantly compromise the mechanical stability of the skin, thereby contributing to the manifestation of ageing symptoms, such as wrinkles. It has been observed that local inflammation often instigates alterations in sWAT; a moderate level of inflammation may facilitate the formation of sWAT, whereas more severe inflammation could potentially result in the degradation of this layer (87).

The ageing of facial features manifests through both the loss and atrophy of fat, which can occur in various facial regions or within the same fat compartment. To provide a generalised observation, the areas that typically undergo fat loss include [60]:

- Periorbital
- Forehead
- Buccal
- Temporal
- Perioral

The persistence of hypertrophy is seen in [60]:

- Submental area
- Jowl
- Lateral nasolabial fold
- Lateral labiomental fold
- Lateral malar regions

The phenomena of atrophy and hypertrophy are not mutually exclusive and can concurrently occur within a singular region. For instance, in the suborbital region, atrophic changes (specifically at the orbital rim) can be observed along with associated concavities. Concurrently, this region may also demonstrate hypertrophy, manifesting as infraorbital fat accumulation and festooning [60].

The adipose compartments within the facial structure are unique entities, presently categorised based on their proximity to the superficial musculoaponeurotic system, either as superficial or deep compartments [61]. A single fat compartment can undergo both hypertrophy and atrophy.

Fat lobules within the superficial adipose compartments are diminutive and consistently dispersed in a compact, homogeneous arrangement [62]. The superficial fat compartments exhibit a high degree of mobility and are susceptible to both static and dynamic muscular stresses. Superficial fat compartments encompass:

1. Upper face
   (a) Forehead: the central and middle

    (b) Lateral-temporal cheek
    (c) Orbital: Superior, lateral inferior
2. Midface
    (a) Medial
    (b) Middle
    (c) Lateral-temporal cheek
    (d) Nasolabial
3. Lower face
    (a) Jowl
    (b) Mental
    (c) Submental

The deep adipose compartments are firmly anchored to the underlying skeletal framework, leading to their immobility. These compartments serve multiple roles, including the provision of contour, support for overlying adipose compartments, and the facilitation of muscle activity by acting as a gliding plane. These deep compartments encompass larger fat lobules that are arranged in a more loosely organised manner, often exhibiting patterns of greater irregularity [62]. Deep adipose compartments, being immobile, include:

- Deep medial cheek fat
- Buccal fat
- Orbital: medial suborbicularis oculi, lateral suborbicularis oculi, and retro-orbicularis oculi

In the superficial planes, which are adjacent to the muscles responsible for facial expression, and in the deeper planes, numerous adipose compartments are observed. Some of these compartments are situated directly atop the facial skeletal structure and include the Nasolabial Fat (NLF), Superficial Medial Cheek (SMC), Middle Cheek, Lateral Temporal Cheek, and the Infraorbital Fat Pad (IOF). The deeper compartments encompass the Deep Medial Cheek (DMC) in the NLF and the Deep Lateral Cheek (DLC).

The facial retaining ligaments are fibrous condensations of an osseocutaneous and musculocutaneous nature, which provide support and maintenance to the various structures of different facial areas. They establish connections between the dermis and soft tissues to the periosteum of the facial skeleton or deep muscle fascia.

The borders of the subcutaneous compartments coincide with the locations of the retaining ligaments that traverse superficially to insert into the dermis. During youth, the transition between these compartments is seamless, rendering them non-detectable. However, with the progression of ageing, a series of concavities and convexities begin to form, distinguishing the various compartments. These morphological alterations have been associated with an array of factors such as minor fat descent, changes in the retaining ligaments (selective atrophy, hypertrophy, and attenuation) leading to ptosis and displacement of the fat compartments [63].

Age-associated alterations in the retaining ligaments have laid the groundwork for one of the most salient hypotheses regarding facial ageing in contemporary research. The progressive extension of these ligaments, combined with the diminution of their supportive capacity over time, collectively contributes to the incidence of soft tissue ptosis. Manifestations include a decrease in rigidity and an increase in laxity. Expansion of the facial spaces extends beyond the weakening of the ligaments, culminating in prototypical age-associated facial bulges and the attenuation of the "multi-linked fibrous system". This phenomenon underscores the multifaceted and interconnected nature of the facial ageing process, with the gradual relaxation of the retaining ligaments playing a pivotal role in the evolution of age-associated facial features [63, 64].

Musculature

The ageing process precipitates an array of changes across all tissues within the orofacial region, inclusive of alterations to muscles, sensorimotor functionality, and associated operations. These shifts encompass degenerative transformations in the Central Nervous System (CNS), modifications in the efferent fibres that supply muscles, variations in certain sensory fibres such as those serving tooth pulp and periodontal tissues, diminished innervation characteristics of muscles and their receptors, along with decreased conduction velocity of trigeminal nerve fibres [65].

Electromyography (EMG) investigations denote a comprehensive array of muscle activation patterns across different age groups. They display heightened electromyographic activity in children and young adults, which gradually wanes in adulthood and old age [66]. Notably, facial skeletal muscles, including masticatory muscles such as the masseter and temporal muscles, undergo atrophy due to lack of use and loss of dentition, reaching up to a reduction of 50% [63, 66] In contrast, muscles of facial expression may not experience comparable degeneration and atrophy due to their frequent utilisation [63]. Illustratively, muscles such as the orbicularis oculi, upper lip elevators, zygomaticus major, and levator labii superioris remain impervious to age-related changes, showing no signs of atrophy or muscle fibre degeneration [63, 67–69]. However, this is not a universal rule; the orbicularis oris fibres of the upper lip have been reported to undergo age-related atrophy, which manifests as reduced muscle thickness, muscle fascicles, and an augmentation of the surrounding epimysium [63, 69].

In youth, muscles of facial expression, predominantly located in perioral and periorbital regions, receive support from deep facial fat pads. This contributes to a uniform facial curvature and facilitates gliding action. With age-related volume loss in various fat pads, these muscles forfeit their support, consequently becoming straighter and shortened over time. The continuous contraction of these muscles, coupled with their increased tonicity at rest, results in the emergence of deep muscle-related lines and wrinkles [70].

Skeleton

The body's bones undergo alterations in mineral composition throughout distinct life stages, such as puberty and ageing. Notably, the mineral composition of the skull presents a unique pattern, with osteoporosis rarely affecting cranial bones [4].

The facial skeleton undergoes substantial transformations with ageing and loss of dentition, leading to a decrease in soft tissue support. This progression instigates significant age-related morphological modifications. The regions most susceptible to resorption encompass areas like parts of the orbital rim, maxilla, piriform area of the nose, and the pre-jowl area of the mandible (Figs. 3.7 and 3.8) [63].

Throughout the later stages of life, distinctive changes are observed within the orbital rim's superomedial region, marked by significant bone resorption in adults over 60 years of age. This ageing process results in a loss of maxilla projection and a 10° decrease in the angle of the jaw. Both the length and height of the mandible diminish, although the breadth remains relatively constant. An increase in the mandibular angle is pronounced with age, apparent in both men and women [63, 66]. Maxillary retrusion contributes to the ageing manifestation of the inferior orbital region and the deepening of nasolabial folds [63].

Premature ageing changes may be observable in those who possess congenital or acquired deficiencies within the relevant skeletal regions. A wealth of experts have observed a clockwise rotation of the maxilla with ageing and an expansion of the bony orbit [72–77]. Owing to the skin being tethered to the bones via retaining ligaments and muscles, which originate from and insert into the skeletal structure, such age-associated transformations in the craniofacial skeleton can considerably impact

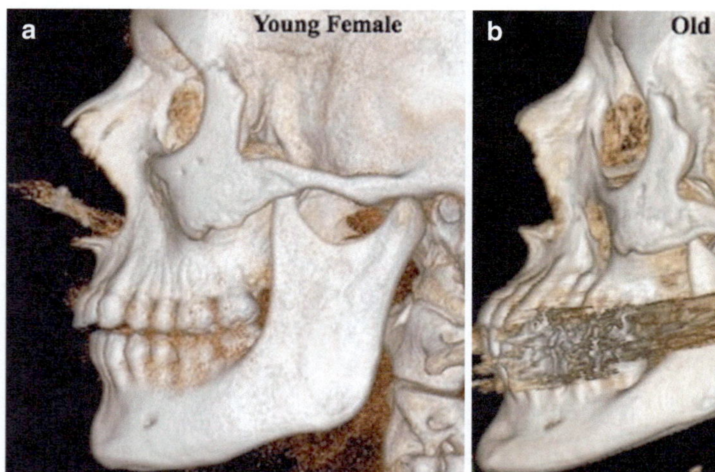
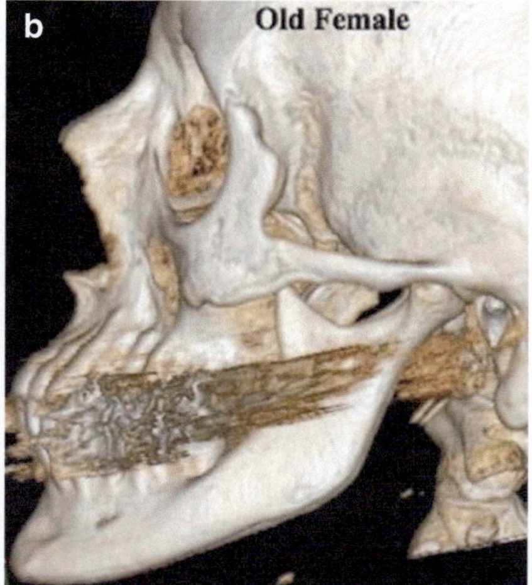

Fig. 3.7 (**a**) Younger profile. Example of a subject in the young age group. Note the position of the orbit, maxilla, and mandible in reference. (**b**) Older profile. Example of a subject in the old age group. Note the retrusion of the orbit and midface with the relative change compared with the mandible. Reproduced with permission from Olivia C. Means, Matthew P. Fahrenkopf, John A. Girotto, 13 - Aging of the facial skeleton, Editor(s): Stephen B. Baker, Pravin K. Patel, Jeffrey Weinzweig, Aesthetic Surgery of the Facial Skeleton, Elsevier, 2022, Pages 104–108 [71]

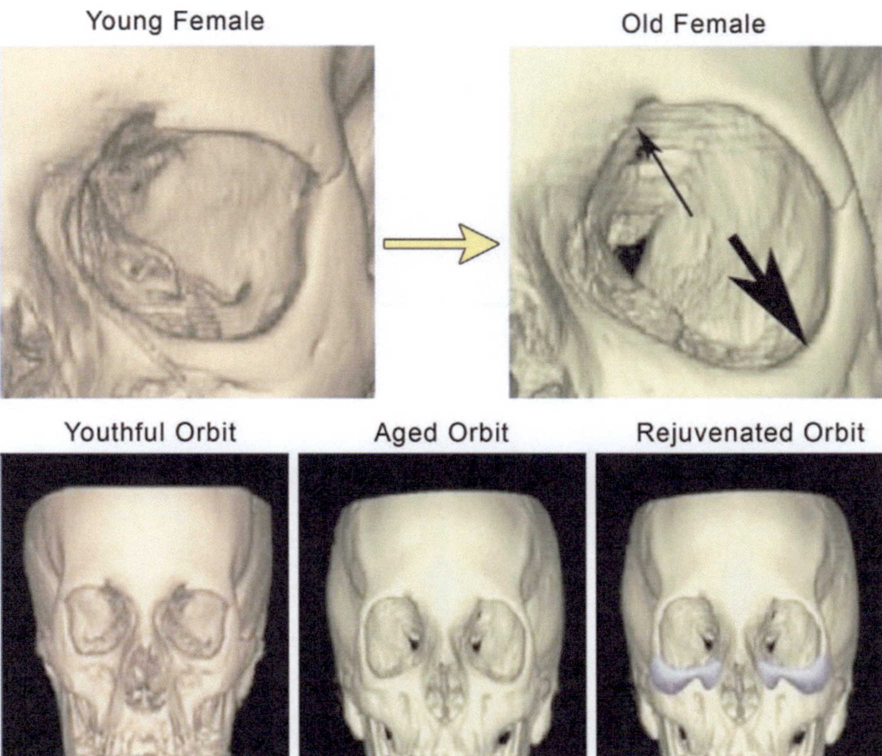

Fig. 3.8 Example images of the bony orbit of a young subject on the left and an old subject on the right (different subject). The aged orbit may be rejuvenated with bony augmentation. Reproduced with permission from Olivia C. Means, Matthew P. Fahrenkopf, John A. Girotto, 13 - Aging of the facial skeleton, Editor(s): Stephen B. Baker, Pravin K. Patel, Jeffrey Weinzweig, Aesthetic Surgery of the Facial Skeleton, Elsevier, 2022, Pages 104–108 [71]

the face's overlying soft tissues. This interaction implies that both the bones and the soft tissues may degrade with ageing, leading to intraorbital fat herniation [78]. Loss of skeletal support further results in the displacement of the ligamentous structure of the face posteriorly, resulting in deep furrows and loss of youthful curvatures of the face [63, 78]. This is particularly noticeable in individuals with congenital or acquired regional bone deficiency.

The ageing of the bony orbit is a significant factor in the development of age-related intraorbital fat herniation (Figs. 3.8 and 3.9) [78].

Ageing leads to a decline in the maxillary angle, which undermines the bony structure of the midface. This exacerbates the nasolabial fold and triggers the formation of tear-trough deformity. With advancing age, the pyriform aperture enlarges, likely driving the morphological transformation of the ageing nose. Such changes encompass relative elongation, a downward-projecting tip, convex shape, and columellar retraction [71, 79].

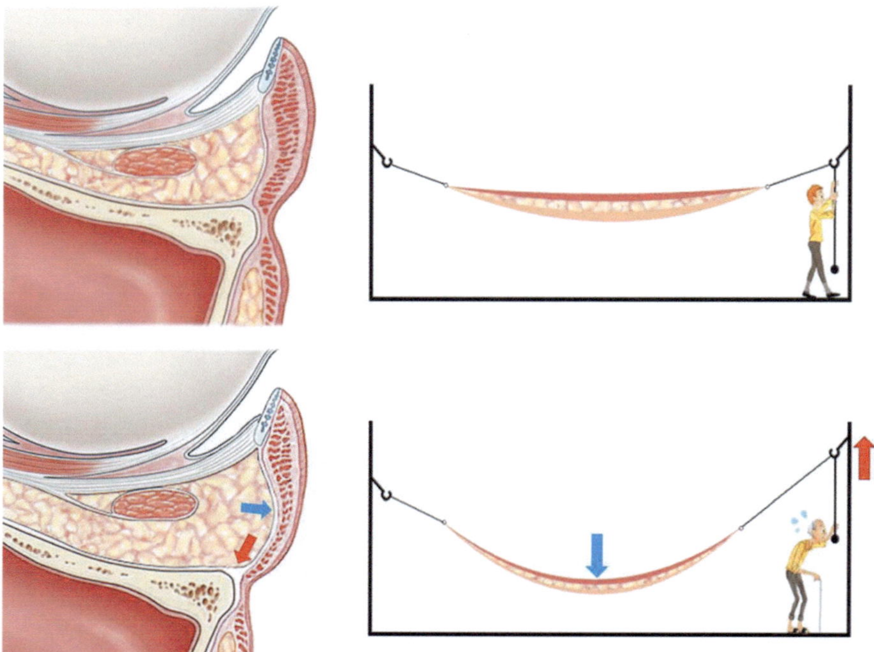

Fig. 3.9 Diagram illustrating our proposed mechanism for infraorbital fat herniation. The red arrow represents the inferior displacement of the inferior orbital rim. The blue arrow represents dermal/fat/muscle atrophy. The ageing man represents the loss of orbicularis oculi muscle tone. Mechanical stretching of the lower eyelid due to the inferior displacement of the inferior orbital rim and weakening of the lower eyelid due to age-related factors such as dermal/fat/muscle atrophy and loss of muscle tone together make the lower eyelid droop anteriorly. Therefore, bulging herniation of the infraorbital fat can be thought of as a "hammock effect". Reproduced with permission from Kim, J., Park, S.W., Choi, J., Jeong, W. and Lee, S., 2018. Ageing of the bony orbit is a major cause of age-related intraorbital fat herniation. Journal of Plastic, Reconstructive & Aesthetic Surgery, 71(5), pp. 658–664

The mandible, much like the maxilla, undergoes reductions in length and height as we age, with little change in its breadth. These alterations contribute to a decrease in chin projection and compromised support to soft tissues, manifested through the laxity of the platysma muscle. An increase in the mandibular angle correlates with a loss in jawline definition (Fig. 3.7) [71].

Classification of Ageing Type

The process of facial ageing exhibits considerable heterogeneity across individuals. For the purpose of effectively evaluating patients and devising appropriate treatment strategies, a classification system can be utilised as a directive reference (Table 3.1).

Table 3.1 Certain parts of the face exhibit fat loss as they age, whereas others exhibit fat persistence or hypertrophy

Type	Appearance	Anatomic changes
Type 1: Hypotrophic	• Cheek appears flat or concave • NLFs and marionette, lines appear due to "pseudoptosis" (i.e., loss of underlying soft tissue) of the skin, which becomes redundant • Jawline skin sags	• Hypotrophy of superficial (SMCF, SLF, MCF, SJF, and IJF) and deep fat compartments (medial and lateral SOOF and DMCF)
Type 2: Hypotrophic/ptotic	• Cheek appears concave at infraorbital areas while appearing convex and ptotic at the nasolabial compartment • Lower cheek slightly convex	• Hypotrophy of deep fat compartments • NLF and SMCF ptosis • Ptosis of MCF, SJF, and IJF
Type 3: Ptotic/hypertrophic	• Infraorbital area appears flat or slightly concave • Convex nasolabial region • Prominent nasolabial fold • Convex lower Cheek	• Hypertrophy and ptosis of SMCF and NLF • Hypertrophy and ptosis of MCF, SJF, and IJF • Slight hypotrophy of deep fat compartments (L-SOOF, M-SOOF, DMCF)
Type 4: Hypertrophic/ptotic	• Cheek appears concave only at the nasojugal groove but convex elsewhere and at the nasolabial region • Convex lower cheek with demarcation of the LTCF	• Hypertrophy with secondary ptosis of the superficial and deep fatty tissues of the cheeks • Ptosis of the nasolabial fold accentuated by hypertrophy • Hypotrophic LTCF

Periorbital, forehead, buccal, temporal, and perioral fat loss occur. However, submental fat hypertrophy is visible in the jowl, lateral nasolabial fold, lateral labiomental crease, and lateral malar regions

DMCF deep medial cheek fat; *IJF* inferior jowl fat; *L-SOOF* lateral suborbicularis oculi fat; *LTCF* lateral temporal-cheek fat; *MCF* middle cheek fat; *M-SOOF* medial suborbicularis oculi fat; *NLF* nasolabial fat; *SJF* superior jowl fat; *SMCF* superficial medial cheek fat

Reproduced with permission Fundaro, S.P., Goh, C.L., Hau, K.C., Moon, H., Lao, P.P. and Salti, G., 2021. Expert consensus on soft-tissue repositioning using absorbable barbed suspension double-needle threads in Asian and Caucasian patients. Journal of Cutaneous and Aesthetic Surgery, 14(1), p. 1 [80]

Facial Balance in Ageing

The harmonious facial proportions and contours are vital in achieving facial balance, a critical aspect of aesthetic perception. The ageing process significantly affects this balance due to inevitable transformations, such as alterations in facial shape, emergence of concavities and convexities, and ptotic (drooping) tissues. Further exacerbating this imbalance is the loss of dentition and consequent dentoalveolar resorption, significantly impacting the structure of the face. Furthermore, hair loss, attributed to hormonal or genetic factors, alters the facial topography, particularly affecting the frontal contour and temple regions. These cumulative changes disrupt the equilibrium of the facial features, leading to the appearance associated with ageing.

Ageing-Ethnic Groups

The process of ageing varies significantly across diverse ethnic groups due to the influence of environmental factors, lifestyle habits, dietary preferences, and genetic characteristics. For instance, skin colour introduces unique elements to the ageing trajectory. Individuals with darker pigmentation often possess higher epidermal melanin concentrations, predisposing them to dyspigmentation, while the presence of a denser, more compact dermis can mask the visibility of facial wrinkles [81]. Comparatively, Caucasian individuals are more likely to display pronounced rhytids, skin laxity, especially in the lower facial region, and facial ptosis [82]. Conversely, Asians tend to be susceptible to inherited or acquired skin pigmentation anomalies [83].

Diverse ethnicities such as Asians, Hispanics, East Asians, and individuals of American ancestry present unique facial structural attributes. Asian individuals typically manifest fewer rhytids in the midface, with ageing primarily resulting in mild to moderate ptosis. East Asians generally have a less anteriorly projected facial skeletal framework compared to Caucasians, causing greater gravitational soft tissue effects in the midface, malar fat pad ptosis, and tear trough formation. Descriptively, the Asian facial morphology often resembles that of an infant, characterised by a wider, rounder face, an elevated brow, a fuller upper lid, a lower nasal bridge with a horizontally flaring ala, a flatter malar prominence and midface, larger, more protuberant lips, and a more retracted chin [81].

In Asian individuals, the occurrence of superficial rhytids is diminished due to increased surface fat and a thicker dermis. Further, Asians have abundant fat and fibre connections between the superficial musculoaponeurotic system and the parotidomasseteric fascia, which aids in decreasing soft tissue ptosis [84].

Wen et al. conducted a study investigating the changes in facial fat compartments among Chinese women of different age groups, with a controlled body mass index. Their findings revealed that as individuals age, the infraorbital area experiences an increase in thickness in both the superficial and deep layers of facial fat. This suggests a redistribution or accumulation of fat in the infraorbital region during the ageing process [84]. Similarly, Jang et al. conducted a study focusing on male patients of different age groups, also with a controlled body mass index. Their research identified a thickening of midfacial fat in the elderly population, particularly in the infraorbital and nasojugal areas. This suggests that as individuals age, there may be a localised increase in fat deposition in these specific regions of the face [85].

African American skin, due to its higher degree of myelinisation, is less prone to UV-induced photoageing compared to other pigmented skin ethnic groups. However, they may exhibit significant degradation of malar fat pads, soft-tissue laxity, and midface jowl formation [81].

Despite the observed differences, research aimed at comprehending the facial ageing process across various ethnic groups remains limited.

Accelerated Ageing Process

Accelerated ageing is a phenomenon characterised by a more rapid progression of the ageing process, resulting in premature manifestations of age-related changes. Several factors have been identified as contributors to this accelerated ageing. Obesity, for instance, has been strongly associated with an expedited ageing process, possibly due to the increased systemic inflammation, oxidative stress, and metabolic dysfunction that accompany excess adiposity. Smoking, another detrimental habit, has also been shown to accelerate ageing, likely through its detrimental effects on cellular function, oxidative stress induction, and impaired repair mechanisms.

Furthermore, environmental factors, such as solar ultraviolet (UV) irradiation, play a significant role in accelerating ageing. Chronic exposure to UV radiation can lead to DNA damage, inflammation, and collagen degradation, contributing to the premature appearance of skin ageing signs. This underscores the importance of sun protection and UV radiation avoidance as preventive measures against accelerated ageing.

Several intrinsic mechanisms contribute to the natural ageing process and its accelerated manifestations. The free-radical oxidative stress hypothesis suggests that cumulative oxidative damage from reactive oxygen species impairs cellular function and accelerates ageing. Mitochondrial dysfunction, characterised by compromised energy production and increased generation of reactive oxygen species, further exacerbates the ageing process. Additionally, telomere shortening, which occurs naturally with each cell division, accelerates cellular ageing and contributes to the overall ageing phenotype.

Understanding the causes and mechanisms underlying accelerated ageing is crucial for developing interventions and preventive strategies to mitigate its impact. By addressing risk factors such as obesity and smoking, and by implementing measures to reduce exposure to environmental stressors like UV radiation, it is possible to mitigate the accelerated ageing process and promote healthier ageing.

Conclusion

In conclusion, facial ageing is a complex and multi-dimensional process involving a combination of intrinsic and extrinsic factors. The ageing process affects both the hard and soft tissues of the face, resulting in a wide range of structural and morphological changes. The skeletal, dental, and cartilaginous structures undergo alterations, leading to loss of volume and support. Fat loss and atrophy, along with the attenuation of the fibro-oseo-cutaneous ligamentous structure, further contribute to facial changes.

Muscular and somatosensory systems are also affected by ageing, leading to changes in facial expressions and sensory perception. These changes can manifest as hollowing in specific regions such as the temporal, buccal, and periorbital areas, deepening of nasolabial folds, concavity of the cheeks, and loss of structural support in the perioral region. The effects of facial muscular contractions can be etched on the skin, resulting in the appearance of facial hypertrophy, ptosis, or skeletonisation.

These age-related morphological changes in the face can have psychological impacts on an individual, as they may project negative emotions and affect personal and social interactions. It is important to understand the multifactorial nature of facial ageing to develop effective interventions and preventive strategies. By addressing factors such as obesity, smoking, sun exposure, and promoting healthy lifestyle choices, it is possible to mitigate the accelerated ageing process and enhance the overall well-being and quality of life for individuals as they age. Further research is needed to elucidate the underlying mechanisms and develop targeted approaches to address the specific needs of individuals from different ethnic backgrounds and cultural contexts.

References

1. Bektas A, Schurman SH, Sen R, Ferrucci L. Aging, inflammation and the environment. Exp Gerontol. 2018;105:10–8.
2. Rodríguez-Rodero S, Fernández-Morera JL, Menéndez-Torre E, Calvanese V, Fernández AF, Fraga MF. Aging genetics and aging. Aging Dis. 2011;2(3):186–95.
3. Christensen K, Iachina M, Rexbye H, Tomassini C, Frederiksen H, McGue M, et al. "Looking old for your age": genetics and mortality. Epidemiology. 2004;15(2):251–2.
4. Marani E, Heida C. Head and neck during puberty and ageing. In: Marani E, Heida C, editors. Head and neck: morphology, models and function. Cham: Springer International Publishing; 2018. p. 493–506.
5. Ilankovan V. Anatomy of ageing face. Br J Oral Maxillofac Surg. 2014;52(3):195–202.
6. Meneghini F, Biondi P. Clinical facial analysis: elements, principles, and techniques. Springer Science & Business Media; 2012.
7. Rexbye H, Petersen I, Johansens M, Klitkou L, Jeune B, Christensen K. Influence of environmental factors on facial ageing. Age Ageing. 2006;35(2):110–5.
8. Warren R, Gartstein V, Kligman AM, Montagna W, Allendorf RA, Ridder GM. Age, sunlight, and facial skin: a histologic and quantitative study. J Am Acad Dermatol. 1991;25(5):751–60.
9. Kennedy C, Bastiaens MT, Willemze R, Bavinck JNB, Bajdik CD, Westendorp RG. Effect of smoking and sun on the aging skin. J Investig Dermatol. 2003;120(4):548–54.
10. Leung W-C, Harvey I. Is skin ageing in the elderly caused by sun exposure or smoking? Br J Dermatol. 2002;147(6):1187–91.
11. Uitto J. Understanding premature skin aging, vol. 337. Mass Medical Soc; 1997. p. 1463–5.
12. Farage MA, Miller KW, Elsner P, Maibach HI. Intrinsic and extrinsic factors in skin ageing: a review. Int J Cosmet Sci. 2008;30(2):87–95.
13. Trojahn C, Dobos G, Lichterfeld A, Blume-Peytavi U, Kottner J. Characterizing facial skin ageing in humans: disentangling extrinsic from intrinsic biological phenomena. Biomed Res Int. 2015;2015:1–9.
14. Gragnani A, Mac Cornick S, Chominski V, de Noronha SMR, de Noronha SAAC, Ferreira LM. Review of major theories of skin aging. Advances in aging. Research. 2014;3:265–84.
15. Mokos ZB, Ćurković D, Kostović K, Čeović R. Facial changes in the mature patient. Clin Dermatol. 2018;36(2):152–8.
16. Stout R, Birch-Machin M. Mitochondria's role in skin ageing. Biology. 2019;8(2):29.
17. Thornton MJ. Estrogens and aging skin. Dermato-endocrinology. 2013;5(2):264–70.

18. Krutmann J, Schikowski T, Morita A, Berneburg M. Environmentally-induced (extrinsic) skin aging: exposomal factors and underlying mechanisms. J Investig Dermatol. 2021;141:1096–103.
19. Marionnet C, Pierrard C, Golebiewski C, Bernerd F. Diversity of biological effects induced by longwave UVA rays (UVA1) in reconstructed skin. PLoS One. 2014;9(8):e105263.
20. Schikowski T, Hüls A. Air pollution and skin aging. Current Environ Health Rep. 2020;7(1):58–64.
21. Nakamura M, Morita A, Seité S, Haarmann-Stemmann T, Grether-Beck S, Krutmann J. Environment-induced lentigines: formation of solar lentigines beyond ultraviolet radiation. Exp Dermatol. 2015;24(6):407–11.
22. Goodman GD, Kaufman J, Day D, Weiss R, Kawata AK, Garcia JK, et al. Impact of smoking and alcohol use on facial aging in women: results of a large multinational, multiracial, cross-sectional survey. J Clin Aesthet Dermatol. 2019;12(8):28.
23. Löffler H. Skin changes induced by alcohol, drug-dependency, and smoking. Braun-Falco's Dermatol. 2020:1–12.
24. Raddatz G, Hagemann S, Aran D, Söhle J, Kulkarni PP, Kaderali L, et al. Aging is associated with highly defined epigenetic changes in the human epidermis. Epigenetics Chromatin. 2013;6(1):36.
25. Characteristics of the aging skin. Adv Wound Care. 2013;2(1):5–10.
26. Farage MA, Miller KW, Elsner P, Maibach HI. Characteristics of the aging skin. Adv Wound Care. 2013;2(1):5–10.
27. Waller JM, Maibach HI. Age and skin structure and function, a quantitative approach (II): protein, glycosaminoglycan, water, and lipid content and structure. Skin Res Technol. 2006;12(3):145–54.
28. Callaghan TM, Wilhelm K-P. A review of ageing and an examination of clinical methods in the assessment of ageing skin. Part I: cellular and molecular perspectives of skin ageing. Int J Cosmet Sci. 2008;30(5):313–22.
29. Tobin DJ. Introduction to skin aging. J Tissue Viability. 2017;26(1):37–46.
30. Farage MA, Miller KW, Maibach HI. Textbook of aging skin. Springer Science & Business Media; 2009.
31. Rossetti D, Kielmanowicz M, Vigodman S, Hu Y, Chen N, Nkengne A, et al. A novel anti-ageing mechanism for retinol: induction of dermal elastin synthesis and elastin fibre formation. Int J Cosmet Sci. 2011;33(1):62–9.
32. Ortonne J, Zartarian M, Verschoore M, Queille-Roussel C, Duteil L. Cellulite and skin ageing: is there any interaction? J Eur Acad Dermatol Venereol. 2008;22(7):827–34.
33. Tsukahara K, Tamatsu Y, Sugawara Y, Shimada K. Morphological study of the relationship between solar elastosis and the development of wrinkles on the forehead and lateral canthus. Arch Dermatol. 2012;148(8):913–7.
34. Jarrar M, Behl S, Shaheen N, Fatima A, Nasab R. Anti-aging effects of retinol and alpha Hydroxy acid on elastin fibers of artificially photo-aged human dermal fibroblast cell lines. Int J Med Health Biomed Pharma Eng. 2015;7:328.
35. Starcher B, Pierce R, Hinek A. UVB irradiation stimulates deposition of new elastic fibers by modified epithelial cells surrounding the hair follicles and sebaceous glands in mice. J Investig Dermatol. 1999;112(4):450–5.
36. Rijken F, Bruijnzeel PL. The pathogenesis of photoaging: the role of neutrophils and neutrophil-derived enzymes. J Investig Dermatol Symp Proc. 2009;14(1):67–72.
37. Coleman S, Saboeiro A, Sengelmann R. A comparison of lipoatrophy and aging: volume deficits in the face. Aesthet Plast Surg. 2009;33(1):14–21.
38. Hall D, Blackett A, Zajac A, Switala S, Airey C. Changes in skinfold thickness with increasing age. Age Ageing. 1981;10(1):19–23.
39. Tan C, Statham B, Marks R, Payne P. Skin thickness measurement by pulsed ultrasound; its reproducibility, validation and variability. Br J Dermatol. 1982;106(6):657–67.
40. Gilhar A, Ullmann Y, Karry R, Shalaginov R, Assy B, Serafimovich S, et al. Ageing of human epidermis: the role of apoptosis, Fas and telomerase. Br J Dermatol. 2004;150(1):56–63.

41. Oriba HA, Bucks DA, Maibach HI. Percutaneous absorption of hydrocortisone and testosterone on the vulva and forearm: effect of the menopause and site. Br J Dermatol. 1996;134(2):229–33.
42. Gilchrest BA, Blog FB, Szabo G. Effects of aging and chronic sun exposure on melanocytes in human skin. J Investig Dermatol. 1979;73(2):141–3.
43. Baumann L. Skin ageing and its treatment. J Pathol. 2007;211(2):241–51.
44. Martini FH, Nath JL, Bartholomew EF, Ober W. Fundamentals of anatomy and physiology. 2001. Pentice Hall; 2015. p. 538–57.
45. Südel KM, Venzke K, Mielke H, Breitenbach U, Mundt C, Jaspers S, et al. Novel aspects of intrinsic and extrinsic aging of human skin: beneficial effects of soy extract. Photochem Photobiol. 2005;81(3):581–7.
46. Chung JH, Eun HC. Angiogenesis in skin aging and photoaging. J Dermatol. 2007;34(9):593–600.
47. Gunin AG, Petrov VV, Golubtzova NN, Vasilieva OV, Kornilova NK. Age-related changes in angiogenesis in human dermis. Exp Gerontol. 2014;55:143–51.
48. McCallion R, Li Wan Po A. Dry and photo-aged skin: manifestations and management. J Clin Pharm Ther. 1993;18(1):15–32.
49. Gniadecka M, Gniadecki R, Serup J, Søndergaard J. Ultrasound structure and digital image analysis of the subepidermal low echogenic band in aged human skin: diurnal changes and interindividual variability. J Investig Dermatol. 1994;102(3):362–5.
50. Uitto J. Connective tissue biochemistry of the aging dermis: age-associated alterations in collagen and elastin. Clin Geriatr Med. 1989;5(1):127–48.
51. Lovell C, Smolenski K, Duance V, Light N, Young S, Dyson M. Type I and III collagen content and fibre distribution in normal human skin during ageing. Br J Dermatol. 1987;117(4):419–28.
52. Lavker RM. Structural alterations in exposed and unexposed aged skin. J Investig Dermatol. 1979;73(1):59–66.
53. Seite S, Zucchi H, Septier D, Igondjo-Tchen S, Senni K, Godeau G. Elastin changes during chronological and photo-ageing: the important role of lysozyme. J Eur Acad Dermatol Venereol. 2006;20(8):980–7.
54. Weihermann AC, Lorencini M, Brohem CA, de Carvalho CM. Elastin structure and its involvement in skin photoageing. Int J Cosmet Sci. 2017;39(3):241–7.
55. Oh J-H, Kim YK, Jung J-Y, Shin J-E, Chung JH. Changes in glycosaminoglycans and related proteoglycans in intrinsically aged human skin in vivo. Exp Dermatol. 2011;20(5):454–6.
56. Stern R, Maibach HI. Hyaluronan in skin: aspects of aging and its pharmacologic modulation. Clin Dermatol. 2008;26(2):106–22.
57. Bernstein E, Underhill C, Hahn P, Brown D, Uitto J. Chronic sun exposure alters both the content and distribution of dermal glycosaminoglycans. Br J Dermatol. 1996;135(2):255–62.
58. Vuillermoz B, Wegrowski Y, Contet-Audonneau J-L, Danoux L, Pauly G, Maquart F-X. Influence of aging on glycosaminoglycans and small leucine-rich proteoglycans production by skin fibroblasts. Mol Cell Biochem. 2005;277(1):63–72.
59. Petrofsky JS, Prowse M, Lohman E. The influence of ageing and diabetes on skin and subcutaneous fat thickness in different regions of the body. J Appl Reliab. 2008;8(1):55.
60. Donofrio LM. Fat distribution: a morphologic study of the aging face. Dermatol Surg. 2000;26(12):1107–12.
61. Wan D, Amirlak B, Rohrich R, Davis K. The clinical importance of the fat compartments in midfacial aging. Plast Reconstr Surg Glob Open. 2013;1(9):e92.
62. Swift A, Liew S, Weinkle S, Garcia JK, Silberberg MB. The facial aging process from the "inside out". Aesthet Surg J. 2020;41:1107–19.
63. Mendelson B, Wong C-H. Anatomy of the aging face. Plast Surgery. 2013;2:78–92.
64. Knize DM. Limited incision submental lipectomy and platysmaplasty. Plast Reconstr Surg. 2004;113(4):1275–8.
65. Sessle BJ. Can you be too old for oral implants? An update on ageing and plasticity in the orofacial sensorimotor system. J Oral Rehabil. 2019;46(10):936–51.

66. Serra-Renom JM, Serra-Mestre JM. Facelift. Atlas of minimally invasive facelift. Springer; 2016. p. 83–97.
67. Penna V, Stark G-B, Eisenhardt SU, Bannasch H, Iblher N. The aging lip: a comparative histological analysis of age-related changes in the upper lip complex. Plast Reconstr Surg. 2009;124(2):624–8.
68. Gosain AK, Amarante M, Hyde JS, Yousif NJ. A dynamic analysis of changes in the nasolabial fold using magnetic resonance imaging: implications for facial rejuvenation and facial animation surgery. Plast Reconstr Surg. 1996;98(4):622–36.
69. Pessa JE, Zadoo VP, Yuan C, Ayedelotte JD, Cuellar FJ, Cochran SC, et al. Concertina effect and facial aging: nonlinear aspects of youthfulness and skeletal remodeling, and why, perhaps, infants have jowls. Plast Reconstr Surg. 1999;103(2):635–44.
70. Le Louarn C. [Muscular aging and its involvement in facial aging: the face recurve concept]. Anna Dermatol Venereol. 2009;136(Suppl 4):S67–72.
71. Means OC, Fahrenkopf MP, Girotto JA. Chapter 13—Aging of the facial skeleton. In: Baker SB, Patel PK, Weinzweig J, editors. Aesthetic surgery of the facial skeleton. London: Elsevier; 2022. p. 104–8.
72. Pessa JE. An algorithm of facial aging: verification of Lambros's theory by three-dimensional stereolithography, with reference to the pathogenesis of midfacial aging, scleral show, and the lateral suborbital trough deformity. Plast Reconstr Surg. 2000;106(2):479–88.
73. Richard MJ, Morris C, Deen BF, Gray L, Woodward JA. Analysis of the anatomic changes of the aging facial skeleton using computer-assisted tomography. Ophthalmic Plast Reconstr Surg. 2009;25(5):382–6.
74. Kahn DM, Shaw RB Jr. Aging of the bony orbit: a three-dimensional computed tomographic study. Aesthet Surg J. 2008;28(3):258–64.
75. Pessa JE, Chen Y. Curve analysis of the aging orbital aperture. Plast Reconstr Surg. 2002;109(2):751–5; discussion 6, 756, 757.
76. Shaw RB Jr, Katzel EB, Koltz PF, Yaremchuk MJ, Girotto JA, Kahn DM, et al. Aging of the facial skeleton: aesthetic implications and rejuvenation strategies. Plast Reconstr Surg. 2011;127(1):374–83.
77. Bartlett SP, Grossman R, Whitaker LA. Age-related changes of the craniofacial skeleton: an anthropometric and histologic analysis. Plast Reconstr Surg. 1992;90(4):592–600.
78. Kim J, Park SW, Choi J, Jeong W, Lee S. Ageing of the bony orbit is a major cause of age-related intraorbital fat herniation. J Plast Reconstr Aesthet Surg. 2018;71(5):658–64.
79. Rohrich R, Hollier L, Gunter J, editors. The aging nose. Dallas rhinoplasty symposium. 2001.
80. Fundaro SP, Goh CL, Hau KC, Moon H, Lao PP, Salti G. Expert consensus on soft-tissue repositioning using absorbable barbed suspension double-needle threads in Asian and Caucasian patients. J Cutan Aesthet Surg. 2021;14(1):1–13.
81. Vashi NA, de Castro Maymone MB, Kundu RV. Aging differences in ethnic skin. J Clin Aesthet Dermatol. 2016;9(1):31–8.
82. Rawlings AV. Ethnic skin types: are there differences in skin structure and function? 1. Int J Cosmet Sci. 2006;28(2):79–93.
83. Yu SS, Pai S, Neuhaus IM, Grekin RC. Diagnosis and treatment of pigmentary disorders in Asian skin. Facial Plast Surg Clin North Am. 2007;15(3):367–80.
84. Wen L-h, Zhong P-h, Wang X-l, An Y, Hu Z-q, Liu D-l, et al. Analysis of age-related changes in midfacial fat compartments in Asian women using computed tomography. J Plast Reconstr Aesthet Surg. 2019;72(11):1839–46.
85. Jang M-S, Kim HY, Dhong H-J, Chung S-K, Hong SD, Cho H-J. An analysis of Asian midfacial fat thickness according to age group using computed tomography. J Plast Reconstr Aesthet Surg. 2015;68(3):344–50.

Facial Assessment in Non-surgical Aesthetic Practice

4

Souphiyeh Samizadeh

Abstract

The escalating interest in non-surgical and minimally-invasive aesthetic procedures underscores the critical role of comprehensive facial assessments in formulating customized treatment plans that align with individual patient profiles and expectations. This chapter explores the multifaceted process of facial evaluation, highlighting the necessity for an exhaustive analysis of facial anatomy and aesthetic objectives to secure desired outcomes. Central to this discourse are the fundamental tenets of facial analysis, such as evaluating facial proportions and symmetry, which are pivotal for a holistic understanding of facial aesthetics. Through detailed exploration of these aspects, the chapter endeavors to furnish aesthetic practitioners with the pivotal knowledge and competencies essential for administering personalized, efficacious, and safe non-surgical aesthetic interventions. This narrative not only enhances the practitioner's diagnostic acumen but also broadens the spectrum of treatment strategies, thereby elevating the standard of patient care in the aesthetic medicine.

Keywords

Facial aesthetics · Facial assessment · Facial shape · Symmetry · Facial type · Facial profile · Dentofacial · Asian aesthetics · Dermal fillers · Botulinum toxin · Mandible · Maxilla · Occlusion

S. Samizadeh (✉)
King's College London, London, UK

University College London, London, UK

Great British Academy of Aesthetic Medicine, London, UK
e-mail: info@baamed.co.uk

© Springer Nature Switzerland AG 2024
S. Samizadeh (ed.), *Thread Lifting Techniques for Facial Rejuvenation and Recontouring*, https://doi.org/10.1007/978-3-031-47954-0_4

This chapter is respectfully dedicated to Dr. Farhad Naini, esteemed consultant orthodontist at St George's University Hospitals NHS Foundation Trust. Dr. Naini's seminal work, Facial Aesthetics: Concepts and Clinical Diagnosis, stands as a cornerstone in our field, offering unparalleled depth and insight [1]. It is a resource I earnestly recommend to all healthcare professionals and practitioners, including those in dermatology, plastic surgery and aesthetic medicine, for its comprehensive exploration of facial aesthetics. Beyond his scholarly contributions, Dr. Naini's dedication to ethical practice and patient care shines brightly, notably through his thoughtful evolution of clinical terminology—from 'lip incompetence' to 'incomplete lip seal.' This change not only reflects a deeper sensitivity towards patient dignity but also exemplifies his profound impact on the language and ethos of our profession.

Facial Assessment in Non-surgical Aesthetics Setting

In non-surgical aesthetic practice, precise facial assessment is pivotal for developing customized treatment plans. This process extends beyond simple observation to a thorough examination that addresses the patient's individual concerns. It involves understanding the multifactorial etiology of facial issues, whether due to aging, volumetric changes, structural deficiencies, or ethnic anatomical characteristics. Such comprehensive evaluations allow practitioners to identify the underlying factors contributing to the patient's aesthetic concerns and devise appropriate treatment strategies.

Reflecting on past practices, the approach to treating manifestations signs of aging lacked this depth of analysis. Historically, treatments such as the filling of nasolabial folds were often approached with a singular focus, without a comprehensive evaluation of the underlying causes. Practitioners might have applied soft tissue fillers directly to these folds without considering the broader anatomical and functional factors contributing to their appearance. This approach overlooks critical elements such as the facial skeletal structure, muscular dynamics, overall facial volume distribution, and the role of dentition in supporting soft tissue. Such oversights underscore the critical need for a holistic assessment that encompasses not only the superficial target areas but also the underlying structural and functional dynamics.

Facial analysis is the first step in patient assessment for facial aesthetics and function prior to treatment planning to define the shape, proportions, volume and contour appearance, symmetry, visible deformities, and relative position of facial features. Such analysis is carried out by direct examination, 2D and 3D photographs under good light, and in case of pre-surgical preparations, radiographs, CT, or MRI imaging. Facial analysis is a process that starts prior to planning for aesthetic procedures and continues throughout the procedure and after. Accurate assessment and analysis play a significant role in treatment planning, evaluation of treatment outcomes, and developing new treatment plans and techniques for successful delivery.

Ensuring consistency and reproducibility in facial analysis is imperative for the reliability of assessments. This goal can be attained by utilizing standardized templates and meticulous documentation of findings. Such systematic approaches to facial analysis empower practitioners to accurately identify suitable candidates for specific procedures, significantly mitigating the risk of post-operative complications that may arise from inappropriate patient selection.

Furthermore, an understanding of the inherent variations in facial anatomy across different ethnicities, genders, and age groups is crucial. These differences, documented through cephalometric studies and clinical observation, influence not only the physical assessment but also the alignment of treatments with culturally and individually varied beauty standards and expectations [2–4]. This initial assessment is fundamental to the success of non-surgical interventions. It ensures that treatments are not only corrective but also tailored to enhance each patient's unique facial architecture. By integrating a detailed understanding of facial anatomy, including the impacts of aging, the specifics of ethnic facial features, and the dynamics of facial musculature and skeletal structure, practitioners can achieve outcomes that are both functionally and aesthetically optimal. This chapter aims to provide a thorough overview of the principles and techniques essential for conducting comprehensive facial assessments in non-surgical aesthetic practice.

Clinical Assessment

Lighting and Background

The significance of lighting and background settings during both consultation and photographic documentation in healthcare settings cannot be overstated. Healthcare facilities, including hospitals, adhere to national standards or codes of practice that dictate specific requirements for lighting. These standards ensure that the levels of illumination, control of glare from light sources, as well as the color and color-rendition properties of these sources, are optimized for clinical environments [5]. It is important to note that the lighting used for patient examinations differs significantly from the more intense surgical lighting found in operating rooms. This distinction is crucial for providing the optimal visibility needed for precise assessments while avoiding the excessive brightness typical of surgical environments. Furthermore, when it comes to clinical photography, the requirements become even more specific. Effective photographic documentation demands steady, high-quality lighting to capture detailed images without distortion. This should be complemented by a non-reflective background, which eliminates potential distractions and focuses attention on the subject of the photograph. Such controlled photographic conditions contribute significantly to the comprehensive evaluation of patients' concerns, offering an invaluable perspective that goes beyond the limitations of direct observation.

Natural Head Position

The Natural Head Position (NHP) is a standardized and reproducible posture of the head when an individual is in an upright stance. It is characterized by the individual's gaze focusing on a distant point directly at eye level (along the horizontal visual axis) or looking into a mirror positioned directly ahead is [6, 7]. This posture is critical for accurate facial evaluation, serving as a fundamental reference in both clinical and research settings.

Improper positioning of the head can significantly compromise the accuracy of facial evaluations. It may result in erroneous observations and measurements, particularly affecting the assessment of the anteroposterior facial angles and the relationships between jaw structures. Given the natural tendency of individuals to assume compensatory postures that mitigate perceived facial asymmetries, careful attention may be required to adjust the head position back to the NHP. This adjustment is crucial for ensuring the integrity of the assessment process, allowing for a more accurate analysis of facial structure and symmetry [7]. Furthermore, during the evaluation, it is imperative to ensure that the peri-oral soft tissues remain relaxed and that there is no contact between the teeth. Common behaviors such as teeth clenching or, in cases of an incomplete lip seal, pressing the lips together can inadvertently lead to mentalis muscle strain. Such actions may distort the observer's perception, falsely suggesting a reduced facial height due to the induced tension in facial musculature.

Craniofacial Soft Tissue Landmarks

Facial analysis can be aided by understanding and using soft tissue and skeletal landmarks (Fig. 4.1). These landmarks, identifiable across individuals, provide a reliable framework for the comprehensive assessment of facial features. They enable the precise measurement of facial lines and angles, thereby facilitating quantitative analysis in aesthetic evaluations. Additionally, the concept of dividing the face into aesthetic units and subunits further refines the assessment process. This division allows for a meticulous examination of each area, both as an independent entity and in its relation to surrounding units. For a thorough evaluation, the following dimensions of each subunit can be evaluated:

- Height: The vertical dimension of the subunit, providing insight into the proportionality of facial features.
- Width: The horizontal extent of the subunit, crucial for understanding facial symmetry and balance.
- Projection: The degree to which a subunit protrudes from the facial plane, influencing the overall facial contour.
- Transition: The manner in which adjacent units blend or demarcate, affecting the harmony and continuity of facial aesthetics.
- Interrelationship: The spatial and proportional relationships among different units, essential for achieving a cohesive understanding of facial structure.

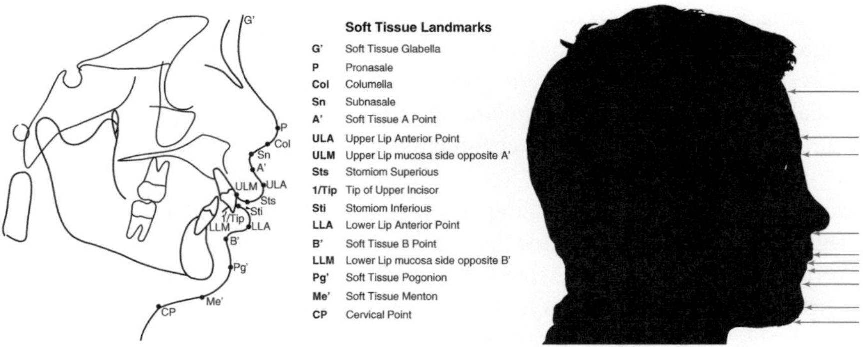

Landmarks	Definition
Tr	Glabella: the most anterior point on the soft tissue outline of the brow ridge
G	Glabella: the most anterior point on the soft tissue outline of the brow ridge
N'	Soft tissue nasion: the deepest point on the soft tissue outline below glabella.
Prn	Pronasale: the most anterior point on the outline of the nose.
Cm	Columella: the most anterior point on the columella of the nose.
Sn	Subnasale: the junction of the upper lip and the columella
A'	Soft tissue A point: the deepest point on the anterior outline of the upper lip below Sn.
Ls	Labrale superius: the muco-cutaneous junction of the upper lip.
Sts	Stomion superius: the lowermost point on the vermillion of the upper lip.
Sto	Stomion: the point of contact, in the midline, between the upper and lower lips, where the lips are competent.
Sti	Stomion inferius: the uppermost point on the vermillion of the lower lip.
Li	Labrale inferius: the muco-cutaneous junction of the lower lip.
B'	Soft tissue B point: the deepest point on the anterior outline of the lower lip, above Pg'.
Pg'	Soft tissue pogonion: the most anterior point on the soft tissue outline of the chin below B'.
Me'	Soft tissue menton: the most inferior point on the soft tissue outline of the chin.

Fig. 4.1 Utilizing Soft Tissue and Skeletal Landmarks in Facial Analysis This figure demonstrates the crucial role of identifiable soft tissue and skeletal landmarks in the comprehensive assessment of facial structure. Reproduced with permission from Bergman, R.T., 1999. Cephalometric soft tissue facial analysis. American Journal of Orthodontics and Dentofacial Orthopedics, 116(4), pp. 373–389 [8]

The Maxillo–Mandibular Relationship: A Critical Consideration in Facial Assessment

The relative position of the maxilla to the mandible can be examined on assessment. The maxillo-mandibular relationship delineates the spatial orientation and interaction between the maxilla (upper jaw) and the mandible (lower jaw), which is pivotal in defining facial structure, aesthetics, and function. This relationship is crucial for assessing the skeletal structure of the face, facial symmetry, and planning both orthodontic and maxillofacial interventions. This relationship can be examined through qualitative observations and quantitative measurements. In orthodontic practice, detailed assessments of the maxilla and mandible's relative positioning are essential for diagnosing malalignments and informing the development of corrective strategies. These assessments encompass:

- Sagittal Relationship: Evaluating the anterior-posterior alignment to identify sagittal discrepancies that affect jaw positioning and occlusion.
- Vertical Relationship: Assessing the vertical dimension for its impact on facial height and profile and identifying vertical growth anomalies.
- Transverse Relationship: Examining lateral alignment to address crossbites or asymmetrical jaw growth that compromises facial balance.
- Centric Relation: Analyzing the neutral, unforced jaw position to assess the jaw's functional dynamics and its implications for the temporomandibular joint (TMJ) and facial aesthetics.

Understanding the maxillo-mandibular relationship is not only fundamental to orthodontic planning but also crucial when devising surgical or non-surgical interventions aimed at enhancing facial harmony and aesthetics. Basic assessments should be conducted to ensure that any non-surgical or minimally invasive aesthetic interventions do not overlook underlying structural considerations that could impact the overall outcome.

Analysis from the Frontal View: Understanding Facial Harmony

Achieving facial harmony significantly depends on the interplay between the face's height and width. It's the proportional relationship of these dimensions, rather than their absolute values, that defines the overall facial type. Additionally, an individual's body composition—whether short and stocky or long and slender—affects the perception of facial proportions and must be considered in the analysis. Accurately assessing these elements requires a systematic approach:

- Vertical Proportions: This focuses on assessing the face's vertical dimensions and detecting any asymmetrical features, crucial for understanding the vertical balance.
  - Facial dimension and proportions
  - Asymmetries
- Transverse Proportions: The analysis of horizontal dimensions emphasizes the importance of assessing the face's width and identifying asymmetries that could affect balance.:
  - Facial dimensions and proportions
  - Asymmetries
- Ears and nose shape and position
- Eyes
  - Scleral show
  - Eyelid shape
- Lip form and symmetry

Further assessments involve analyzing the relationships between various facial widths, including:

- Bitemporal distance: The distance across the temporal regions.
- Bizygomatic distance: The broadest distance across the zygomatic arches.
- Bigonal distance: The breadth across the mandibular angles.
- Mental width: The width of the mandible at the chin.

The comparison of these widths against the face's height, as detailed in Fig. 4.2, provides a framework for defining the facial shape (Fig. 4.2).

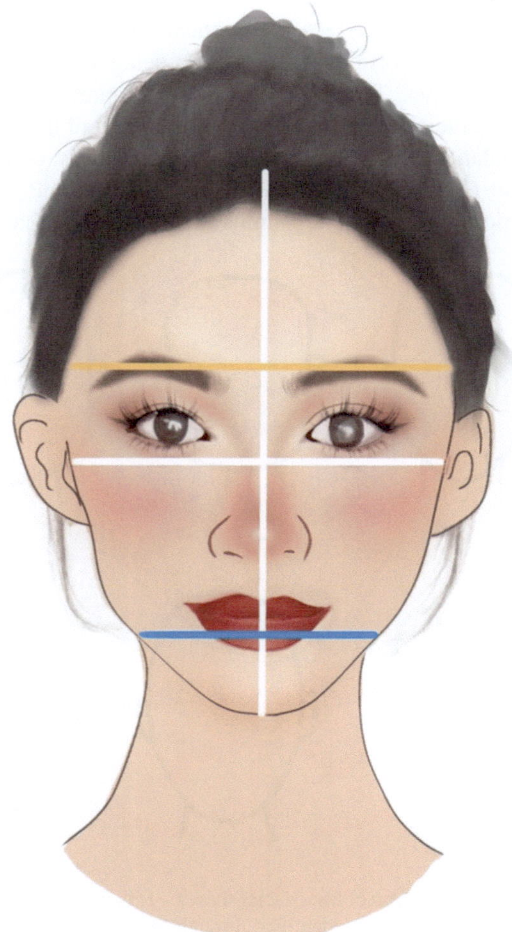

Fig. 4.2 Facial shape is defined through a comparative analysis of specific facial widths relative to overall facial height. This methodical approach allows for the categorization of facial types by assessing dimensional proportions that contribute to the unique contour and structure of the face

Basic Facial Shape: Frontal View

The following table outlines the primary facial shapes based on these dimensions:

Basic facial shape (frontal view)	
Overall facial shape	Square Round Triangular
Vertical facial height	Reduced Normal Increased
Transverse facial width	Broad (wide) Normal Narrow

Examples of various facial and head shapes can be seen below (Fig. 4.3):

Vertical Proportions

The division of the face into vertical thirds offers a structured approach to evaluating facial proportions, facilitating a detailed comparison of the upper, middle, and lower sections. This method allows for a precise assessment of the relative heights of these facial thirds (Fig. 4.4). A key aspect of this analysis is determining the vertical balance of the face, which is achieved by comparing the lower anterior face height (measured from the subnasale to the soft tissue menton) against the total anterior face height (spanning from the glabella to the menton). For practical

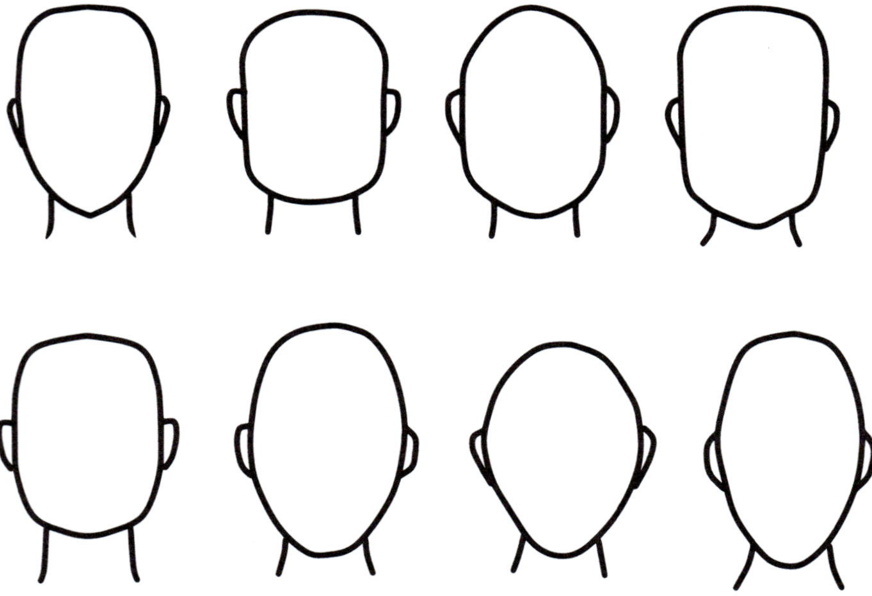

Fig. 4.3 Illustration of basic facial shapes - This figure showcases examples of square, round, and triangular facial shapes identified through frontal view analysis, providing a visual reference for understanding the impact of vertical facial height and transverse facial width on overall facial aesthetics [9, 10]

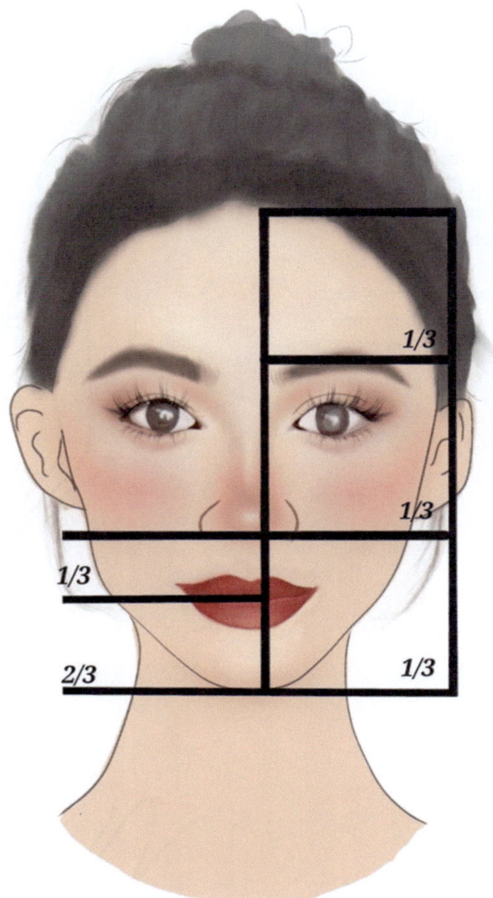

Fig. 4.4 Vertical Proportions of the Face- This figure illustrates the division of the face into vertical thirds, with an additional focus on the further subdivision of the lower face to evaluate the vertical proportions of the upper and lower lips facilitating assessment of facial balance and symmetry

measurement, the vertical dimension of the face can be gauged using simple tools such as a ruler. Specifically, the upper facial height and the lower facial height are critical metrics. Typically, these two measurements are found to be equivalent, providing a harmonious vertical balance that is essential for facial aesthetics [11].

The lower anterior face height, juxtaposed with the overall anterior face height, is instrumental in determining the face's vertical equilibrium. This measurement aids in distinguishing between different facial types based on their vertical dimension ratios: (Fig. 4.5).

- Equal: Indicates an average facial type, where the vertical proportions are harmoniously balanced.
- Reduced ratio: Characterizes a short-faced type, suggesting a shorter lower facial third relative to the overall facial height.
- Increased ratio: Identifies a long-faced type, indicating a longer lower facial third in comparison to the overall facial height.

Fig. 4.5 Lower Anterior Face Height and Classification of Facial Types - This figure illustrates the method of determining the lower anterior face height relative to the overall anterior face height, enabling the classification of facial types into average, short-faced, and long-faced categories based on their vertical dimension ratios

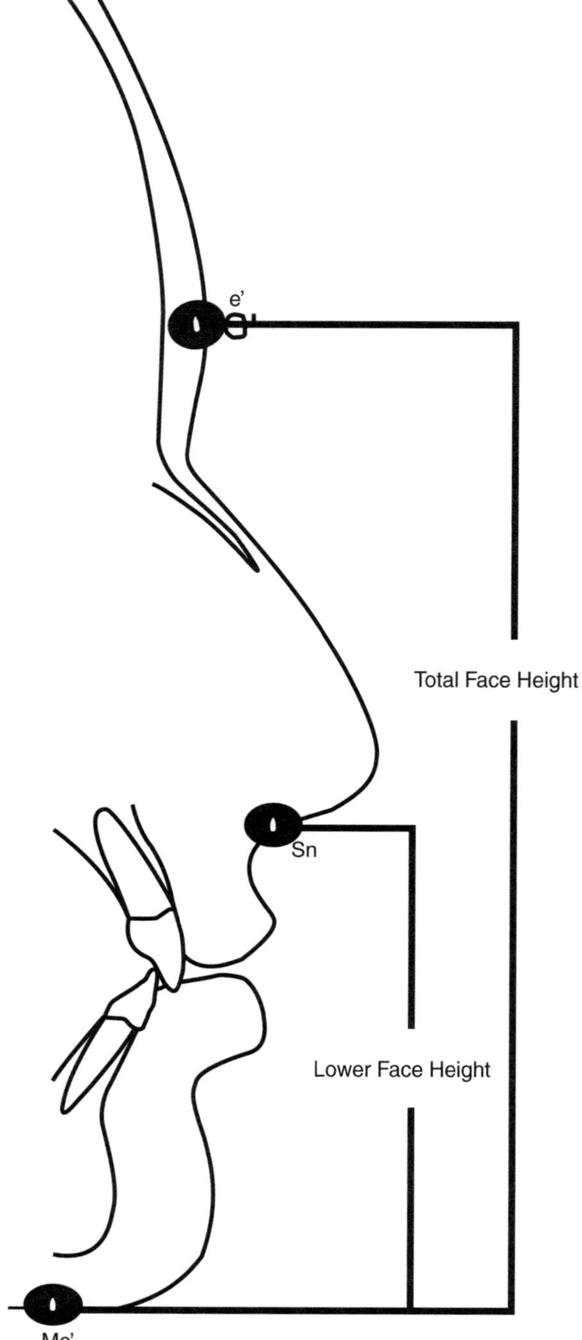

The lower anterior facial third is meticulously segmented, facilitating an in-depth examination of the vertical proportions of both the upper and lower lips. This detailed approach necessitates individual measurements of the lengths of the upper and lower lips, as well as a comprehensive assessment of the proportional heights within the lower facial segment. Specifically, the measurement process involves:

The upper lip length: subnasale to stomion superius.
The lower lip length: stomion inferius to soft tissue menton.

Symmetry

Symmetry is a component of face attractiveness. Mild asymmetry is generally considered normal and often acceptable within the natural variance observed in human faces. Research consistently shows that symmetry is closely associated with the perception of facial beauty, with faces that are more symmetrical and closer average proportions being perceived as more attractive [12–15]. Direct anthropometry, digital photography, and three-dimensional surface imaging techniques may be used to analyse craniofacial surface morphology and symmetry. For accurate symmetry assessment, it is crucial to evaluate the patient in an upright position [16]. Transverse asymmetries are best assessed with the patient's head in NHP and a relaxed stance. This standard positioning mitigates the potential for gravity-induced distortion of facial features, ensuring a more reliable evaluation of the facial balance. Furthermore, it's important to recognize that individuals often unconsciously adjust their head position to minimize the visual impact of asymmetries. These compensatory poses can significantly alter the appearance of facial symmetry and are frequently observed in social media pictures and videos, where individuals may present themselves in angles that are most flattering. This tendency underscores the need for a structured approach to facial assessment in clinical settings, where controlled conditions can provide a more objective view of symmetry without the influence of self-adjusted poses.

Vertical Asymmetries

Facial Midline

Vertical asymmetries are discerned by employing the inter-pupillary line as a benchmark. This strategy ensures a reliable reference, especially in the absence of conditions such as ocular dystopia. Establishing the facial midline is crucial for a comprehensive analysis of asymmetries, with the inter-pupillary line providing the initial point of reference. This guideline extends through the central forehead, intersects the inter-pupillary space, and continues along the nose's dorsum to the philtrum of the upper lip, facilitating a thorough assessment of vertical alignment.

Vertical Mandibular Asymmetry

Vertical mandibular asymmetry, indicative of conditions such as condylar hyperplasia, hypoplasia, or agenesis, presents unique challenges in facial symmetry assessment. Identifying these asymmetries requires careful observation and measurement, often necessitating advanced diagnostic imaging to determine the underlying skeletal discrepancies accurately.

Transverse Proportions

To accurately assess the transverse dimensions of the face, a frontal evaluation is essential. This approach allows for the identification of any deviations in facial midline symmetry. The facial structure is segmented into fifths, utilizing the width between the inner corners of the eyes (inter-canthal distance) as a key reference point for measuring transverse proportions. This methodical division aids in the precise determination of facial width and the identification of any lateral asymmetries that may impact overall facial harmony (Fig. 4.6).

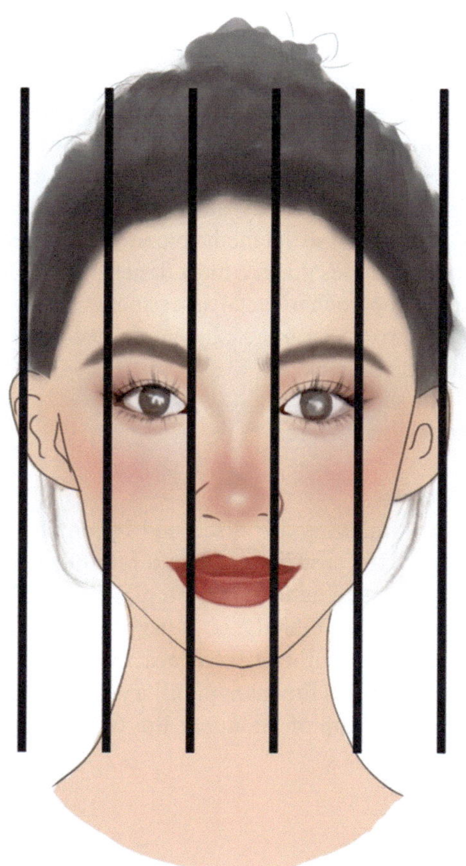

Fig. 4.6 The 'Rule of Fifths' in Measuring Transverse Facial Proportions-The 'Rule of Fifths' is a standardized method for evaluating the transverse proportions of the face, wherein the face is conceptually divided into five vertical segments of equivalent width, each approximately equal to the width of the patient's eye. The central fifth is defined by the inner canthi, which are the medial junctures where the upper and lower eyelids converge, encompassing the lacrimal ducts. This proportional analysis is a tool in identifying asymmetries or deviations from ideal facial symmetry, facilitating a more precise assessment of facial balance and aesthetic harmony

Analysis: Oblique View

The oblique perspective offers a nuanced examination of facial features, providing insight into their three-dimensional contours and interrelations. This angle allows for the assessment of:

- Forehead: Observing contour and frontal hairline.
- Temporal: Evaluating the concavity or convexity and soft tissue fullness.
- Orbital: Inspecting the eye shape, eyelid position, and periorbital volume.
- Zygomatic and malar regions: Assessing prominence, volume, and the transition to adjacent areas.
- Paranasal: Noting any concavities or convexities adjacent to the nasal base.
- Preauricular: Inspecting the anterior to the ear and the blending into the cheek.
- Mandibular angle and jawline: Assessing angle definition, jawline contour, and symmetry.
- Submental area: Evaluating the fullness, definition, and continuity with the neck.

Analysis: Lateral

Examining each side of the face separately is crucial, as asymmetry often manifests uniquely on each side. From a lateral viewpoint, the following can be delineated:

- Forehead projection: Analyzing the protrusion or recession relative to the facial planes.
- Infra-orbital rims: Assessing prominence or retrusion in relation to the globe.
- Nose: Evaluating shape, size, and the nasolabial angle for harmony with the face.
- Paranasal regions: Identifying support or deficiency affecting nasolabial folds.
- Nasolabial Angle: Assessing the angle between the philtrum and the upper lip to gauge the aesthetic relationship between the nose and the upper lip.
- Jaw relationship: Examining the mandibular projection and its relation to the maxilla.
- Facial profile: Classifying as straight, convex, or concave based on the overall contour.
- Lips: Assessing the fullness, symmetry, and position relative to each other and the face.
- Lower lip and chin: Assessing the relationship between the lower lip, chin projection, and the lower facial contour.
- Lower lip to submental plane angle: Evaluating the angle for insights into lower facial contour.
- Mandibular plane angle: Observing the angle formed by the mandibular plane with other reference planes offers clues about facial height and lower jaw alignment.

Infra-orbital Rims

The anatomical configuration of the infraorbital rims serves as a critical marker for evaluating the orbital and midfacial volumetric attributes. Deviations or deficiencies in these rims can be diagnostic of underlying skeletal retrusions, notably affecting the orbital and periorbital aesthetic zones. Such conditions often reflect a broader skeletal insufficiency that may necessitate comprehensive aesthetic or reconstructive strategies. The relative position of the anteroposterior position of the infraorbital rim can be assessed to:

- The globe of the eye
- The supra-orbital ridge

An underdeveloped infra-orbital rim usually accompanies a high-level deficiency of the maxilla and a hypoplastic midface.

Para-nasal Region

Parallelly, the presence of paranasal hollowing is a significant indicator of skeletal underpinning inadequacies, primarily denoting anteroposterior deficiencies in the maxillary region. This phenomenon not only disrupts the facial aesthetic equilibrium but also signals potential functional implications, necessitating a multidimensional approach to restore facial harmony and structural integrity.

Skeletal Pattern

The skeletal architecture forms the foundational structure upon which facial aesthetics are built, making its comprehensive assessment indispensable. Understanding the positional relationship between the mandible and maxilla is a cornerstone of aesthetic evaluation and treatment planning. This relationship is pivotal because it directly influences the facial profile, symmetry, and balance, which are essential elements of perceived beauty and harmony. The maxilla and mandible form the basis of the lower facial third, dictating the contour of the jawline, the prominence of the chin, and the overall facial structure. An accurate assessment of the maxilla-to-mandible relationship allows practitioners to identify underlying skeletal discrepancies that can affect facial aesthetics. For instance, a retruded mandible (mandibular retrusion) or a protruded mandible (mandibular prognathism) significantly alters the facial profile, impacting the aesthetic balance. Moreover, the maxilla-mandible relationship is crucial for determining the optimal approach to enhance facial proportions and symmetry. Recognizing and addressing these skeletal relationships can lead to more natural and harmonious outcomes. It enables practitioners to tailor treatments that not only address superficial signs of aging or enhance specific features but also consider the underlying skeletal structure for comprehensive facial rejuvenation. This approach ensures that non-surgical interventions contribute positively to the facial harmony, reinforcing the importance of a deep understanding of the maxilla-mandible relationship in aesthetic medicine. The skeletal pattern, defined by the relative positioning of the maxilla to the mandible, significantly impacts the alignment and interrelationship of the maxillary and mandibular teeth. This spatial orientation between the two major jawbones is a key determinant in the occlusal relationship and dental arch congruity, affecting not only the functional aspects of mastication and speech but also the aesthetic presentation of the lower facial third. Accurate assessment and understanding of this relationship are crucial for diagnosing dental malocclusions and planning effective orthodontic, maxillofacial, and aesthetic interventions (Fig. 4.6). Given the inherently three-dimensional nature of the human face, a comprehensive assessment of this pattern necessitates examining the interrelations across multiple planes:

- Anterior-posterior: This aspect examines the spatial positioning of the maxilla in relation to the mandible, delineating the sagittal balance critical for facial harmony and function.
- Vertical Proportions: Assessment of each segment's relative height is paramount in establishing the overall vertical harmony of the face. It is instrumental in diagnosing disproportionate vertical growth or deficiency.
- Transverse relationships: Evaluating facial width at key anatomical landmarks helps identify lateral asymmetries or disproportions, offering insights into potential skeletal imbalances.

To ensure the accuracy of these assessments, it is imperative to observe the patient in NHP, as compensatory head postures can lead to misinterpretations of skeletal and soft tissue relationships. For example, when tilting the head back, the chin tends to come further forward and appear more prominent. By carefully analyzing the skeletal architecture, specifically the positional relationship between the maxilla and mandible, practitioners can achieve a comprehensive diagnostic and formulate a tailored treatment strategy to enhance facial aesthetics [1, 11].

The following outlines a method for clinically evaluating skeletal relationships without the need for radiographic imaging. To accurately assess the anteroposterior (AP) skeletal pattern, it's essential to maintain the patient's head in a natural head position—upright, relaxed, and gazing at a distant point at eye level. Additionally, having the teeth lightly occluded during the assessment aids in identifying the natural relationship between the maxilla and mandible. To evaluate this relationship, the most anterior points of the maxilla and mandible are palpated through the base of the lips at the midline. The most concave point on the upper lip is called point A, and on the lower lip, it is called point B. This palpation helps in determining the relative positioning of the lower jaw to the upper jaw, classified into three major skeletal classes:

- Class I Skeletal Relationship: This is identified when the mandible lies 2–3 mm posterior to the maxilla. The facial profile observed in this class is typically straight, indicating a harmonious anteroposterior relationship between the maxilla and mandible.
- Class II Skeletal Relationship: In this class, the mandible appears retrusive relative to the maxilla, resulting in a convex facial profile. The degree of mandibular retrusion relative to the maxilla is further categorized into mild, moderate, or

  S. Samizadeh

severe, based on the extent of the discrepancy. This classification is crucial for planning treatment strategies aimed at correcting or camouflaging the retrusive mandible to achieve a more balanced facial profile.

- Class III Skeletal Relationship: Characterized by a retrusive maxilla relative to the mandible, this class presents with a concave facial profile. Similar to Class II, the discrepancy in Class III can be mild, moderate, or severe. Understanding the degree of discrepancy is essential for determining the appropriate aesthetic approach, whether it involves augmenting the maxilla, addressing the mandibular prominence, or a combination of both to restore facial harmony (Fig. 4.7). Although the soft tissue outline is examined, this indicates the underlying skeletal pattern. Variations in soft tissue thickness may mask the true skeletal pattern or its severity. It's essential to differentiate between dento-alveolar protrusion or retrusion and the skeletal conditions known as maxillary and mandibular prognathism or retrognathism. The former concerns the alignment of teeth and their supporting alveolar bone, not necessarily indicative of the jaw's overall spatial orientation. In contrast, prognathism or retrognathism relates to the anterior or posterior positioning of the jawbones themselves, underscoring a fundamental aspect of the skeletal architecture of the face. This systematic assessment provides invaluable insights into the structural underpinnings of facial aesthetics, enabling practitioners to tailor their non-surgical treatments to each patient's unique skeletal characteristics. By accurately classifying the skeletal relationship, clinicians can enhance facial harmony, improve profiles, and ensure that aesthetic enhancements are congruent with the patient's overall facial structure.

Upper Lip: Anatomical and Aesthetic Evaluation

The aesthetic evaluation of the upper lip encompasses a detailed analysis of its form, contour, and the nasolabial angle, which plays a significant role in facial harmony. This evaluation involves assessing the columella's inclination, the curvature of the upper lip, and the nasolabial angle, providing insights into the underlying maxillary structure and lip aesthetics. Different methodologies can be employed to measure these aspects, each offering unique advantages and potential limitations. The nasolabial angle, a critical parameter in this assessment, is defined by two lines: one extending from the subnasale to the columella's most anterior point, and the other from the subnasale to the labialis superior, the most anterior point of the upper lip's vermilion border. This angle offers valuable information about the upper lip's projection and the columella's slope, directly influencing the overall facial profile. An increased nasolabial angle (Fig. 4.8) could result from maxillary deficiency.

Evaluating Lower Facial Contours in Aesthetic Practice: From Labiomental Fold to Chin

The assessment of the lower lip and chin region plays an integral role in the comprehensive facial evaluation, especially crucial for planning aesthetic treatments

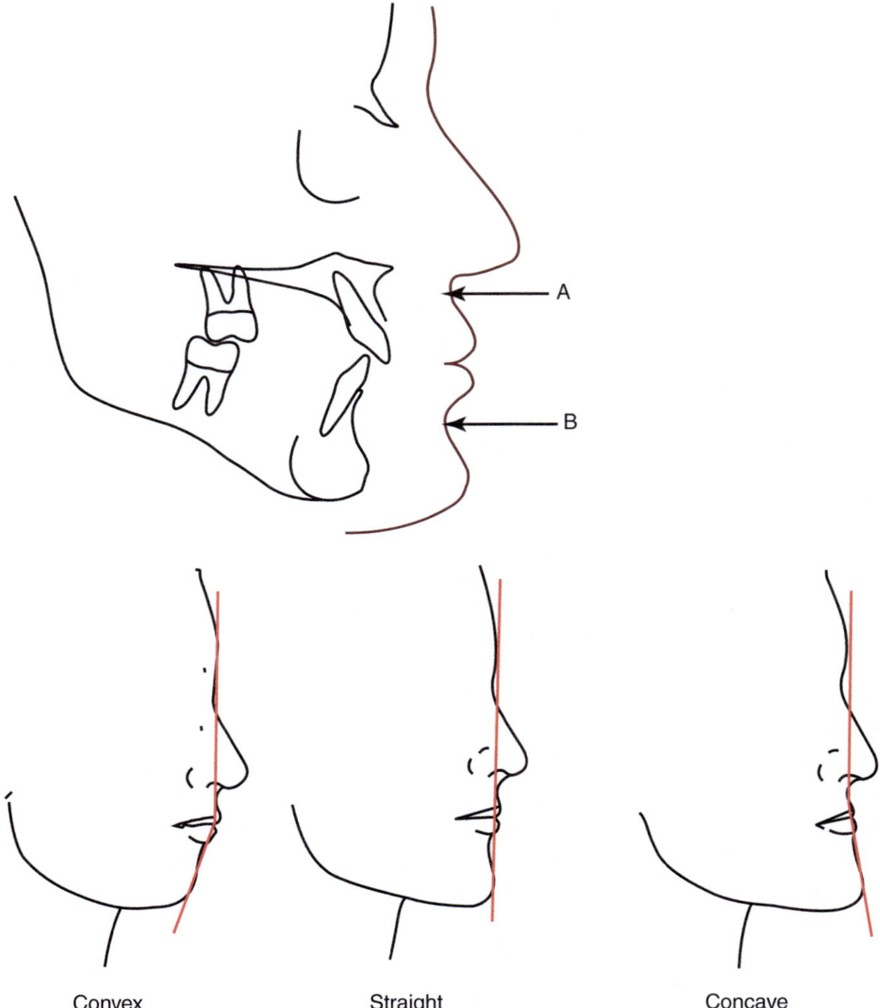

Fig. 4.7 Analysis of Maxillo-Mandibular Relationships and Facial Profiles-This image demonstrates the technique for assessing the maxillo-mandibular relationship by palpation through the midline at the base of the lips, identifying key points A (maxilla) and B (mandible). It visually categorizes the skeletal classifications based on this relationship: Class II: Depicts a retrusive mandible relative to the maxilla, leading to a convex facial profile, with variations from mild to severe. Class I: Illustrates a normative alignment where the mandible lies 2–3 mm posterior to the maxilla, resulting in a straight facial profile. Class III: Shows a retrusive maxilla relative to the mandible, culminating in a concave facial profile, which can range from mild to severe. This palpation and visual examination serve as a baseline for initial assessment. For a more comprehensive analysis and accurate diagnosis, radiographic evaluations, such as lateral cephalograms, are commonplace in orthodontic examinations. These radiographs provide in-depth insights into skeletal relationships, essential for formulating precise treatment plans in aesthetic and orthodontic interventions

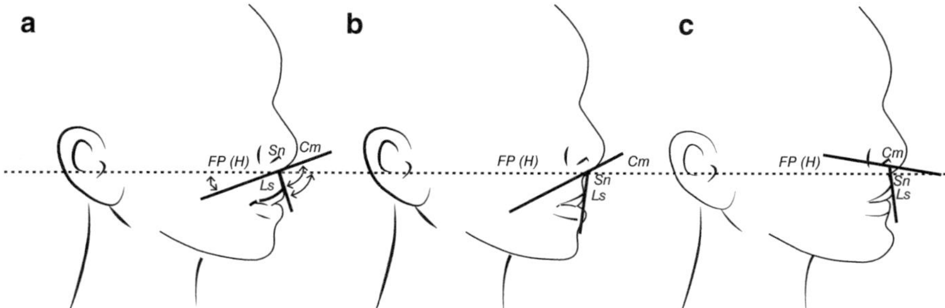

Fig. 4.8 Illustration of the Nasolabial Angle: Measurement and Clinical Significance-This figure illustrates the precise method for measuring the nasolabial angle, a key aesthetic marker of the facial profile. The angle is delineated by two critical lines: one extending from the subnasale to the columella's most anterior point, and another from the subnasale to the labialis superior, marking the upper lip's vermilion border's most anterior point. The angle these lines form with a horizontal reference provides insight into the columella's inclination and the upper lip's projection. Highlighted variations include: (**a**) The angles created by these lines and the horizontal reference line used can be utilised to account for the columella's slope-the standard nasolabial angle, providing a baseline for comparison; (**b**) An increased nasolabial angle, often observed in Class III skeletal profiles, indicative of potential maxillary retrusion; and (**c**) A reduced nasolabial angle, suggesting different aesthetic considerations. These measurements are instrumental in diagnosing structural imbalances and guiding corrective aesthetic interventions

targeting the lower face. This analysis not only delineates the aesthetic contours and volumes of these areas but also uncovers structural relationships and potential imbalances that could influence treatment choices. Labio-mental fold, a key anatomical feature offers insights into the structural and aesthetic characteristics of the lower face. The depth and contour of the labio-mental fold can significantly influence the perceived harmony and balance of the facial profile, serving as an indicator of various underlying anatomical considerations. By analysing the labio-mental fold, the curvature of the lower lip, and the projection of the chin, practitioners can make informed decisions on interventions that harmonize facial proportions, enhance aesthetic appeal, and address patient-specific concerns effectively. The curvature of the lower lip is directly influenced by the depth of the labio-mental fold (Fig. 4.9). Consequently, the characteristics of the labio-mental fold can reveal important anatomical insights:

- Inclination of the Lower Incisors: The orientation of the lower teeth directly impacts the labio-mental fold's prominence and, subsequently, the curvature of the lower lip.
- Anteroposterior Position of the Chin (Soft Tissue Pogonion): This parameter is essential in defining the lower facial profile.
- Lower Anterior Face Height: Correlates with the lower anterior face height, indicating vertical proportions of the face.

A pronounced labio-mental fold often signifies a reduced lower anterior facial height, typically associated with progenia, while a flatter fold suggests retrogenia or an increase in vertical facial dimensions.

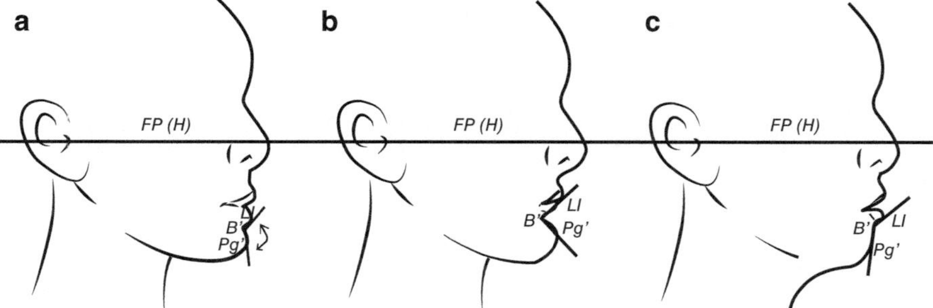

Fig. 4.9 Labio-Mental Angle Variations-This figure illustrates the influence of labio-mental fold depth and lower lip curvature on facial aesthetics. The labio-mental angle, delineated by points Li-B' and B'-Pg', showcases how variations in facial height affect this critical aesthetic zone, underlining its importance in facial analysis and corrective planning (**a**) Demonstrates the angle between the lower lip's most inferior point (Li), the labio-mental fold's deepest point (B'), and the most anterior point on the chin (Pg'), indicative of lower lip curvature. In (**b**), a reduced angle is observed in individuals with a shorter facial height, resulting in a more pronounced curvature. Conversely, (**c**) shows an increased angle in individuals with a longer facial height, leading to a less pronounced curvature

Lips

Following the analysis of the labio-mental fold, the aesthetic evaluation extends to include the relationship between the lips, chin, and nose. Several methods facilitate this assessment, each with its unique perspective and specific considerations, aiding in the comprehensive understanding of the lips' relationship to the chin and nose (Fig. 4.10). This analysis should be performed with the patient in a natural head position, facilitates a precise assessment of facial aesthetics, contributing to the formulation of tailored treatment plans that enhance facial harmony. Some examples include [1]:

- E-line (Ricketts): This approach assesses the relative prominence of the upper and lower lips against an Esthetic line extending from the tip of the nose to the soft tissue pogonion. Variations across age, gender, and ethnicity significantly influence this assessment, highlighting the necessity for a customized approach in treatment planning.
- The Holdaway/H-line and H-Angle/Harmony line: H-line, extending from the soft tissue pogonion to the upper lip, and the H-angle, formed by the H-line and the nasion-pogonion profile line. This method assesses lower lip position relative to the H-line, ideally within −1 to +2mm, and determines the upper lip prominence via the H-angle, ideally between 7 to 15 degrees.
- Steiner S-line. Steiner's S-line analysis involves drawing a line from the chin to mid-columella. Lips positioned on the S-line are considered ideally aligned, while those behind or in front of it indicate retrusive or protrusive lips, respectively.

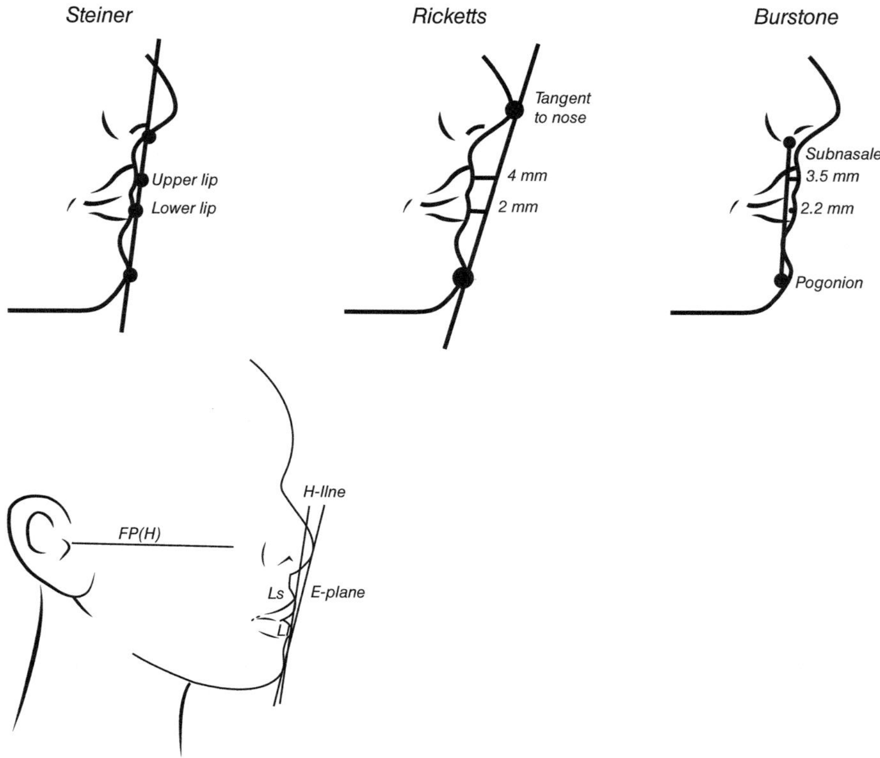

Fig. 4.10 The anteroposterior position of the chin can be assessed in relation to the forehead and the upper face. The line at the level of the chin will alter dramatically with any upward or downward inclination. The Ricketts "E" Plane is tangential to the chin and nasal tip. The Holdaway "H" line is tangential to the chin and upper lip

- Burstone: In Burstone's technique, the trajectory extending from the subnasale to the soft tissue pogonion is used to quantitatively analyze the protrusion levels of the upper and lower lips, intentionally excluding nasal prominence from the assessment.

Chin

The assessment of the chin is a crucial aspect of facial aesthetic evaluation, focusing on its structural and positional attributes relative to the overall facial harmony. The chin, a distinctive feature of Homo sapiens, plays a significant role in defining the lower facial contour and profile. Its projection, symmetry, and alignment with the facial midline directly influence perceived attractiveness and character traits. Anatomically, the chin encompasses the anterior mandibular projection (mental symphysis) and its overlying soft tissue [1].

Assessment [1]

Key considerations include the chin's relationship with the lower lip, its contribution to facial profile aesthetics, and the impact of its size and position on facial harmony.

- Sagittal Projection: Evaluation of the chin's forward or backward projection in relation to the mandible and maxilla, considering both soft tissue (pogonion) and skeletal landmarks.
- Vertical Height: Determination of the chin's height, addressing vertical excess or deficiency, which affects facial proportions.
- Symmetry and Midline Alignment: Examination of the chin's symmetry and its alignment with the facial midline, identifying deviations that impact overall facial balance.
- Soft Tissue Analysis: Inspection of the soft tissue thickness and contour overlying the bony chin, which contributes to the chin's aesthetic appearance.

The Ricketts zero-meridian line technique is an instrumental method in evaluating the anteroposterior position of the chin (soft tissue pogonion, Pg') relative to the facial profile. This approach offers a precise analysis of the chin's projection by drawing a vertical line from the soft tissue nasion, perpendicular to the Frankfort Horizontal plane. The position of Pg' along this line provides insights into whether the chin is protrusive or retrusive, impacting facial harmony and aesthetics significantly (Fig. 4.11).

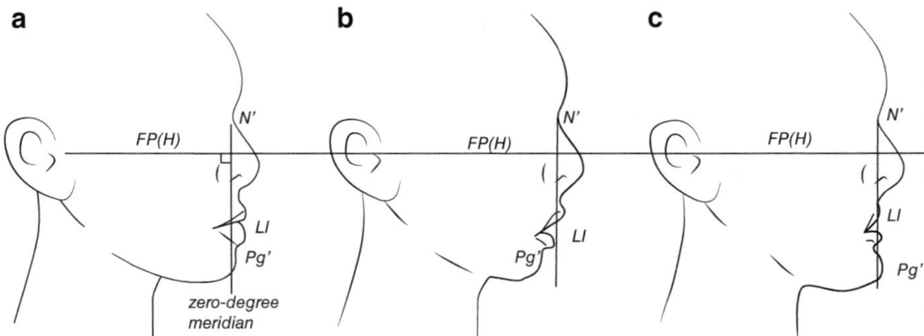

Fig. 4.11 Ricketts Zero-Meridian Line Assessment of Chin Projection- Illustrated here is the Ricketts zero-meridian line method that can be used for assessing the anteroposterior position of the chin in relation to the facial skeleton. This vertical line, drawn perpendicularly from nasion to the Frankfort Plane, serves as a baseline for evaluating chin projection. In this analysis, (**a**) represents a Class I scenario where the soft tissue chin point (Pg') is ideally aligned with the line, indicating balanced chin projection. Scenario (**b**) shows a Class II condition with the chin point falling behind the line, signifying retrusion, while (**c**) displays a Class III condition, where the chin point advances ahead of the line, indicating prognathism. This measurement aids in the diagnosis and planning of corrective treatments for achieving facial harmony

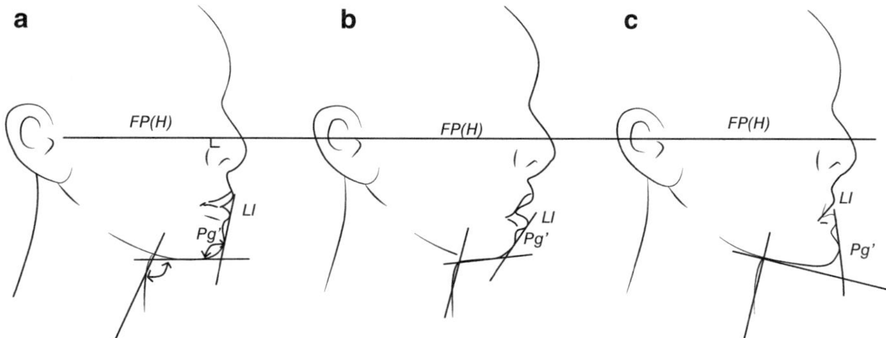

Fig. 4.12 Evaluating the Lower Lip to Submental Plane Angle-This figure demonstrates the measurement of the lower lip to submental plane angle, a critical assessment in determining facial balance and aesthetics. The angle is gauged between the labialis inferior (the most anterior point on the lower lip's outline) and soft tissue pogonion, extending tangentially to the submental plane. (**a**) The standard measurement technique, highlighting the angle's relevance to aesthetic evaluation. This angle is measured between the lines labialis inferior (most anterior point on outline of the lower lip/vermillion border) and soft tissue pogonion and a tangent to the submental plane. (**b**) An enlarged angle observed in a Class II scenario, indicative of increased vertical facial dimension and retrognathia. (**c**) A diminished angle in a Class III case, suggesting a more harmonious facial profile

Lower Lip to Submental Plane Angle Analysis

The Lower Lip to Submental Plane Angle is a critical metric in facial aesthetics, indicating the harmonious alignment of the lower lip relative to the neck's contour. An ideal angle closely approximates a right angle, signifying aesthetic balance. This angle's determination is influenced by several factors, including the lower lip's orientation, the submental plane's inclination, chin positioning, facial vertical proportions, and submental adipose tissue presence (Fig. 4.12).

Mandibular Plane Angle

The mandibular plane angle is a fundamental orthodontic measurement that reflects the vertical facial growth pattern and has significant implications for both orthodontic diagnosis and aesthetic facial assessments. To measure this angle, align a straight edge or digital caliper along the inferior border of the mandible, extending it to intersect with the Frankfort Horizontal Plane. The intersection point typically lies near the posterior aspect of the skull, establishing the mandibular plane angle (Fig. 4.13). Asymmetries between the right and left sides of the mandibular plane can occur and are essential to identify for a complete facial analysis. Consequently, each side should be evaluated independently to ensure accurate diagnosis and treatment planning.

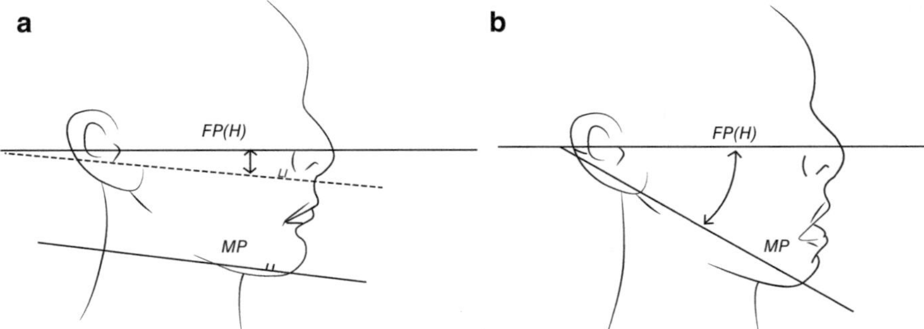

Fig. 4.13 Frankfort-Mandibular Plane Angle-This figure illustrates the clinical assessment of the Frankfort-mandibular plane angle, a key metric in determining facial type. (**a**) Demonstrates a reduced angle characteristic of short-faced individuals, where the vertical dimension of the face is less pronounced. (**b**) Shows an increased angle found in long-faced individuals, indicating a more pronounced vertical facial dimension. This angle assessment is crucial for diagnosing facial structure variations and planning appropriate treatments

Soft Tissues and Classification Systems

In facial aesthetic practice, the evaluation of skin and soft tissues, along with the identification of signs of aging or pathology, is critical. The facial soft tissue assessment involves a systematic approach that leverages various classification systems. These systems are crucial for the detailed examination and categorization of soft tissue characteristics, encompassing aspects such as texture, elasticity, volume, and aging signs. The application of these classification frameworks facilitates a comprehensive understanding of facial soft tissues, aiding in the formulation of targeted treatment strategies. Each classification method brings unique insights, yet they collectively contribute to a holistic evaluation of the patient's facial aesthetics. This section delineates the principal classification systems, enabling practitioners to achieve a nuanced assessment and improve aesthetic intervention outcomes. By presenting a selection of these systems, this chapter serves as a primer, guiding clinicians through the intricacies of facial soft tissue assessment. It is important to note that the myriad of available classifications extends beyond the scope of this chapter. Each system has its particular strengths and constraints, and their thorough exploration and application are vital in advancing clinical practice in facial aesthetics.

The Skin

The Fitzpatrick Skin Phototype

The Fitzpatrick skin phototype is a widely accepted and frequently used system among professionals to describe a person's skin type regarding the amount of

Table 4.1 Fitzpatrick skin type

Skin type	Typical features	Tanning ability
I	Pale white skin Blue/green eyes Blond/red hair	Always burns Does not tan
II	Fair skin Blue eyes	Burns easily Tans poorly
III	Darker white skin	Minimal burn Tans evenly
IV	Light brown skin	Burns minimally Tans moderately and easily
V	Brown skin	Rarely burns Tans easily
VI	Dark brown Black skin	Never burns Always tans excessively

melanin pigment in the skin and its response to ultraviolet radiation exposure. Thomas B. Fitzpatrick developed this system in 1975. It is established on an individual's (Table 4.1) [17]:

1. Skin colour
2. Responses to the sun (degree of burning and tanning)

This classification can aid clinicians in treatment planning for various cosmetic procedures, such as light and laser devices, chemical peels, and tolerance to different topical agents.

Skin Quality

Humphrey and colleagues have proposed a framework of attributes contributing to skin quality in healthy skin rooted in three fundamental categories: visual, mechanical, and topographical, with crepiness, laxity, and hydration shared in all three categories [18].

Visual:
- Redness
- Dullness
- Sallowness
- Radiance
- Shine
- Uneven pigmentation

Mechanical:
- Elasticity
- Pliability
- Firmness
- Thickness

Topographical:
- Roughness
- Fine lines
- Coarse lines
- Dryness
- Pores

Various devices and tools can be used for the subjective and objective assessment of the skin and its various attributes, including [18]:

Objective:
- Image analysis
- 3D fringe projection
- Antera 3D
- Stephens Wrinkle Analysis Raking Light
- Silicone replicas
- VISIA-CR
- Dermaspectrophotometer (L*, ITA), Colourimeters
- Chromameters
- Mexameters
- Reflectance confocal microscopy
- Optical coherence tomography
- Colourimeters
- Ultrasound

Subjective:
- Melasma Area and Severity Index
- Mottled Pigmentation Area and Severity Index
- Melasma Quality of Life
- Clinician's Erythema Assessment
- A four-point Erythema Scale
- A ten-point Skin Tone Evenness Scale
- Modified Fitzpatrick Wrinkle Scale
- A ten-point dryness scale
- Allergan Skin Roughness Scale
- Tactile Roughness Scale

Rhytids

Lines, wrinkles, furrows, and folds are all used interchangeably. However, these can be better defined and classified (Table 4.2) [19]. The increase in the number of wrinkle evaluation systems and classifications makes it very difficult to compare the success of cosmetic procedures. Numerous systems have been shown to be effective in measuring a variety of skin ageing processes.

Table 4.2 Facial rhytid-Nomenclature- Adapted from Lemperle, Gottfried. "A classification of facial wrinkles" (2015)

Classification	Sub-classification	Characteristics	Depth	Aetiology	Treatment options
Superficial wrinkles		Textural changes of the skin surface	Limited to superficial dermal creasing	Intrinsic ageing Photoaging	Respond to chemical peeling, dermabrasion, and laser resurfacing
Mimetic wrinkles	Lines (partial thickness) Furrows (full thick ness)	Deep creasing Perpendicular to underlying facial muscles	Deep dermal creasing	Repeated facial movement and expression Dermal elastosis	Botulinum toxin Dermal fillers Surgical options such as skin/muscle resection
Folds		Overlapping skin/soft tissues due to genetic laxity, intrinsic ageing, loss of tone, bony atrophy, gravity, and resultant sagging			Tightening procedures Correction of skeletal and soft tissue volume loss Surgical resection and tightening
Combination		Combination		Combination	Multi-disciplinary treatment is required

Glogau Classification

Glogau developed the traditional rhytide/photoaging classification scheme that is used most frequently:

- Mild (age 28–35 years)
  - Little wrinkles
  - No keratosis
  - Requires little or no makeup for coverage
- Moderate (age 35–50 years)
  - Early wrinkling
  - Sallow complexion with early actinic keratosis
  - Requires little makeup
- Advanced (age 50–60 years)
  - Persistent wrinkling
  - Discolouration of the skin with telangiectasias and actinic keratosis
  - Always wears makeup

- Severe (age 65–70 years)
  - Severe wrinkling
  - Photoaging
  - Gravitational and dynamic forces affecting the skin
  - Actinic keratosis with or without cancer
  - Wears makeup with poor coverage

Atrophic and Hypertrophic

Although the clinical aspects of photoaging vary significantly across people, two major types are reported: atrophic and hypertrophic (Figs. 4.14 and 4.15). These types have specific clinical, histological, and molecular characteristics. Therefore, each type requires specific treatment modalities.

Skin quality assessment systems and devices have limitations. Objective measurements are frequently utilised in isolation and are primarily used to research the effects of ageing, which lack support in total skin quality assessments. Additionally, because skin qualities vary according to the facial region, and probe-based techniques can only examine small areas of the skin, the information obtained may not offer an accurate depiction of overall facial skin quality.

Moreover, objective assessment instruments may be limited to assessing a single characteristic of the skin at a time. This assessment can detect statistically significant changes but may overlook clinically insignificant changes in skin quality. Future research is required and should be inclusive of all ethnicities [18, 22, 23]. The photographic and descriptive scale/classification systems shown below can be used as a guide.

Various authors, institutions, and pharmaceutical companies have many different classifications for lines, wrinkles, and folds on the face. Some examples are shown below, and each has its limitations and advantages.

Area-Specific: Rhytids Classification

There are many different classifications for the lines, wrinkles, and folds on the face. One of the examples is the zero-point photographic and descriptive scale by Zhang et al. (Fig. 4.16) for lateral canthal lines, forehead, glabella, and nasolabial folds [24].

Area-Specific: Topographic Changes

Forehead

Carruthers and colleagues have published a 5-point photonumeric rating scale to objectively quantify resting (static) and hyperkinetic (dynamic) forehead lines [25]:

0: No wrinkles
1: No wrinkles present at rest but fine lines with facial expression
2: Fine wrinkles present at rest and deep lines with facial expression
3: Fine wrinkles present at rest and deeper lines with facial expression
4: Deeper wrinkles at rest and deeper furrows with facial expression

Atrophic

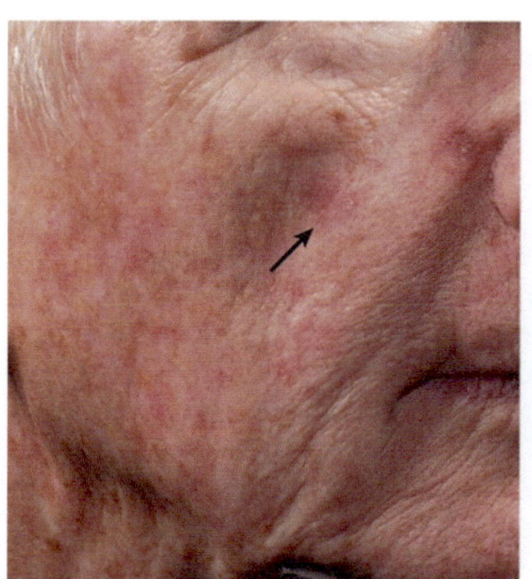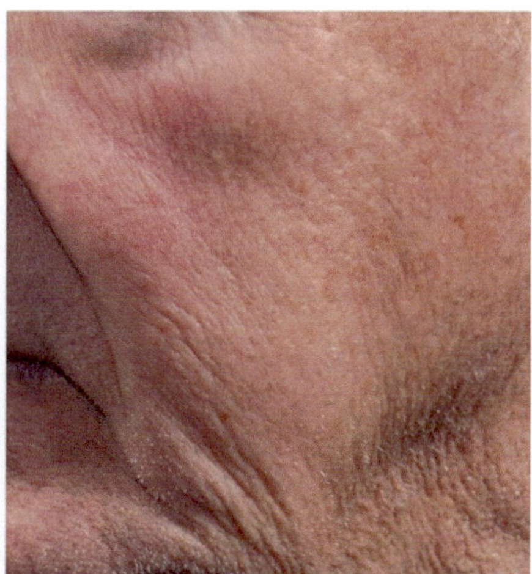

Hypertrophic

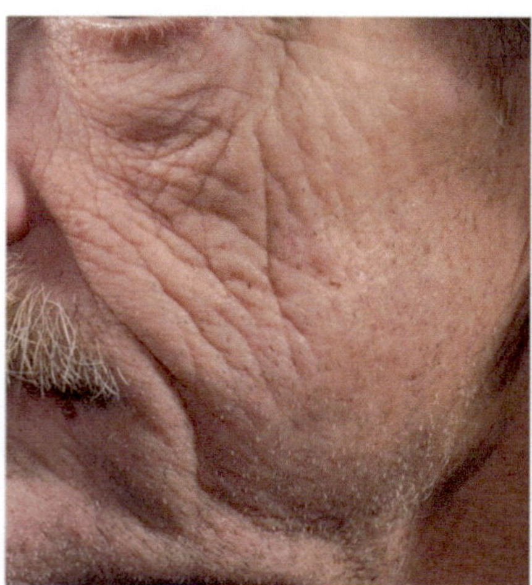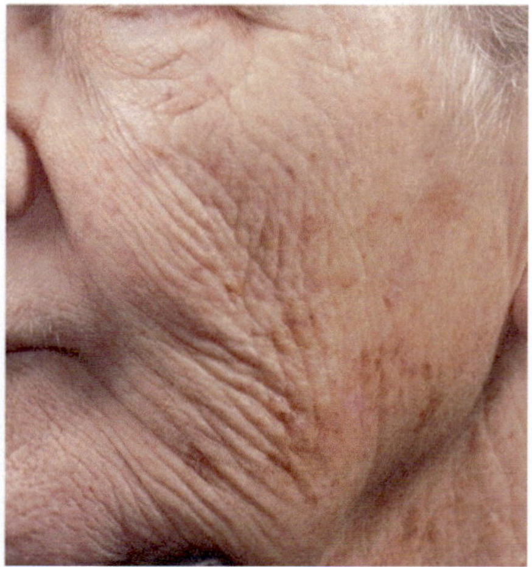

Fig. 4.14 Representative photographs of participants with atrophic or hypertrophic photoaging. Top row, two participants with atrophic photoaging demonstrate salient features, including fine wrinkles inferior to the eye and around the mouth, the paucity of coarse wrinkles, patchy erythema, a slightly shiny quality to the skin's appearance, and scattered light brown lentigines. Actinic keratosis is indicated (arrow). Bottom row, two participants with hypertrophic photoaging demonstrate deep, coarse wrinkling of the central cheek. The skin colour is homogeneous with a sallow hue, and there is minimal to absent erythema and telangiectasia. Reproduced with permission from Sachs, D.L., Varani, J., Chubb, H., Fligiel, S.E., Cui, Y., Calderone, K., Helfrich, Y., Fisher, G.J. and Voorhees, J.J., 2019. Atrophic and hypertrophic photoaging: clinical, histologic, and molecular features of 2 distinct phenotypes of photoaged skin. Journal of the American Academy of Dermatology, 81(2), pp. 480–488 [20]

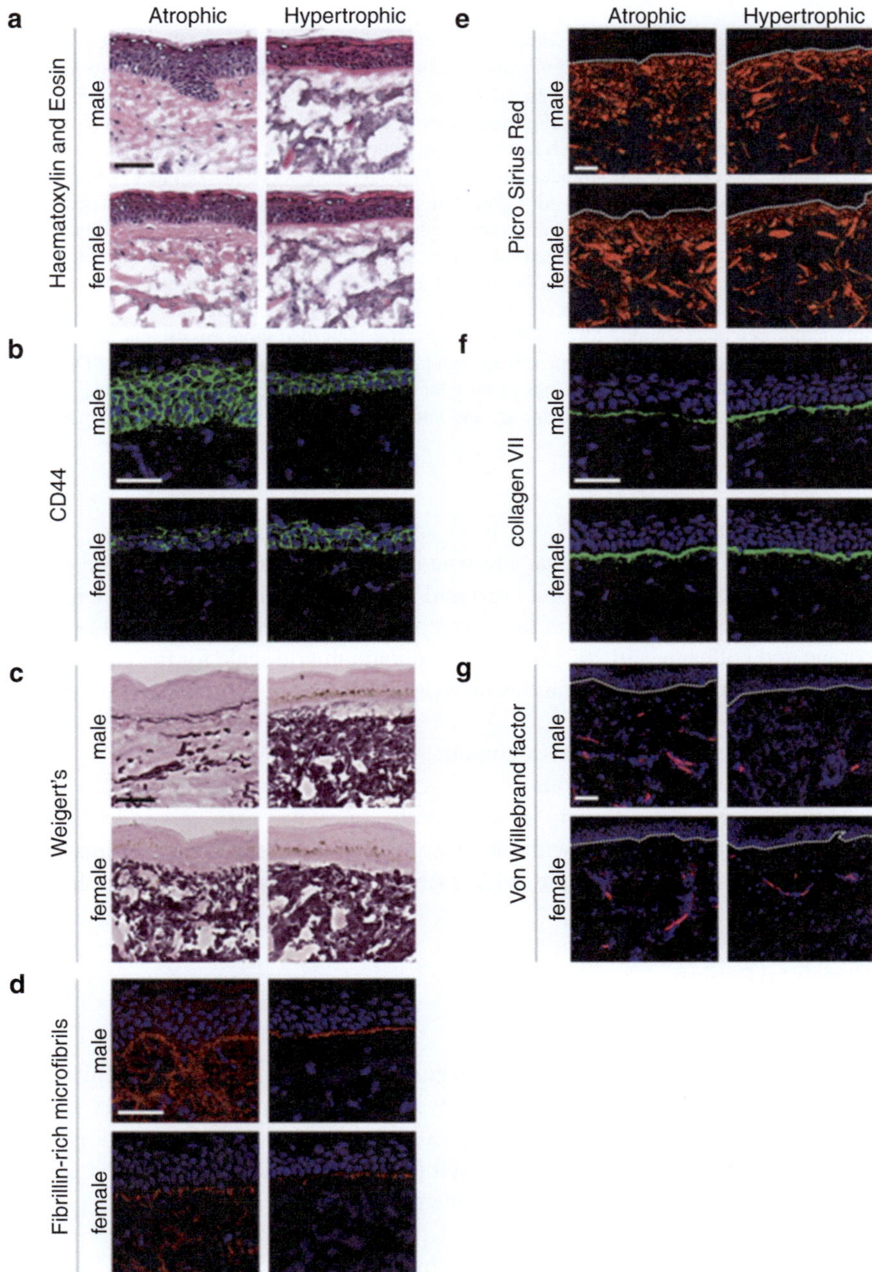

Fig. 4.15 Differential histological features are present in atrophic photoaging and hypertrophic photoaging. All data refer to facial skin, and all volunteers, regardless of their phenotypic status, exhibited characteristic flattening of the dermal-epidermal junction (DEJ). Epidermal thickness was maintained in male AP skin, but significantly thinned in AP females and all HP facial skin (**a**).

(continued)

Gender differences were apparent within the AP cohort for CD44, a major cell surface receptor of hyaluronic acid; AP females had significantly reduced CD44 abundance as compared to AP males. In contrast, no gender differences were identified for HP (**b**). Weigert's resorcin fuchsin staining identified severe solar elastosis in AP females and in both males and females with HP. Solar elastosis was not detected in AP males; however, the amount of elastic fibres was significantly depleted (**c**). Immunofluorescence staining identified that in all HP, there was a marked loss of fibrillin-rich microfibrils (FRMs) at the DEJ. In AP facial skin, a reduction in FRM at the DEJ was observed in females, whilst FRM morphology was preserved in AP males (**d**). Picrosirius red staining for organised fibrillar collagens identified no significant difference within the papillary dermis for either AP or HP cohorts (**e**). The distribution and intensity of collagen VII immunofluorescence at the DEJ were significantly reduced for male AP as compared to female AP and HP (**f**). Immunofluorescence staining for von Willebrand factor identified more vascular structures in AP than HP (**g**). Scale bars: 50 μm. Reproduced with permission from Langton, A K et al. "Distinctive clinical and histological characteristics of atrophic and hypertrophic facial photoageing". Journal of the European Academy of Dermatology and Venereology: JEADV vol. 35, 3 (2021): 762–768. doi:10.1111/jdv.17063 [21]

Temporal Fossa Atrophy

The temporal fossa loses its characteristic convex shape and becomes sunken with ageing. As a result, the temporal crest and zygomatic arch are exposed, lending to the skeletal appearance of the face. Temple Volume Rating Scale, published by Lorenc and colleagues in 2021, is a useful photonumeric scale for the classification of loss of volume and ageing in this area [26]:

0: Convex: Temple with a convex contour
1: Flat: Temple with flat contour
2: Moderate concavity: Temple with moderate concavity
3: Severe concavity: Temple with severe concavity and visible bony landmarks
4: Extreme concavity: Temple with extreme concavity and pronounced bony landmarks

Periorbital Region

Eyebrows

One of the first facial areas that display signs of ageing is the periorbital region, with the brow malposition contributing to the overall impression of age. In 2008, Alastair Carruthers and colleagues published a validated brow positioning grading scale. This five-point photonumeric scale developed spans the placement of the form of eyebrow that most usually needs adjustment [27]:

0: Youthful, refreshed look and high-arch eyebrows
1: Medium-arch eyebrow
2: Slight arch of the eyebrow
3: Flat arch of the eyebrow, visibility of folds, and tired appearance
4: Flat eyebrow with barely any arch, marked visibility of folds, and fatigued appearance

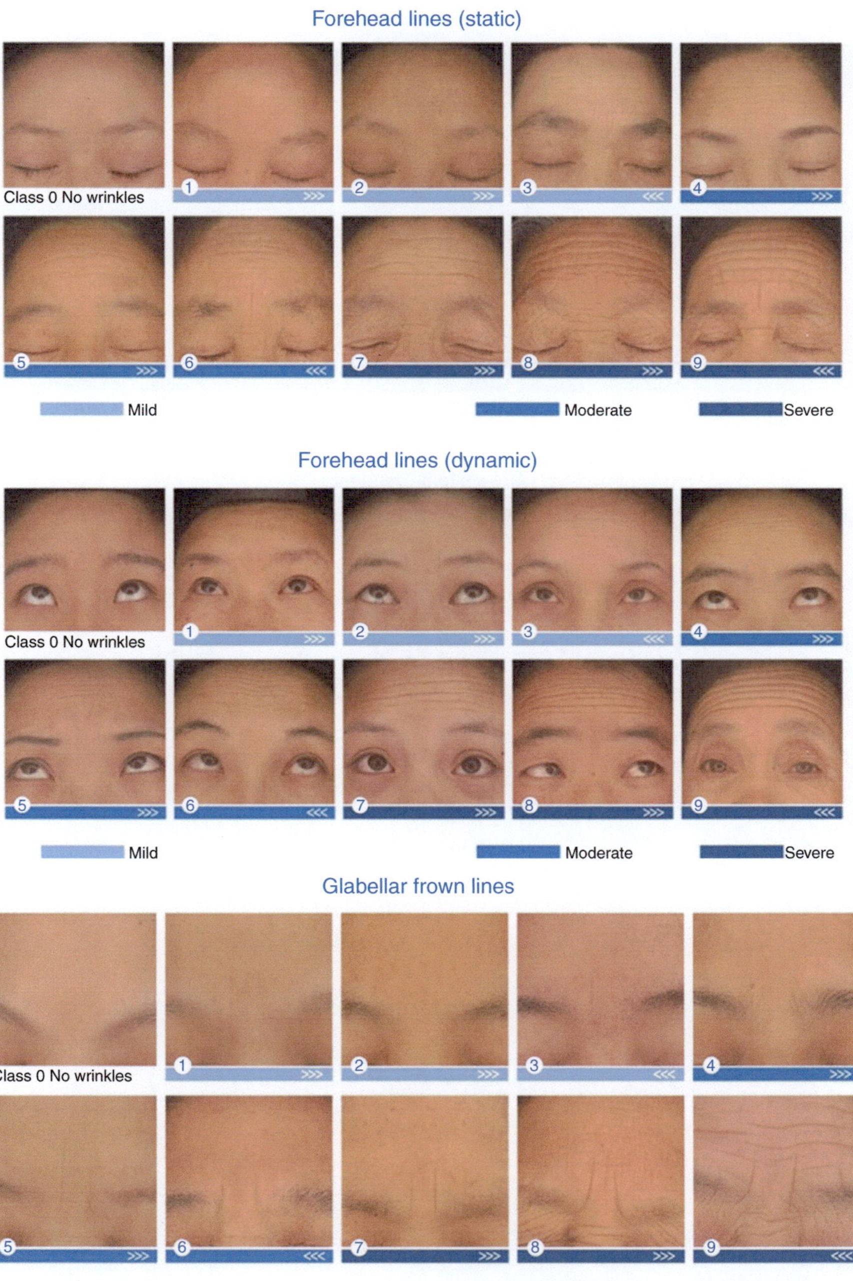

Fig. 4.16 Wrinkle classification for forehead lines, glabella lines, lateral canthal lines and naso-labial folds. Reproduced with permission from Zhang, J., Hou, W., Feng, S., Chen, X., Wang, H. Classification of facial wrinkles among Chinese women. Journal of Biomedical Research 2017; 31(2): 108 [This is an open-access article distributed under the terms of the Creative Commons Attribution License, which permits unrestricted use, distribution, and reproduction in any medium, provided the original author and source are credited.] [24]

　　　　　　　　　　　　　　　　　　　　S. Samizadeh

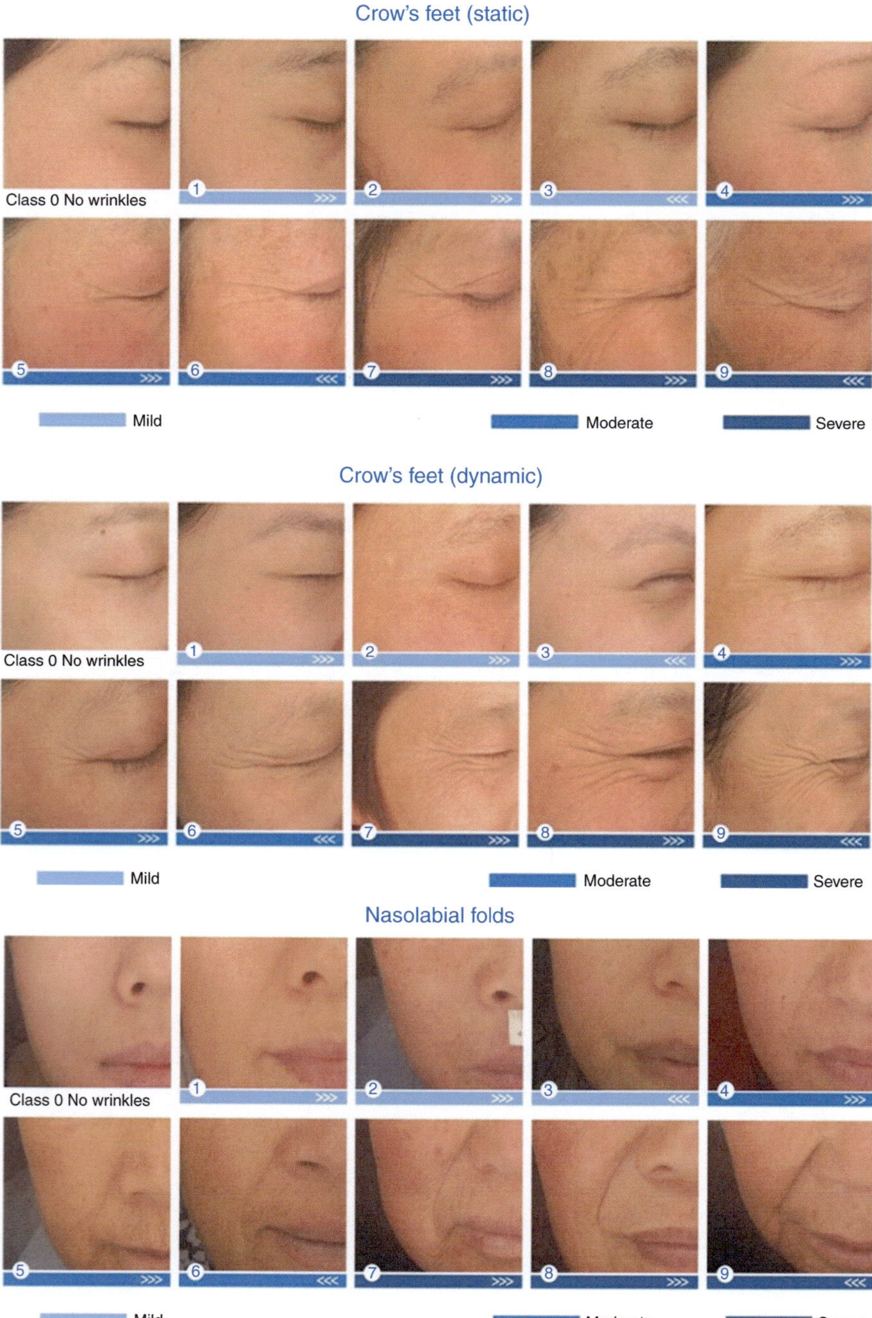

Fig. 4.16 (continued)

Tear Trough Deformity

The literature uses definitions and classifications of infraorbital grooves and hollowness interchangeably. The classifications should be based on aetiology, anatomical features, and presentation [28].

Depending on the anatomical features, infraorbital grooves are characterised as:

- Nasojugal grooves (or folds)
- Tear trough deformities
- Palpebromalar grooves

Contributing factors include (Fig. 4.17) [28]:

- Intraorbital fat herniation
- Skin and subcutaneous fat atrophy
- Orbital orbicularis oculi muscle contraction or squinting
- Malar bone resorption

Turkamani has classified tear trough deformity into five different categories (Fig. 4.18):

- "Hill" due to the superficial infraorbital fat pad herniation
- "Valley" caused by fat reduction and skin changes

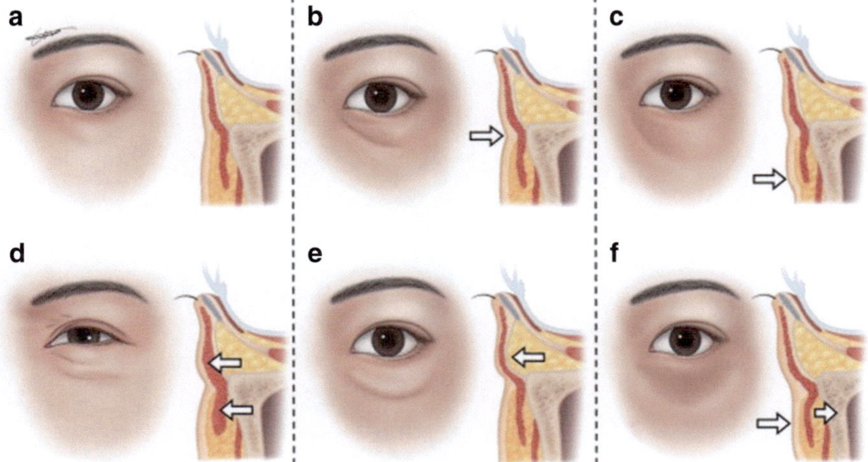

Fig. 4.17 Causes of groove or hollowness: (**a**) Normal condition. (**b**) The appearance of tear trough deformity (TTD) through the atrophy of the skin and subcutaneous fat in the suborbital area. (**c**) The formation of the nasojugal groove in the skin and subcutaneous fat in the suborbital area. (**d**) The appearance of TTD is due to the contraction of the orbital part of the orbicularis oculi muscle or squinting. (**e**) The appearance of TTD is due to herniation of intraorbital fat. (**f**) The appearance of infraorbital hollowness through malar bone resorption with soft tissue atrophy. Reproduced with permission from Lee, J. H., & Hong, G. (2018). Definitions of groove and hollowness of the infraorbital region and clinical treatment using soft-tissue filler. Archives of plastic surgery, 45(3), 214–221 [28]

Fig. 4.18 The new classification of tear trough deformity. Type 1: Hill; Type 2: Valley; Type 3: Hill-Valley; Type 4: Hill-Valley-Hill-Valley; and Type 5: Mixed. Reproduced with permission from Turkmani, M.G., 2017. New classification system for tear trough deformity. Dermatologic Surgery, 43(6), pp. 836–840 [29]

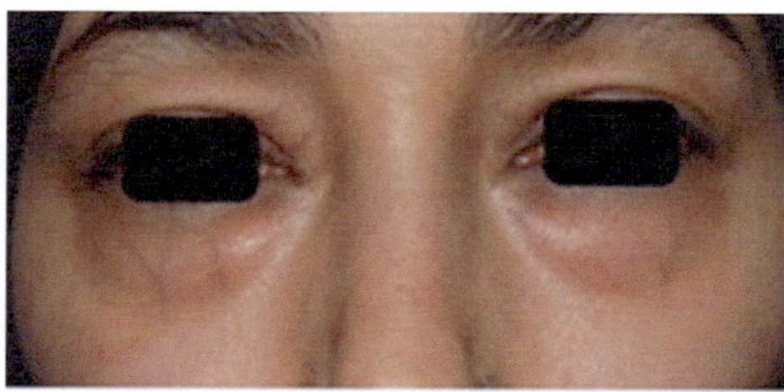

Type 1

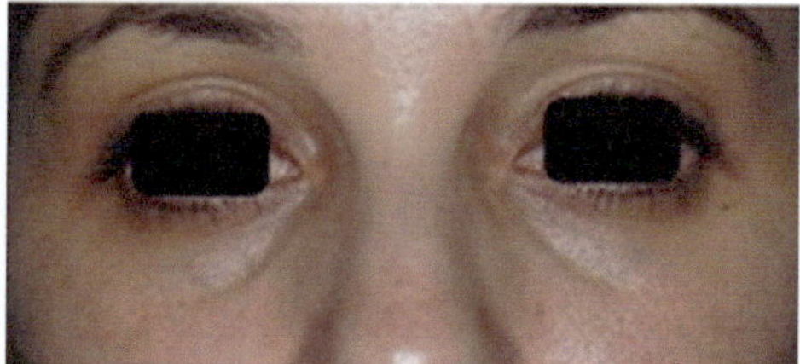

Type 2

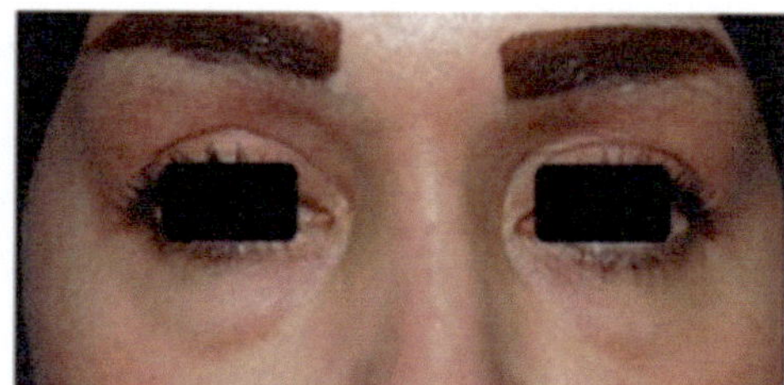

Type 3

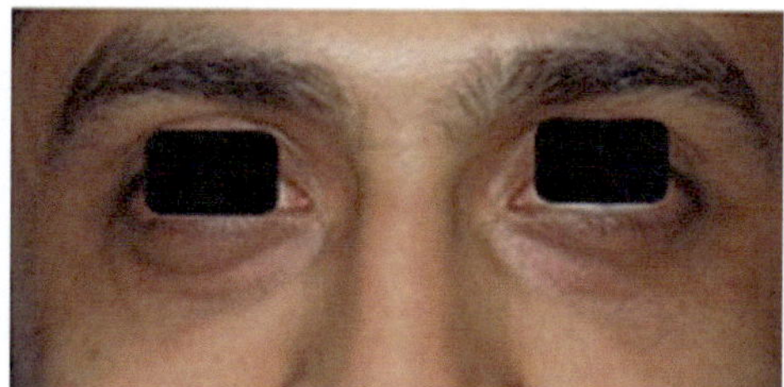

Type 4

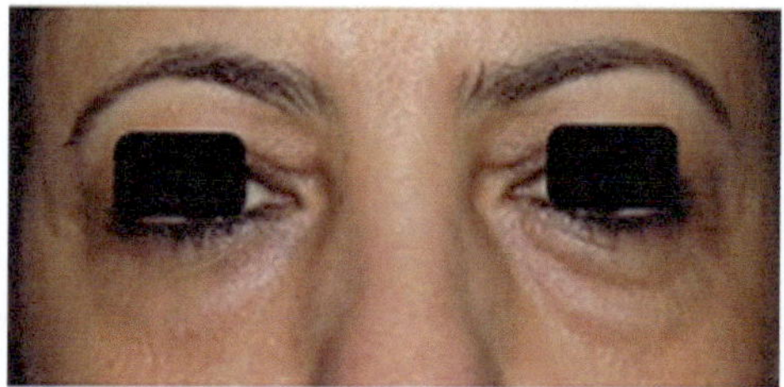

Type 5

- "Hill-valley" resulting due to weakening of the orbital portion of the orbicularis oculi muscle and its retaining ligaments, followed by fat reduction and skin changes
- "Hill-valley-hill-valley" due to a series of changes in portions of the orbicularis oculi muscle and its retaining ligaments
- "Mixed" form depicting a range of any of the four deformities

Peng and Peng have developed a three-classification system for tear trough deformity and a six-step evaluation procedure (Tilt, Snap, Smile, Squint, Pull, Push) to treat tear trough using dermal fillers [30].

Classification [30]
- Category A (atrophy)
  - A0: No tear troughs nor volume loss of the anteromedial cheek
  - A1: Medial tear troughs only
  - A2: Medial tear troughs and visible palpabromalar grooves
  - A3: Medial tear troughs, visible palpabromalar grooves, and anteromedial cheek volume deficiency
- Category B (bulging)
  - B0: No lower eyelid bags or malar festoons
  - B1: Only lower eyelid bags
  - B2: Only malar festoons
  - B3: Lower eyelid bags and malar festoons
- Category L (laxity)
  - L0: No lower eyelid laxity nor cheek laxity
  - L1: Only cheek laxity
  - L2: Only lower eyelid laxity
  - L3: Lower eyelid and cheek laxities
- Combination

The aim of this six-step evaluation procedure is as follows (Fig. 4.19) [30]:

1. To check for laxity
2. To assess the regional anatomical impact of patient expressions
3. To visualise the extent and degree of attachment of the tear trough ligament to aid in treatment planning
4. To simulate a post-treatment appearance and facilitate patient decisions

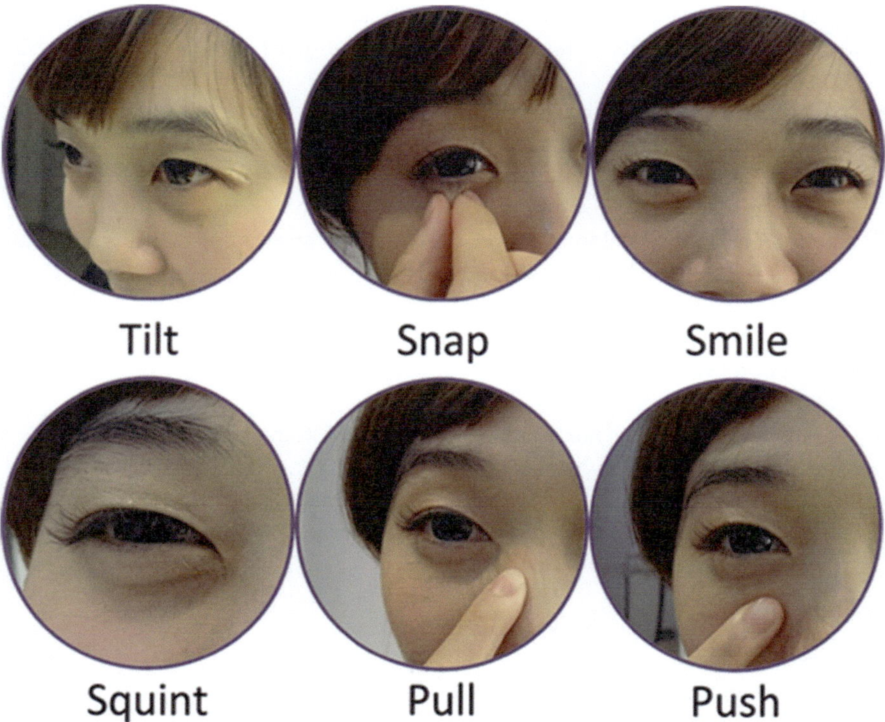

Fig. 4.19 A six-step evaluation procedure developed by Peng and Peng. Reproduced with permission from Peng, P.H.L. and J.H. Peng, Treating the tear trough: a new classification system, a six-step evaluation procedure, hyaluronic acid injection algorithm, and treatment sequences. Journal of cosmetic dermatology, 2018. 17(3): p. 333–339 [30]

Midface

Nasolabial Folds
Classification of nasolabial folds as described by Zhang et al. can be seen in Table 4.3 [31]:

- Skin type
- Fat pad type
- Muscular type
- Bone retrusion type
- Hybrid/combination type

Lower Face

Marionette Lines
The deepening of the pre-jowl sulcus and marionette lines/folds results from bone resorption, tissue atrophy, hyperactivity of regional muscles, and descent of soft

Table 4.3 Clinical types and properties of nasolabial folds

Type	Standing upright and still (I)	Standing upright with smile (II)	Laying supine and still (III)	Laying supine with smile (IV)	Hand lifting of facial tissue when standing upright and still (V)
Skin type	(1) Simple skin type: appearance of fine wrinkles (2) Sagging type: apparent wrinkles, tissue contracted, and skin area relatively increased; nasolabial fold exhibited as a deep furrow	Deepening of the deep fold	(1) Nasolabial fold disappeared or became unapparent (2) Wrinkles remained or mitigated	(1) Nasolabial fold clearly smoothed compared to condition in state II (2) Wrinkles smoothed compared to conditions in state II	Excellent improvement of nasolabial fold (+++)
Fat pad type	Thick fat pad or plump zygomatic area, nasolabial fold manifested as a concave	Deepening of the concave	Nasolabial fold became slightly shallower, but the concave remained	Nasolabial fold was slightly shallower than in state II	Significant improvement (+ +)
Muscular type	High tension resulting from muscle contraction; nasolabial fold displayed as a deep furrow	Deepening of the deep fold	Nasolabial fold showed no clear change	Nasolabial fold was no shallower than in state II	Significant improvement (+ +)
Bone retrusion type	Retrusion of the bone tissue around the pyriform aperture; the upper segment of the nasolabial fold manifested as a concave	Deepening of the concave	Nasolabial fold showed no change or became slightly shallower	Nasolabial fold showed no change or became slightly shallower than in state II	Slight improvement (+)
Hybrid type	Combination of two or more of the above type	Deepening	Differed among individual subtypes	Differed among individual subtypes	Differed among individual subtypes

Reproduced with permission from Zhang L, Tang MY, Jin R, Zhang Y, Shi YM, Sun BS, Zhang YG. Classification of nasolabial folds in Asians and the corresponding surgical approaches: By Shanghai 9th People's Hospital. J Plast Reconstr Aesthet Surg. 2015 Jul;68(7):914–9 [31]

tissue against the fixed ligaments in the area. Marionette Lines Grading Scale for objective quantification of the severity of melomental folds was published by Alastair Carruthers and colleagues in 2008. The scale ratings are [32]:

0: No visible fold, continuous skin line
1: Shallow but visible fold with a slight indentation
2: Moderately deep folds with apparent features at normal appearance but not when stretched
3: Very long and deep folds, prominent facial features
4: Extremely long and deep folds detrimental to facial appearance

Jawline

Jawline Contour Rating Scale is a photonumeric scale published by Lorenc and colleagues and can be used for assessment and classification of this area [26]:

0: None: Smooth, uninterrupted jawline contour
1: Mild: Mildly visible anterior and/or posterior jowl sulcus
2: Moderate: Moderate volume loss of anterior and/or posterior jowl sulcus
3: Severe: Severe volume loss of anterior and/or posterior jowl sulcus
4: Extreme: Extreme volume loss of anterior and/or posterior jowl sulcus with pronounced jowl laxity

Chin Ptosis and Chin Retrusion

Chin Retrusion Rating Scale, published by Lorenc and colleagues in 2021, is a useful photonumeric tool [26]:

0: None: No chin retrusion
1: Mild: Minimal chin retrusion
2: Moderate: Moderate chin retrusion
3: Severe: Severe chin retrusion

Cervicomental Angle

Ageing can result in an increased cervicomental angle.

Décolletage

The décolletage area is particularly susceptible to ageing indications. The epidermis and dermis of this area are thinner than those of other parts of the face [33, 34]. Furthermore, subcutaneous adipose tissue and sebaceous glands are decreased [34, 35]. Additionally, the platysma muscle frequently solicits the décolletage, contributing to the formation of lines and wrinkles in this area [36]. Skin laxity, lines/wrinkles, hyperpigmentation, erythema, tactile roughness, atrophy, and telangiectasias are all characteristics of photodamaged skin in this area [34]. Fabi–Bolton 5-point chest wrinkle scale (F–B scale) can be used for the decolletage area (Fig. 4.20) [37].

Grade	Wrinkle description	Chest
1	Wrinkles absent	
2	Shallow, but visible lines	
3	Moderately deep lines	
4	Deep with well-defined lines	
5	Very deep with redundant folds	

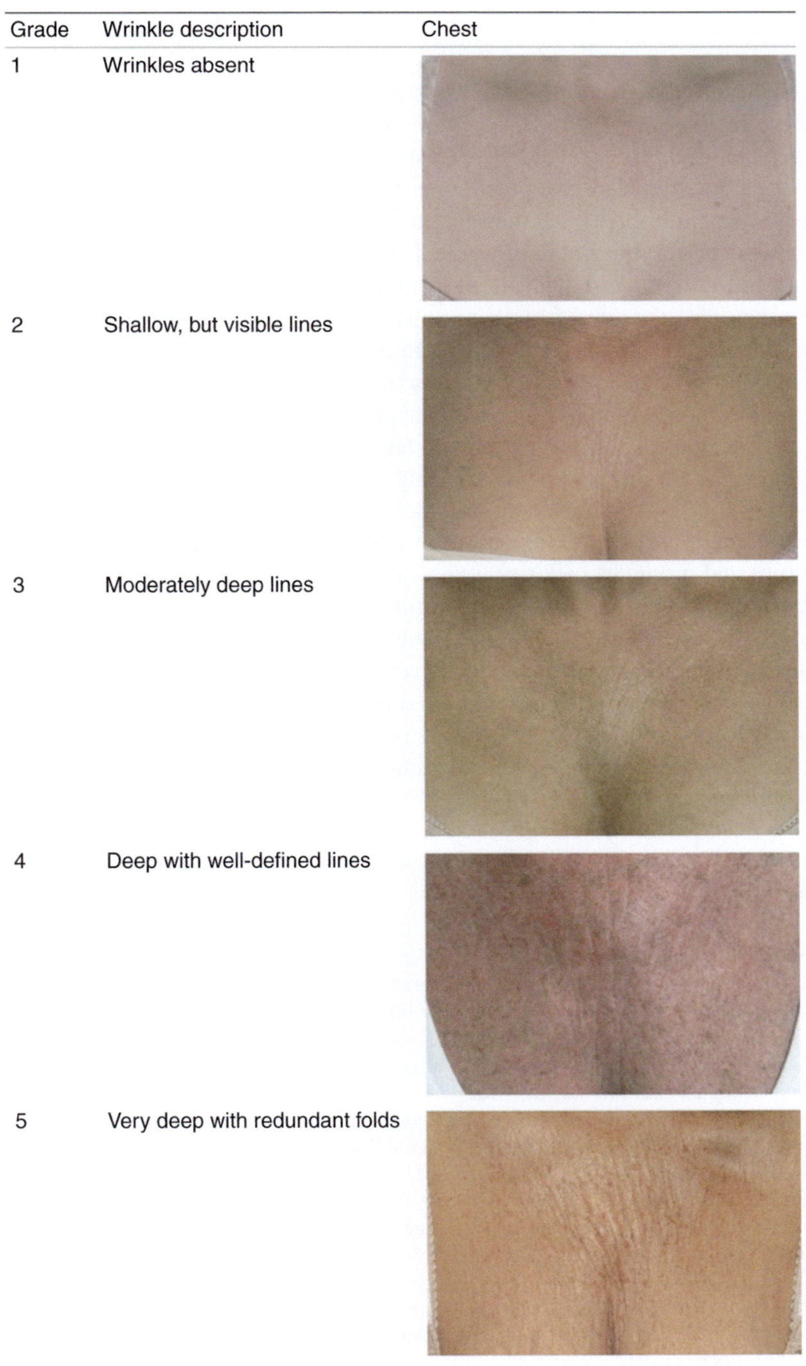

Fig. 4.20 Fabi–Bolton 5-point chest wrinkle scale (F–B scale) can be used for the decolletage area. Reproduced with permission from Fabi, S., et al., The Fabi–Bolton chest wrinkle scale: a pilot validation study. Journal of cosmetic dermatology, 2012. 11(3): p. 229–234 [37]

Conclusion

In conclusion, the chapter on facial assessment in non-surgical aesthetic practice underscores the critical role that a comprehensive facial evaluation plays in delivering personalised, safe, and effective treatments. To excel in this vital aspect of aesthetic practice, clinicians and practitioners must continually expand their knowledge base and stay informed about the latest advancements in the field. This commitment to continuous learning and improvement enables them to make well-informed decisions when designing individualised treatment plans.

Furthermore, the art of facial assessment necessitates repetition and practice. By consistently evaluating diverse patient profiles and refining their skills, practitioners can develop a keen artistic eye that discerns subtle variations in facial anatomy, proportions, and age-related changes. This level of expertise allows for more accurate assessments and ultimately leads to better patient outcomes.

Cultivating an artistic eye also enables practitioners to approach each patient holistically, taking into account each individual's unique features, concerns, and expectations. This empathetic approach fosters stronger patient-practitioner relationships and promotes better communication, which is essential in understanding patients' desires and achieving their aesthetic goals.

In essence, mastering facial assessment is a dynamic and ongoing process that requires dedication, practice, and the development of an artistic eye. By embracing these principles and remaining committed to excellence, aesthetic practitioners can ensure that they consistently deliver high-quality, personalised care that meets the evolving needs of their patients and maintains the highest standards in non-surgical aesthetic practice.

References

1. Naini FB. Facial aesthetics: concepts and clinical diagnosis. Wiley; 2011.
2. Larrabee W, Makielski K, Henderson J. Variations in facial anatomy with race, sex, and age. In: Larrabee W, Makielski K, Henderson J, editors. Surgical anatomy of the face. Philadelphia: Lippincott Williams & Wilkins; 2004. p. 22–8.
3. Zhuang Z, et al. Facial anthropometric differences among gender, ethnicity, and age groups. Ann Occup Hyg. 2010;54(4):391–402.
4. Freitas LMAd, et al. A comparison of skeletal, dentoalveolar and soft tissue characteristics in white and black Brazilian subjects. J Appl Oral Sci. 2010;18:135–42.
5. Soltic S, Chalmers A. Optimization of LED lighting for clinical settings. J Healthcare Eng. 2019;2019:5016013.
6. Lundström A, et al. Natural head position and natural head orientation: basic considerations in cephalometric analysis and research. Eur J Orthod. 1995;17(2):111–20.
7. Naini FB, Naini FB. Clinical diagnostic records, natural head position and craniofacial anthropometry. In: Facial aesthetics: concepts & clinical diagnosis. Wiley; 2011. p. 71–85.
8. Bergman RT. Cephalometric soft tissue facial analysis. Am J Orthod Dentofac Orthop. 1999;116(4):373–89.
9. Samizadeh S, Wu W. Ideals of facial beauty amongst the Chinese population: results from a large national survey. Aesthet Plast Surg. 2018;43:1–11.
10. Samizadeh S. The ideals of facial beauty among Chinese aesthetic practitioners: results from a large National Survey. Aesthet Plast Surg. 2018;43:1–13.

11. Roberts-Harry D, Sandy J. Orthodontics. Part 2: patient assessment and examination I. Br Dent J. 2003;195(9):489–93.
12. Baudouin J-Y, Tiberghien G. Symmetry, averageness, and feature size in the facial attractiveness of women. Acta Psychol. 2004;117(3):313–32.
13. Fink B, et al. Facial symmetry and judgements of attractiveness, health and personality. Personal Individ Differ. 2006;41(3):491–9.
14. Jones BC, DeBruine LM, Little AC. The role of symmetry in attraction to average faces. Percept Psychophys. 2007;69(8):1273–7.
15. Komori M, Kawamura S, Ishihara S. Averageness or symmetry: which is more important for facial attractiveness? Acta Psychol. 2009;131(2):136–42.
16. Jackson TH, et al. Face symmetry assessment abilities: clinical implications for diagnosing asymmetry. Am J Orthod Dentofac Orthop. 2013;144(5):663–71.
17. Sachdeva S. Fitzpatrick skin typing: applications in dermatology. Indian J Dermatol Venereol Leprol. 2009;75(1):93–6.
18. Humphrey S, et al. Defining skin quality: clinical relevance, terminology, and assessment. Dermatol Surg. 2021;47(7):974–81.
19. Lemperle G. A classification of facial wrinkles. 2015.
20. Sachs DL, et al. Atrophic and hypertrophic photoaging: clinical, histologic, and molecular features of 2 distinct phenotypes of photoaged skin. J Am Acad Dermatol. 2019;81(2):480–8.
21. Langton AK, et al. Distinctive clinical and histological characteristics of atrophic and hypertrophic facial photoageing. J Eur Acad Dermatol Venereol. 2021;35(3):762–8.
22. Mayrovitz HN, et al. Skin indentation firmness and tissue dielectric constant assessed in face, neck, and arm skin of young healthy women. Skin Res Technol. 2017;23(1):112–20.
23. van der Wal M, et al. Objective color measurements: clinimetric performance of three devices on normal skin and scar tissue. J Burn Care Res. 2013;34(3):e187–94.
24. Zhang J, et al. Classification of facial wrinkles among Chinese women. J Biomed Res. 2017;31(2):108.
25. Carruthers A, et al. A validated grading scale for forehead lines. Dermatol Surg. 2008;34(Suppl 2):S155–60.
26. Lorenc ZP, et al. Validating a series of photonumeric rating scales for use in facial aesthetics using statistical analysis of intra- and inter-rater reliability. Aesthet Surg J Open Forum. 2021;3(4):ojab039.
27. Carruthers A, et al. A validated brow positioning grading scale. Dermatol Surg. 2008;34:S150–4.
28. Lee J-H, Hong G. Definitions of groove and hollowness of the infraorbital region and clinical treatment using soft-tissue filler. Arch Plast Surg. 2018;45(3):214–21.
29. Turkmani MG. New classification system for tear trough deformity. Dermatol Surg. 2017;43(6):836–40.
30. Peng PHL, Peng JH. Treating the tear trough: a new classification system, a 6-step evaluation procedure, hyaluronic acid injection algorithm, and treatment sequences. J Cosmet Dermatol. 2018;17(3):333–9.
31. Zhang L, et al. Classification of nasolabial folds in Asians and the corresponding surgical approaches: by Shanghai 9th People's hospital. J Plast Reconstr Aesthet Surg. 2015;68(7):914–9.
32. Carruthers A, et al. A validated grading scale for marionette lines. Dermatol Surg. 2008;34:S167–72.
33. Peterson JD, Goldman MP. Rejuvenation of the aging chest: a review and our experience. Dermatol Surg. 2011;37(5):555–71.
34. Peterson JD, Kilmer SL. Three-dimensional rejuvenation of the décolletage. Dermatol Surg. 2016;42:S101–7.
35. Otberg N, et al. Variations of hair follicle size and distribution in different body sites. J Investig Dermatol. 2004;122(1):14–9.
36. Becker-Wegerich PM, Rauch L, Ruzicka T. Botulinum toxin A: successful décolleté rejuvenation. Dermatol Surg. 2002;28(2):168–71.
37. Fabi S, et al. The Fabi–Bolton chest wrinkle scale: a pilot validation study. J Cosmet Dermatol. 2012;11(3):229–34.

Facial Beauty: A Different Perspective

Souphiyeh Samizadeh

Abstract

This chapter explores the multifaceted concept of "facial beauty and attractiveness," a subject that has captivated scientists, artists, philosophers, and anthropologists alike. The quest for beauty, often manifesting in the pursuit of cosmetic enhancements, is not a modern phenomenon but a timeless human preoccupation, deeply rooted in the history and literature of every culture and ethnicity. Historical evidence underscores how societies across ages have endeavored to align their appearance with the prevailing beauty ideals of their time. Facial aesthetics and attractiveness represent a complex interplay of various disciplines including neuroscience, psychology, sociology, biology, and mathematics. This complexity is indicative of the cognitive intricacies involved in the perception of integrated beauty, which cannot be fully understood through a singular lens focusing solely on aesthetic appeal. The analysis of beauty standards, influenced by both intrinsic biological factors and extrinsic cultural and social norms, reveals a dynamic interplay between the objective and subjective determinants of beauty. Cross-cultural studies highlight the variability in beauty standards, yet also point to an underlying unity, suggesting a collective human inclination towards certain aesthetic qualities. Understanding facial beauty extends beyond the superficial, engaging with the neurological responses elicited by aesthetically pleasing features, such as the activation of the medial orbitofrontal cortex in

S. Samizadeh (✉)
King's College London, London, UK

University College London, London, UK

Great British Academy of Aesthetic Medicine, London, UK
e-mail: info@baamed.co.uk

© Springer Nature Switzerland AG 2024
S. Samizadeh (ed.), *Thread Lifting Techniques for Facial Rejuvenation and Recontouring*, https://doi.org/10.1007/978-3-031-47954-0_5

response to attractive faces and expressions. This chapter seeks to provide aesthetic practitioners with a deeper insight into the complex dimensions of beauty, illuminating the integrated nature of facial aesthetics as it intersects with human psychology, societal influences, and biological imperatives.

Keywords

Ageing · Facial ageing · Facial rejuvenation · Ligaments · Musculature · Skin ageing · Facial beauty · Cosmetic procedures · Non-surgical aesthetics · Facial symmetry

Over the past three decades, research on facial beauty has revealed several breakthroughs. These insights are crucial for aesthetic practitioners across various disciplines and specialties. Social, developmental, cognitive, and evolutionary psychologists have conducted extensive research, resulting in findings published in peer-reviewed, esteemed psychology journals. However, these findings are not always accessible to those in the aesthetic field [1]. Recently, there has been a heightened focus among medical aesthetic organizations, surgeons, and researchers on understanding how attractiveness is perceived and evaluated.

Greek mythology narrates the tale of Helen of Troy, whose beauty was so profound that it is said to have "launched a thousand ships," leading King Menelaus to wage war against Prince Paris to reclaim her. In modern times, our understanding of beauty is informed by a multitude of factors that our brains process daily. These include youth, health, body composition, skin tone, color, averageness, symmetry, gender expression, and personality traits, among others. This multidimensional approach to beauty underscores the complex nature of aesthetic perception and its significance in the field of aesthetic medicine [2, 3].

Aligned with the notion that "beauty is in the eye of the beholder," perceptions of attractiveness vary among individuals and cultures. However, there exists a significant consensus across diverse cultures when evaluating the same faces, suggesting universal criteria for what is deemed attractive [3].

These criteria include both physical characteristics—such as facial shape (e.g., adiposity, averageness, masculinity/femininity, symmetry) and color (e.g., complexion)—and other attributes inferred from these visual cues (e.g., youthfulness, health, personality). The connection between these traits and attractiveness is likely mediated by complex, genotype-dependent biological processes [3].

Although the definition of beauty itself is not universal, attractive faces have been shown to be more favourably perceived since childhood. Studies show that people perceived as attractive have a more favourable life [4]. Research indicates that attractiveness can confer numerous societal advantages, facilitating easier progress in social hierarchies, employment, relationships, friendships, and even financial earnings. Moreover, attractiveness appears to influence political success, with more visually appealing candidates often enjoying a competitive advantage, being perceived as more competent, sociable, intelligent, healthy, and possessing superior interpersonal skills [5–10]. These benefits extend to greater media coverage, public attention, and leniency in the face of controversies [11, 12]. Such conclusions are supported by observational and experimental research from across the globe, including the USA, France, Germany, and the UK [8, 13–15].

The perception of attractiveness is not merely superficial but imbued with assumptions about a person's intellect, sociability, friendliness, and overall desirability [16]. This raises intriguing questions about human nature: Are our judgments deeply influenced by appearance? Does the "beautiful is good" stereotype actually hold true in our society?

The Brain and Chemicals

A Tiny Snapshot

The fascination with beauty finds its roots deep within our brains and the complex chemical interactions that occur.

The Reward System: "Visual Reward"

Face perception is mediated by a distributed neural network within the brain [17]. The sight of a beautiful face triggers pleasure sensations. Activation of the brain's dopaminergic reward system occurs in response to aesthetically pleasing faces, with increased responsiveness when such faces engage in direct eye contact with the observer [18]. Extensive functional neuroimaging studies have shown that attractive faces activate the brain's reward processing centers (notably the orbitofrontal cortex and nucleus accumbens) more intensely compared to those deemed less attractive [17, 19–24]. This response is both linear and non-linear and is influenced by facial expressions. For instance, functional MRI (fMRI) studies reveal that a smile can amplify the activity in the orbitofrontal cortex, suggesting that a smile directed at the viewer enhances the perceived attractiveness of a face [23, 25].

Cognitive Functions and Memory

Behavioral studies corroborate that attractive faces are more easily remembered. fMRI scans highlight several key findings [26]:

1. The right orbitofrontal cortex shows increased activity in direct proportion to the perceived beauty of a face. This finding is consistent with the role of the orbitofrontal cortex in processing reward and valuing stimuli. The linear increase in activity as a function of attractiveness ratings supports the idea that the brain assigns greater value or reward to faces it deems more attractive, influencing cognitive processes such as attention and memory encoding.
2. Increased activity in the left Hippocampus related to memory success. The hippocampus is critically involved in memory formation and retrieval. The observation that activity in the left hippocampus increases with the memory performance underscores the hippocampus's role in successfully encoding and recalling faces, with better performance for attractive faces.

3. Stronger functional connectivity between orbitofrontal and hippocampal regions for attractive faces. This point highlights the interaction between the brain's reward system (orbitofrontal cortex) and its memory encoding system (hippocampus) specifically in the context of processing attractive faces. The enhanced functional connectivity suggests that the perception of attractiveness not only engages reward pathways but also effectively mobilizes memory systems, leading to better memory encoding and retrieval of attractive faces.

These insights demonstrate that the improved recall of attractive faces is due to enhanced collaboration between the orbitofrontal cortex, associated with reward processing, and the hippocampus, crucial for efficient memory encoding [26]. This effect of facial attractiveness is pervasive, affecting all stages of facial processing in the brain—from initial perception to memory retrieval regardless of facial expression [27]. Consequently, the preferential memory for attractive faces influences cognitive functions, notably memory, by leveraging the reward-based activation in the orbitofrontal cortex to boost memory-encoding processes in the hippocampus [26, 27]. Such neural responses to facial stimuli thereby influence key cognitive domains, including attention, memory, and emotional regulation [22].

Innate

Preference for attractive faces is innate.

The innate preference for attractive faces has been a subject of study since the 1980s, with research indicating that infants spend more time looking at faces deemed attractive [28]. Further investigation into whether this "attractiveness effect" is present from birth involved showing newborns (14–151 hours post-birth) pairs of attractive and unattractive female faces, with results indicating that newborns consistently focused more on the attractive faces [29]. This inclination towards attractive features is evident from a very young age, with subsequent studies confirming that babies aged 2 months and older also exhibit a preference for staring at faces considered attractive by adult standards [29, 30].

Additional research explored newborns' visual preferences for faces based on beauty and symmetry. Using computer-generated chimeric faces blending elements of attractive and unattractive female faces, it was found that babies significantly favored looking at the average and chimerically beautiful faces over the unattractive ones, regardless of the faces' vertical symmetry. This preference was consistent among infants as young as 4 months, indicating an early development of "aesthetic perception" similar to adults [31].

Further studies extended these findings to infant preferences across different facial types, including white and black adult male and female faces, as well as infant faces. Through visual preference experiments where infants were presented with pairs of faces rated for attractiveness by adults, a marked preference for attractive faces was observed across all types. These results not only reaffirm the innate nature of this phenomenon but also reveal its universality across races, genders, and ages [32]. Importantly, these preferences emerge before babies are significantly influenced by environmental and cultural factors, underscoring the innate aspect of beauty perception.

Psychology and Sociology of Beauty

1. First impressions matter.
2. Facial attractiveness significantly influences social interactions and decision-making processes.
3. Self-perception of beauty profoundly influences one's quality of life.

Drawing on evolutionary and socialization theories, it's evident that beauty plays a crucial role in both personal development and social interactions [33]. Facial attractiveness has a critical function in human social and affective behaviour. It acts as a strong social signal, steering mate selection and various other social evaluations [23].

Studies reveal that individuals, often unconsciously, form first impressions based on facial attributes. These initial assessments reflect automatic generalizations from adaptive categorizations of faces that share structural similarities, such as "babies, familiar or unfamiliar people, evolutionarily unfit people, and a variety of emotions" [34]. There is a notable consensus in these impressions, which carry meaningful social implications. Appearance holds considerable importance as certain facial attributes significantly influence adaptive behaviors, where even minimal expression of these traits can make a lasting impression. This phenomenon represents an overgeneralization based on initial perceptions. Specifically, facial characteristics suggesting low evolutionary fitness, infantile features (baby face), distinct emotions, and identity discernible through facial cues lead to broad generalizations about familiar and unfamiliar faces [34].

Ecological theory posits that humans possess an innate ability to anticipate another individual's behavior in social contexts through facial observation alone. This can be succinctly described by the principle that "prototypes are attractive because they require less cognitive effort to process." [35].

Averageness, Symmetry, Sexual Dimorphism

Averageness, symmetry, sexual dimorphism, and youthfulness are identified as four pivotal factors in determining facial beauty [1]. These traits are associated with genetic quality indicators, though the validity of such associations is often debated [3, 36–40].

Humans are innately attracted to facial symmetry, which is interpreted as a marker of genetic diversity and overall fitness [34]. The role of symmetry in the perception of facial attractiveness has been extensively studied, with the findings showing that symmetrical features are more attractive to both sexes. Although facial symmetry is closely linked to perceptions of beauty, the element of averageness within symmetrical features introduces a layer of complexity to this association [41]. Facial symmetry appears to be advantageous in sexual competitiveness; it is thought to reflect an individual's genotypic and phenotypic characteristics [42, 43]. In comparison, asymmetrical or atypical facial features might signify genetic or developmental problems, such as foetal alcohol syndrome. These attributes are often subconsciously associated with reduced intelligence and competence, irrespective of the accuracy of these perceptions [44]. Although symmetry is commonly linked to beauty, it is not universally accepted as the primary determinant of attractiveness [1]. Fluctuating asymmetry, or slight deviations from perfect symmetry, is considered an indicator of developmental stability, reflecting an organism's resilience to mutations, parasites, and toxins. Attractiveness may be influenced by features other than symmetry, with symmetry possibly correlating with these traits rather than serving as the direct cue for attractiveness. This leads to the proposition that the human preference for facial symmetry might not stem from evolved psychological adaptations but could be a byproduct of the perceptual system's inherent design [18].

Asymmetry has an unfavourable impact due to the deviation from the norm. This perspective underscores the complexity of attractiveness, suggesting that factors beyond mere symmetry contribute to our perceptions of beauty. Therefore, averageness might hold a more pivotal role in the perception of beauty [41].

Bashour (2006) emphasizes the critical role of averageness in facial attractiveness, describing it as the fundamental element that both explains the preference for attractive faces and uniquely satisfies the criteria necessary and sufficient for facial beauty" [1]. Studies have illustrated a preference for averageness in both naturally occurring and digitally generated faces [45, 46]. Faces that deviate from the average possess more pronounced traits compared to the general population, whereas average faces bear resemblance to the common facial characteristics within society. The attractiveness of average faces could stem from their feature alignment mirroring the population's average, which is linked to biological diversity [2]. Thus, in any given group, the faces deemed most attractive are those that approximate the population's mathematical average [47]. Langlois suggests this preference aligns with evolutionary tendencies favoring traits that are representative of the population's mean.

Moreover, this preference aligns with cognitive processes that gravitate towards prototypical examples within a category [48]. Faces that are digitally averaged by merging multiple individuals' features are universally found to be appealing across various ethnicities, with symmetry enhancing the allure of these average faces [45, 49–52]. Although averageness is favoured, it is noteworthy that attractive faces are not always average [53].

Sexual dimorphism, which refers to the observable physical differences between males and females, significantly influences perceptions of beauty across different cultures. These distinctions, often attributed to the differing ratios of estrogen to testosterone, play a crucial role in shaping beauty and attractiveness standards for both genders [54]. Sexual dimorphism, along with characteristics that distinguish between genders, significantly influences how beauty and attractiveness are perceived in both men and women.

Facial attractiveness is key in attracting a mate, with studies showing facial beauty as a trait selected for its reflection of hormonal health during adolescence. These hormone-based indicators must trigger cognitive or emotional responses in others to be effective. Pubertal hormones influence facial beauty in both men and women, suggesting that our brains, shaped by early hormonal events and activated by hormones during puberty, respond emotionally to these cues of sexual selection [55].

Female faces displaying pronounced feminine features, such as high cheekbones, a smaller jawline, and fuller lips, are typically found attractive [56]. These features are thought to signal youth and fertility [57–60]. An individual's perception of beauty can also be influenced by parental attributes, personal experiences, and traits similar to one's own. Preferences for certain male and female facial characteristics may be shaped by the ages and features of one's parents, like hair and eye color [61, 62].

Women's preferences for masculine facial features vary and have been linked to hormonal fluctuations across the menstrual cycle. Recent studies suggest women show a heightened attraction to more masculine faces during their most fertile periods, although this finding has been subject to debate [63–67].

Following this, men exhibiting high testosterone levels display distinct masculine features such as dense hair, pronounced eyebrows, smaller lips, and a defined jawline with a prominent chin, which are associated with health, immunocompetence, and preferred by potential mates [68–71]. Bearded men are often viewed as more mature, authoritative, and aggressive compared to those who are clean-shaven [72–77]. However, while high testosterone may signal dominance, it doesn't necessarily enhance attractiveness in the eyes of the opposite sex [78]. Indeed, excessive dominance can detrimentally impact reproductive success, with a preference often shown for moderate masculinity [79, 80]. Women may seek more masculine features in partners for short-term relationships, while opting for softer and not hypermasculine traits in long-term partners. Several studies in evolutionary psychology and mate preference research, suggesting that women might prefer more masculine features in partners for short-term relationships due to the associated signals of genetic fitness and health. In contrast, for long-term relationships, women might favor men with softer, less hypermasculine traits, which are often associated with perceived stability, cooperation, and parenting ability [71]. Additionally, faces with hypermasculine features are often linked to perceptions of dominance, aloofness, and untrustworthiness [81]. Research findings suggest that women in the United Kingdom and Japan demonstrate a marked preference for men with feminized facial attributes [81]. Research on beauty standards within Chinese populations and among aesthetics professionals has found a consensus preference among both genders for a softer jawline and a slender, rounded chin in individuals of both sexes [82, 83].

The association between female facial beauty and hormonal signals is straightforward, but the correlation with male facial attractiveness is nuanced. Female preferences for masculine features in men vary, especially across the menstrual cycle. During ovulation, when the likelihood of conception is higher, women show a stronger preference for masculine facial traits. Additionally, women engaged in long-term relationships tend to exhibit a more pronounced shift towards favoring masculinity around mid-cycle [84]. While this phenomenon has been subject to scrutiny, evidence persists that hormonal fluctuations during the menstrual cycle significantly impact women's attractiveness ratings, skewing preferences towards more masculine faces during their fertile phases [63–67].

Youthfulness and Ageing

A youthful facial appearance is often perceived as more attractive in women [85]. Individuals generally retain their relative level of attractiveness throughout their lifespan [85].

Features reminiscent of infancy, such as large eyes, small noses, pronounced foreheads, and compact, narrow facial dimensions, tend to evoke attraction and caregiving responses originally intended for children [1]. Infant-like traits have been shown to suggest exuberance, amicability, and open-mindedness [41]. These infantile features, indicative of vitality, friendliness, and openness, are part of what is known as the baby schema. The primary aspects of this schema are concentrated in the head and facial area, engaging fundamental aspects of human social cognition. This engagement likely underpins caregiving behaviors and affects infant-caretaker dynamics [86]. Furthermore, a Japanese study reported that moderately juvenile faces and those with an augmentation of femininity are highly attractive [87].

The evolutionary hypothesis discusses the role of beauty and its component elements in mate selection. It is centred on the predictive power of these components in predicting the characteristics of prospective mates [2]. For instance, preferences for a youthful appearance in female faces may focus courtship efforts on females with high reproductive potential. In another example, complexion and obesity may indicate one's current state of health [3, 36, 88].

With ageing, the face and skin morphology exhibits distinct alterations. Dermatological aging manifests as wrinkles, skin laxity and the emergence of hyperpigmentation and lentigines [89]. Volume depletion in facial regions, such as the mid-face, and the presence of jowls, along with a descending brow line, can alter the perceived dimensions of the eyes and impart an impression of fatigue or melancholy [90]. These phenotypic changes are subliminally recognized as indicators of aging and, by extension, diminished reproductive capability, detracting from overall attractiveness [55].

Overall, younger faces are universally found more attractive, and perceived age plays a crucial role in assessments of attractiveness. The ability to use facial cues to gauge age is consistent across different cultures and ethnicities because facial aging follows similar patterns across diverse ethnic backgrounds. However, the significance of specific aging signs may vary among different cultures and civilizations [89].

Mathematics

The inherent beauty observed in the human body, facial features, and the natural world can be attributed to their mathematical composition. This chapter has highlighted the pivotal role of symmetry in the aesthetic appreciation of facial beauty. Leonardo da Vinci's illustrative studies of the human form accentuated its proportional harmony, employing mathematical ratios to delineate structural balance (Fig. 5.1).

Fig. 5.1 Leonardo da Vinci's drawings of the human body emphasised its proportions and used ratios to define balance in structures. Image Credit: Pixabay

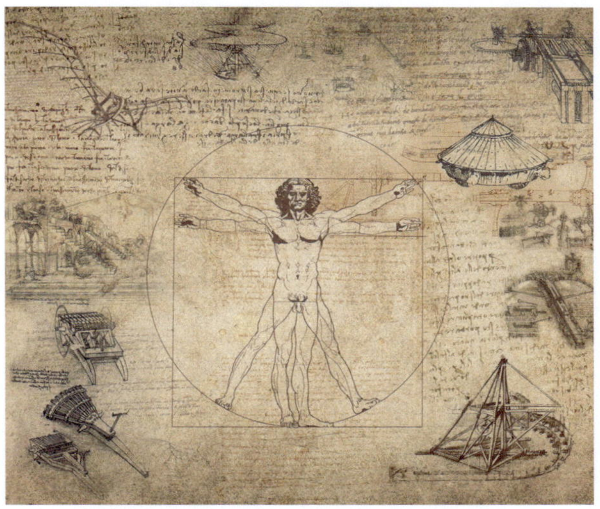

The Golden Ratio, or phi (approximately 1:1.618), epitomizes symmetry and balance, a concept revered by the ancient Greeks as the epitome of perfect harmony (Fig. 5.1) [91]. This ratio, reflective of a universal pattern, is prevalent in the natural world and ancient human creations, including Egyptian art and architecture where the Fibonacci sequence illustrates a similar convergence around phi. Beyond human anatomy, the Golden Ratio's presence extends to architectural marvels and artistic endeavors, observable in nature's spirals like those in seashells and floral arrangements, and celebrated artworks such as Leonardo da Vinci's Mona Lisa. The human brain is wired to find the Golden Ratio aesthetically pleasing, favoring forms that adhere to these proportions [92]. Brian Bejan, a professor of mechanical engineering, highlights that images framed within a Golden Ratio rectangle allow for the most efficient visual processing, suggesting an inherent synergy between vision, cognition, and the natural movement observed across animal species. This ratio underscores the coexistence of pattern and diversity as fundamental aspects of nature's evolutionary blueprint. He states, "It is the oneness of vision, cognition and locomotion as the design of the movement of all animals on earth. The phenomenon of the golden ratio contributes to this understanding of the idea that pattern and diversity coexist as integral and necessary features of the evolutionary design of nature" [93].

Orthodontics has led advancements in analyzing facial parameters and profiles, utilizing cephalometric radiography [67, 78–80]. Ricketts highlighted this in 1982 in "Clinics in Plastic Surgery," and Moss et al. further developed the concept in 1995 within "Semin Orthod" [81]. In 1982, Ricketts published, "The normal face and the occlusion of the teeth have a majestic beauty. The study strongly suggests that aesthetics can indeed be made scientific rather than the need to resort to subjective perceptions as in the past" [81]. He demonstrated the application of a "golden divider" for assessing facial features and proportions [81]. Intriguingly, the growth ratio of the mandible's condylar to corpus axis mirrors that observed in spiral seashells, illustrating a recurring pattern in nature [18].

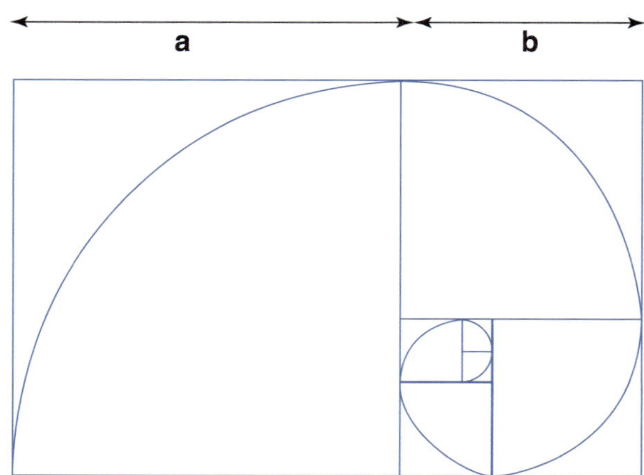

Fig. 5.2 The Golden Ratio is a mathematical concept that arises when a line is divided into two parts, with the ratio of the longer part (a) to the shorter part (b) equal to the ratio of the sum of the two parts (a + b) to the longer part (a). This ratio is approximately equal to 1.618. The Golden Ratio: $\Phi = 1.618033\ldots$

The Golden Ratio, also known as the Fibonacci ratio or the "divine proportion," is a mathematical relationship detailing the ratio between two segments and their combined length, often manifested in nature's spirals through the Fibonacci sequence (Fig. 5.2).

Mack published on the practical use of ideal proportions while treating the dentition and the lower part of the face to enhance facial aesthetics in 1991 [69]. The correlation between the Golden Ratio, facial beauty, and attractiveness has seen a resurgence in interest. When analyzing facial profiles through the lens of the Golden Ratio by overlaying this mathematical form, Fibonacci spirals of different scales emerge, revealing sequences of Fibonacci curves across varied square dimensions (Fig. 5.3) [94].

A comprehensive review of the literature and empirical studies indicates that neoclassical canons and the Golden Ratio do not universally predict beauty or how it is perceived. Wang et al. conducted a comparative analysis on the adherence to four neoclassical facial proportion canons among Caucasian subjects (103 North Americans) and Chinese participants (106 individuals from the Han Chinese ethnic group, which is predominant in China). This study highlighted racial differences and challenged the applicability of Renaissance scholars' facial canons, historically used as guidelines for artists, as universal standards of beauty [81]. The most attractive faces may not conform to Marquardt's Golden Ratio facial mask [82, 83]. Further research involving Southern Chinese subjects revealed discrepancies between actual facial proportions and the anthropometric neoclassical canons [84]. Extensive studies across diverse ethnic groups, including Asian, African American, North American, and Turkish populations, have similarly demonstrated the limited relevance of neoclassical canons to accurately reflect or predict facial beauty across different demographics [81, 85–88].

While the canons of beauty and the Golden Ratio hold significance and are utilized in assessment and treatment planning within fields such as aesthetic medicine and orthodontics, recent evidence suggests that these classical measures do not reliably predict beauty on a global scale [95–105]. The facial features, including

Fig. 5.3 Fibonacci spirals

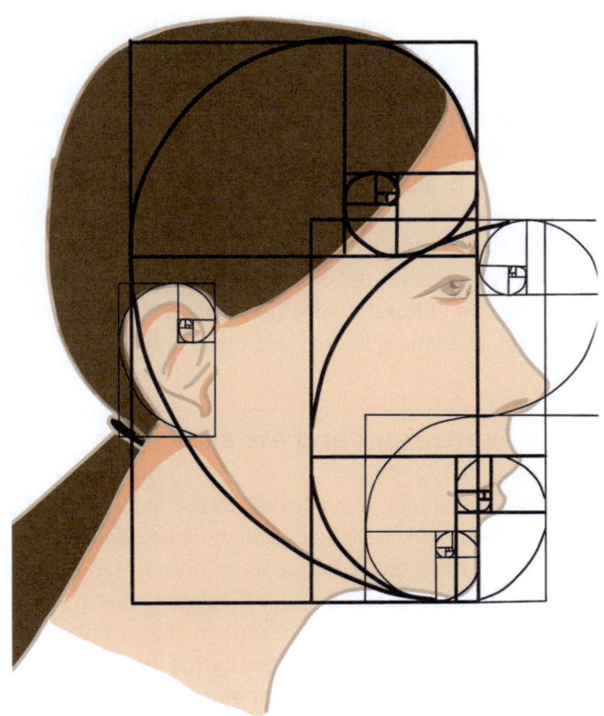

dimensions, angles, curves, and contours, exhibit variations influenced by factors such as age, gender, and ethnicity [106].

Facial Aesthetics Across Cultures

Across various ethnicities, countries, and age groups, there is a remarkable consistency in the perception of facial beauty. Research has indicated that certain facial features universally influence perceptions of attractiveness. Evolutionary psychologists propose that these characteristics are indicators of health, suggesting a natural selection process where humans have developed an innate preference for traits associated with healthy individuals [18]. There is a notable cross-cultural consensus on the standards of attractiveness and beauty, with several studies confirming such agreement [33, 56, 107]. The evaluation of facial shape and its aesthetic appeal remains constant across different cultural contexts. For example, studies have shown that Japanese and Caucasian men and women alike find similar female facial features attractive, such as high cheekbones, a narrow lower face, and large eyes [56].

The study "Changing Trends, Attitudes, and Concepts of Asian Beauty" by Liew et al. highlights a consensus that, although attractive individuals from various races exhibit unique ethnic features, they often possess similar facial traits [93]. This suggests that the foundational principles of beauty and aesthetic enhancement are largely universal, with aesthetic ideals being slightly adapted based on cultural, environmental, and media influences. Following this, Samizadeh's research into the beauty ideals among Chinese laypersons and aesthetic practitioners reveals that the standards of beauty in East Asia diverge significantly from Western norms. This study underscores the variability in aesthetic preferences and challenges the notion of a singular, global standard of beauty, highlighting the cultural specificity of beauty ideals in different regions [82, 83]. However, this distinction does not negate the fact that individuals of different ethnicities can be universally recognized as beautiful by people from other cultural backgrounds. This suggests a complex interplay between culturally specific ideals and a broader, perhaps innate, appreciation of certain aesthetic qualities that transcend regional preferences.

Facial Expressions and Attractiveness

The impact of facial expressions on the perception of facial beauty and attractiveness is substantial, with scientific evidence underscoring their influence. Research has demonstrated that individuals exhibiting sad facial expressions are perceived as less attractive compared to those displaying neutral or happy expressions, which are regarded similarly in terms of attractiveness [108]. Specifically, smiling has been identified as a factor that enhances the perceived attractiveness of women [85]. Neuroscientific studies have pinpointed the medial orbitofrontal cortex (mOFC) as a critical brain region engaged in evaluating the reward value of stimuli, including attractive faces. It has been observed that happy facial expressions, such as smiles, elicit heightened activity in the mOFC. This suggests that smiles directed towards an observer increase the perceived attractiveness of a face by enhancing its reward value in the observer's brain, as indicated by increased mOFC activity [23]. This observation is grounded in both psychological and neurobiological research, which suggests that smiling can trigger positive emotional responses in observers due to its association with happiness, sociability, and good health. From a biological standpoint, smiling releases neuropeptides along with neurotransmitters like dopamine and serotonin in the brain of the observer, which are associated with feelings of well-being and reduced stress levels. Furthermore, evolutionary psychology proposes that smiling may signal cooperative tendencies and genetic fitness, making individuals appear more appealing and trustworthy to potential mates. The positive impact of smiling on attractiveness is thus multifaceted, involving complex interactions between observer perception, emotional response, and evolutionary predispositions.

Conclusion

The human fascination with beauty, a constant throughout history, has evolved into a formidable industry valued in the billions. Empirical evidence from both observational studies and controlled laboratory settings confirms a pervasive bias favoring individuals deemed beautiful. While perceptions of attractiveness are shaped by a mosaic of personal preferences and cultural influences, a remarkable consensus emerges when diverse groups evaluate a common set of faces—clear patterns of universal appeal transcend cultural boundaries, revealing a shared understanding of what constitutes facial beauty. This chapter has explored the nuanced interplay between evolutionary biology, psychology, and societal norms in shaping our perceptions of attractiveness. From the role of symmetry and the Golden Ratio in denoting health and reproductive potential to the impact of facial expressions on attractiveness ratings, the scientific inquiry into beauty unravels complex layers of human cognition and social interaction. Notably, the positive effect of smiling on perceived attractiveness highlights the intertwining of emotional expression with evolutionary and neurobiological mechanisms, reinforcing the importance of interpersonal dynamics in attractiveness assessments. Moreover, cross-cultural studies, such as those involving Chinese laypersons and aesthetic practitioners, underscore the variability, with other research highlighting an underlying unity in beauty standards globally. In summary, while individual and cultural variations in the perception of beauty persist, underlying principles—rooted in evolutionary biology, psychology, and a collective human experience—guide a universal recognition of beauty. This convergence suggests a fundamental aspect of human nature in the appreciation of aesthetics, bridging diverse perspectives through a common visual language of attractiveness. Continuing to unravel the complexities of beauty, the interplay of science, culture, and personal preference enriches the understanding of this age-old preoccupation, reaffirming its significance in human society.

References

1. Bashour M. History and current concepts in the analysis of facial attractiveness. Plast Reconstr Surg. 2006;118(3):741–56.
2. Little AC, Jones BC, DeBruine LM. Facial attractiveness: evolutionary based research. Philos Trans R Soc B Biol Sci. 2011;366(1571):1638–59.
3. White JD, Puts DA. Genes influence facial attractiveness through intricate biological relationships. PLoS Genet. 2019;15(4):e1008030.
4. Wigginton M, Stockemer D. The limits of the attractiveness premium in elections. Elect Stud. 2021;70:102274.
5. Pfeifer C. Physical attractiveness, employment and earnings. Appl Econ Lett. 2012;19(6):505–10.
6. Berggren N, Jordahl H, Poutvaara P. The right look: conservative politicians look better and voters reward it. J Public Econ. 2017;146:79–86.
7. Praino R, Stockemer D, Moscardelli VG. The lingering effect of scandals in congressional elections: incumbents, challengers, and voters. Soc Sci Q. 2013;94(4):1045–61.
8. Milazzo C, Mattes K. Looking good for election day: does attractiveness predict electoral success in Britain? Br J Polit Int Rel. 2016;18(1):161–78.
9. Stockemer D, Praino R. Physical attractiveness, voter heuristics and electoral systems: the role of candidate attractiveness under different institutional designs. Br J Polit Int Rel. 2017;19(2):336–52.
10. White AE, Kenrick DT, Neuberg SL. Beauty at the ballot box: disease threats predict preferences for physically attractive leaders. Psychol Sci. 2013;24(12):2429–36.

11. Stockemer D, Praino R. The good, the bad and the ugly: do attractive politicians get a 'break' when they are involved in scandals? Polit Behav. 2019;41(3):747–67.
12. Tsfati Y, Markowitz Elfassi D, Waismel-Manor I. Exploring the association between Israeli legislators' physical attractiveness and their television news coverage. Int J Press/Polit. 2010;15(2):175–92.
13. Lev-On A, Waismel-Manor I. Looks that matter: the effect of physical attractiveness in low- and high-information elections. Am Behav Sci. 2016;60(14):1756–71.
14. Antonakis J, Dalgas O. Predicting elections: child's play! Science. 2009;323(5918):1183.
15. Jäckle S, Metz T. Beauty contest revisited: the effects of perceived attractiveness, competence, and likability on the electoral success of German MPs. Polit Policy. 2017;45(4):495–534.
16. Harrar H, Myers S, Ghanem AM. Art or science? An evidence-based approach to human facial beauty a quantitative analysis towards an informed clinical aesthetic practice. Aesthet Plast Surg. 2018;42(1):137–46.
17. Kranz F, Ishai A. Face perception is modulated by sexual preference. Curr Biol. 2006;16(1):63–8.
18. Fink B, Neave N. The biology of facial beauty. Int J Cosmet Sci. 2005;27(6):317–25.
19. Aharon I, et al. Beautiful faces have variable reward value: fMRI and behavioral evidence. Neuron. 2001;32(3):537–51.
20. Bray S, O'Doherty J. Neural coding of reward-prediction error signals during classical conditioning with attractive faces. J Neurophysiol. 2007;97(4):3036–45.
21. Cloutier J, et al. Are attractive people rewarding? Sex differences in the neural substrates of facial attractiveness. J Cogn Neurosci. 2008;20(6):941–51.
22. Ishai A. Sex, beauty and the orbitofrontal cortex. Int J Psychophysiol. 2007;63(2):181–5.
23. O'Doherty J, et al. Beauty in a smile: the role of medial orbitofrontal cortex in facial attractiveness. Neuropsychologia. 2003;41(2):147–55.
24. Winston JS, et al. Brain systems for assessing facial attractiveness. Neuropsychologia. 2007;45(1):195–206.
25. Liang X, Zebrowitz LA, Zhang Y. Neural activation in the "reward circuit" shows a nonlinear response to facial attractiveness. Soc Neurosci. 2010;5(3):320–34.
26. Tsukiura T, Cabeza R. Remembering beauty: roles of orbitofrontal and hippocampal regions in successful memory encoding of attractive faces. NeuroImage. 2011;54(1):653–60.
27. Marzi T, Viggiano MP. When memory meets beauty: insights from event-related potentials. Biol Psychol. 2010;84(2):192–205.
28. Samuels CA, Ewy R. Aesthetic perception of faces during infancy. Br J Dev Psychol. 1985;3(3):221–8.
29. Slater A, et al. Newborn infants prefer attractive faces. Infant Behav Dev. 1998;21(2):345–54.
30. Slater A, et al. Newborn infants' preference for attractive faces: the role of internal and external facial features. Infancy. 2000;1(2):265–74.
31. Samuels CA, et al. Facial aesthetics: babies prefer attractiveness to symmetry. Perception. 2013;42(11):1244–52.
32. Langlois JH, et al. Facial diversity and infant preferences for attractive faces. Dev Psychol. 1991;27(1):79–84.
33. Langlois JH, et al. Maxims or myths of beauty? A meta-analytic and theoretical review. Psychol Bull. 2000;126(3):390–423.
34. Zebrowitz LA, Montepare JM. Social psychological face perception: why appearance matters. Soc Personal Psychol Compass. 2008;2(3):1497–517.
35. Winkielman P, et al. Prototypes are attractive because they are easy on the mind. Psychol Sci. 2006;17(9):799–806.
36. De Jager S, Coetzee N, Coetzee V. Facial adiposity, attractiveness, and health: a review. Front Psychol. 2018;9:2562.
37. Thornhill R, Gangestad SW. Human facial beauty. Hum Nat. 1993;4(3):237–69.
38. Van Dongen S, Gangestad SW. Human fluctuating asymmetry in relation to health and quality: a meta-analysis. Evol Hum Behav. 2011;32(6):380–98.

39. Zaidi AA, et al. Facial masculinity does not appear to be a condition-dependent male ornament and does not reflect MHC heterozygosity in humans. Proc Natl Acad Sci. 2019;116(5):1633–8.
40. Lee AJ, et al. Facial averageness and genetic quality: testing heritability, genetic correlation with attractiveness, and the paternal age effect. Evol Hum Behav. 2016;37(1):61–6.
41. Baudouin J-Y, Tiberghien G. Symmetry, averageness, and feature size in the facial attractiveness of women. Acta Psychol. 2004;117(3):313–32.
42. Thornhill R, et al. Major histocompatibility complex genes, symmetry, and body scent attractiveness in men and women. Behav Ecol. 2003;14(5):668–78.
43. Mealey L, Bridgstock R, Townsend GC. Symmetry and perceived facial attractiveness: a monozygotic co-twin comparison. J Pers Soc Psychol. 1999;76(1):151–8.
44. Zebrowitz LA, Montepare JM. Appearance DOES matter. Science. 2005;308(5728):1565–6.
45. Apicella CL, Little AC, Marlowe FW. Facial averageness and attractiveness in an isolated population of hunter-gatherers. Perception. 2007;36(12):1813–20.
46. Valentine T, Darling S, Donnelly M. Why are average faces attractive? The effect of view and averageness on the attractiveness of female faces. Psychon Bull Rev. 2004;11(3):482–7.
47. Langlois JH, Roggman LA, Musselman L. What is average and what is not average about attractive faces? Psychol Sci. 1994;5(4):214–20.
48. Langlois JH, Roggman LA. Attractive faces are only average. Psychol Sci. 1990;1(2):115–21.
49. Rhodes G, et al. The attractiveness of average faces: cross-cultural evidence and possible biological basis. 2002.
50. Pollard J. Attractiveness of composite faces: a comparative study. Int J Comp Psychol. 1995;8(2):77–83.
51. Rhee SC, Lee SH. Attractive composite faces of different races. Aesthet Plast Surg. 2010;34(6):800–1.
52. Jones BC, DeBruine LM, Little AC. The role of symmetry in attraction to average faces. Percept Psychophys. 2007;69(8):1273–7.
53. DeBruine LM, et al. Dissociating averageness and attractiveness: attractive faces are not always average. J Exp Psychol Hum Percept Perform. 2007;33(6):1420–30.
54. Hicks KE, Thomas JR. The changing face of beauty: a global assessment of facial beauty. Otolaryngol Clin N Am. 2020;53(2):185–94.
55. Johnston VS. What do women want? Trends Cogn Sci. 2006;1(10):9–13.
56. Perrett DI, May KA, Yoshikawa S. Facial shape and judgements of female attractiveness. Nature. 1994;368(6468):239–42.
57. Jones D, et al. Sexual selection, physical attractiveness, and Facial Neoteny: cross-cultural evidence and implications [and comments and reply]. Curr Anthropol. 1995;36(5):723–48.
58. Johnston VS, Franklin M. Is beauty in the eye of the beholder? Ethol Sociobiol. 1993;14(3):183–99.
59. Buss DM. Sex differences in human mate preferences: evolutionary hypotheses tested in 37 cultures. Behav Brain Sci. 2010;12(1):1–14.
60. Cunningham MR. Measuring the physical in physical attractiveness: quasi-experiments on the sociobiology of female facial beauty. J Pers Soc Psychol. 1986;50(5):925–35.
61. Perrett D, et al. Facial attractiveness judgements reflect learning of parental age characteristics. Proc R Soc London B Biol Sci. 2002;269(1494):873–80.
62. Little AC, et al. Investigating an imprinting-like phenomenon in humans: partners and opposite-sex parents have similar hair and eye colour. Evol Hum Behav. 2003;24(1):43–51.
63. Johnston VS, et al. Male facial attractiveness: evidence for hormone-mediated adaptive design. Evol Hum Behav. 2001;22(4):251–67.
64. Penton-Voak IS, Perrett DI. Female preference for male faces changes cyclically: further evidence. Evol Hum Behav. 2000;21(1):39–48.
65. Penton-Voak IS, et al. Menstrual cycle alters face preference. Nature. 1999;399(6738):741–2.
66. Puts DA, et al. Women's attractiveness changes with estradiol and progesterone across the ovulatory cycle. Horm Behav. 2013;63(1):13–9.

67. Jones BC, et al. No compelling evidence that preferences for facial masculinity track changes in women's hormonal status. Psychol Sci. 2018;29(6):996–1005.

68. Penton-Voak IS, Chen JY. High salivary testosterone is linked to masculine male facial appearance in humans. Evol Hum Behav. 2004;25(4):229–41.

69. Rhodes G, et al. Does sexual dimorphism in human faces signal health? Proc R Soc Lond B Biol Sci. 2003;270(Suppl 1):S93–5.

70. Thornhill R, Gangestad SW. Facial attractiveness. Trends Cogn Sci. 1999;3(12):452–60.

71. Kruger DJ. Male facial masculinity influences attributions of personality and reproductive strategy. Pers Relat. 2006;13(4):451–63.

72. Addison WE. Beardedness as a factor in perceived masculinity. Percept Mot Skills. 1989;68(3):921–2.

73. Geniole SN, McCormick CM. Facing our ancestors: judgements of aggression are consistent and related to the facial width-to-height ratio in men irrespective of beards. Evol Hum Behav. 2015;36(4):279–85.

74. Dixson BJ, Vasey PL. Beards augment perceptions of men's age, social status, and aggressiveness, but not attractiveness. Behav Ecol. 2012;23(3):481–90.

75. Dixson BJ, Brooks RC. The role of facial hair in women's perceptions of men's attractiveness, health, masculinity and parenting abilities. Evol Hum Behav. 2013;34(3):236–41.

76. Saxton TK, et al. A lover or a fighter? Opposing sexual selection pressures on men's vocal pitch and facial hair. Behav Ecol. 2016;27(2):512–9.

77. Dixson B, et al. The masculinity paradox: facial masculinity and beardedness interact to determine women's ratings of men's facial attractiveness. J Evol Biol. 2016;29(11):2311–20.

78. Swaddle JP, Reierson GW. Testosterone increases perceived dominance but not attractiveness in human males. Proc R Soc London B Biol Sci. 2002;269(1507):2285–9.

79. Mueller U, Mazur A. Reproductive constraints on dominance competition in male Homo sapiens. Evol Hum Behav. 1998;19(6):387–96.

80. Cunningham MR, Barbee AP, Pike CL. What do women want? Facialmetric assessment of multiple motives in the perception of male facial physical attractiveness. J Pers Soc Psychol. 1990;59(1):61–72.

81. Perrett DI, et al. Effects of sexual dimorphism on facial attractiveness. Nature. 1998;394(6696):884–7.

82. Samizadeh S. The ideals of facial beauty among Chinese aesthetic practitioners: results from a large National Survey. Aesthet Plast Surg. 2018;43:1–13.

83. Samizadeh S, Wu W. Ideals of facial beauty amongst the Chinese population: results from a large national survey. Aesthet Plast Surg. 2018;43:1–11.

84. Penton-Voak I, et al. Symmetry, sexual dimorphism in facial proportions and male facial attractiveness. Proc R Soc London B Biol Sci. 2001;268(1476):1617–23.

85. Tatarunaite E, et al. Facial attractiveness: a longitudinal study. Am J Orthod Dentofac Orthop. 2005;127(6):676–82.

86. Glocker ML, et al. Baby schema in infant faces induces cuteness perception and motivation for caretaking in adults. Ethology. 2009;115(3):257–63.

87. Ishi H, et al. Analyses of facial attractiveness on feminised and juvenilised faces. Perception. 2004;33(2):135–45.

88. Stephen ID, et al. Facial skin coloration affects perceived health of human faces. Int J Primatol. 2009;30(6):845–57.

89. Porcheron A, et al. Influence of skin ageing features on Chinese women's perception of facial age and attractiveness. Int J Cosmet Sci. 2014;36(4):312–20.

90. Knoll BI, Attkiss KJ, Persing JA. The influence of forehead, brow, and periorbital aesthetics on perceived expression in the youthful face. Plast Reconstr Surg. 2008;121(5):1793–802.

91. Prokopakis EP, et al. The golden ratio in facial symmetry. Rhinology. 2013;51(1):18–21.

92. Di Dio C, Macaluso E, Rizzolatti G. The golden beauty: brain response to classical and renaissance sculptures. PLoS One. 2007;2(11):e1201.

93. Bejan A. The golden ratio predicted: vision, cognition and locomotion as a single design in nature. Int J Design Nat Ecodyn. 2009;4(2):97–104.

94. Schwind V. The golden ratio in 3D human face modeling. Stuttgart: Stuttgart Media University; 2011.
95. Jayaratne YSN, et al. Are neoclassical canons valid for southern Chinese faces? PLoS One. 2012;7(12):e52593.
96. Farkas LG, et al. Vertical and horizontal proportions of the face in young adult north American Caucasians: revision of neoclassical canons. Plast Reconstr Surg. 1985;75(3):328–38.
97. Dawei W, et al. Differences in horizontal, neoclassical Facial canons in Chinese (Han) and north American Caucasian populations. Aesthet Plast Surg. 1997;21(4):265–9.
98. Farkas L, Forrest C, Litsas L. Revision of neoclassical facial canons in young adult Afro-Americans. Aesthet Plast Surg. 2000;24(3):179–84.
99. Borman H, Ozgür F, Gürsu G. Evaluation of soft-tissue morphology of the face in 1,050 young adults. Ann Plast Surg. 1999;42(3):280–8.
100. Le TT, et al. Proportionality in Asian and north American Caucasian faces using neoclassical facial canons as criteria. Aesthet Plast Surg. 2002;26(1):64–9.
101. Al-Sebaei MO. The validity of three neo-classical facial canons in young adults originating from the Arabian peninsula. Head Face Med. 2015;11(1):1–7.
102. Sepehr A, et al. The Persian Woman's face: a photogrammetric analysis. Aesthet Plast Surg. 2012;36(3):687–91.
103. Edler R. Background considerations to facial aesthetics. J Orthod. 2001;28(2):159–68.
104. Choe KS, et al. The Korean American Woman's face: anthropometric measurements and quantitative analysis of Facial aesthetics. Arch Facial Plast Surg. 2004;6(4):244–52.
105. Torsello F, et al. Do the neoclassical canons still describe the beauty of faces? An anthropometric study on 50 Caucasian models. Prog Orthod. 2010;11(1):13–9.
106. Prendergast PM. Facial proportions. In: Erian A, Shiffman MA, editors. Advanced surgical facial rejuvenation: art and clinical practice. Berlin, Heidelberg: Springer Berlin Heidelberg; 2012. p. 15–22.
107. Rhodes G. The evolutionary psychology of facial beauty. Annu Rev Psychol. 2006;57:199–226.
108. Mueser KT, et al. You're only as pretty as you feel: facial expression as a determinant of physical attractiveness. J Pers Soc Psychol. 1984;46(2):469–78.

Thread Lifting Excellence: Aligning with East Asian Facial Characteristics and Beauty Ideals

6

Souphiyeh Samizadeh

Abstract

In the pursuit of aesthetic excellence, professionals specializing in facial re-contouring and rejuvenation must consider the unique anthropometric, anatomical, and cultural factors that characterize East Asian patients. The inherent differences in facial structure between East Asian and Caucasian populations require a tailored approach to both surgical and non-surgical cosmetic procedures, including thread lifting. Additionally, the rich cultural context of East Asia, with its deep-rooted beliefs in facial physiognomy and distinct beauty ideals, plays a critical role in shaping patient aspirations and expectations for aesthetic treatments. A thorough understanding of these critical differences ensures that aesthetic enhancements are not only effective from a clinical perspective but also align with the cultural and personal ideals of beauty held by patients. This chapter discusses the complexities of adapting aesthetic procedures to meet the specific needs of East Asian individuals, emphasizing the importance of a holistic, culturally sensitive, and scientifically grounded approach in the field of aesthetic medicine.

Keywords

Thread lift · Thread lifting · Facial contouring · Facial rejuvenation · Non-surgical lift · Threads · Non-surgical · Minimally invasive · Aesthetics · Asian beauty

S. Samizadeh (✉)
King's College London, London, UK

University College London, London, UK

Great British Academy of Aesthetic Medicine, London, UK
e-mail: info@baamed.co.uk

© Springer Nature Switzerland AG 2024
S. Samizadeh (ed.), *Thread Lifting Techniques for Facial Rejuvenation and Recontouring*, https://doi.org/10.1007/978-3-031-47954-0_6

Individuals seeking cosmetic treatments increasingly favour non-surgical options with less downtime. Thread lifting is a prevalent minimally invasive procedure in Asia for facial contouring and rejuvenation [1]. The market is abundant with various types of sutures/threads, and more are being developed and introduced as the demand keeps increasing. Threads are mainly used for facial contouring and prevention in young adults and soft tissue repositioning and rejuvenation in those with signs of facial ageing.

It is pertinent to understand that the facial morphology of East Asians is very different from that of Caucasians. This is inclusive of hard tissue and soft tissue morphology. Furthermore, cultural beliefs and treatment goals vary in Asia and directly influence treatment planning. With globalisation, ideals of beauty are becoming closer to each other. However, there are significant differences in the attractive and ideal faces among Asians and Caucasians. These differences reflect cultural differences and distinctive treatment expectations and goals.

Asian women prefer an oval facial shape with obtuse jaw angles and a rounded, pointy chin. The oval facial shape, with a continuous even line laterally from the forehead to the chin, is considered ideal for younger and older women [2–6]. Prominent malar eminence and zygomatic arch with subzygomatic hollowing are not regarded as beautiful. An ideal midface would have a full and rounded anterior cheek and not prominent zygomatic arches. Hence, techniques that increase the zygomatic arch width or height, including injection of dermal fillers and threads that cross the malar eminence, are not ideal for Asian faces.

Differences in facial dimensions, morphology and skeletal characteristics between ethnic groups, particularly between Caucasians and Asians, necessitate a tailored approach in thread lifting techniques and the strategic placement of threads. Caucasians and Asians, for example, have distinct facial structures that influence the choice of aesthetic treatments. These differences affect not just the cosmetic outcome but also the techniques and strategies clinicians use to achieve desired results. Tailoring these approaches ensures that procedures like thread lifting are both effective and harmonious with the individual's ethnic and cultural aesthetics.

Asians, in general, have brachycephalic head shapes, where the breadth of the head is greater than the length [7]. In both sexes, the Chinese have the greatest cephalic index values (maximum head size multiplied by maximum head length ×100) and the smallest head circumference [8]. As a result, the face is wide and short [5, 9]. Examination of the faces of young adult Chinese, Vietnamese, and Thai has revealed that the Asian face possesses the following dominant characteristics (Figs. 6.1 and Table 6.1) [5, 10, 11]:

- Wide intercanthal distance relative a shorter palpebral fissure
- Wide soft nose
- Wide facial contours
- Small mouth width
- The lower face is smaller than the forehead height.

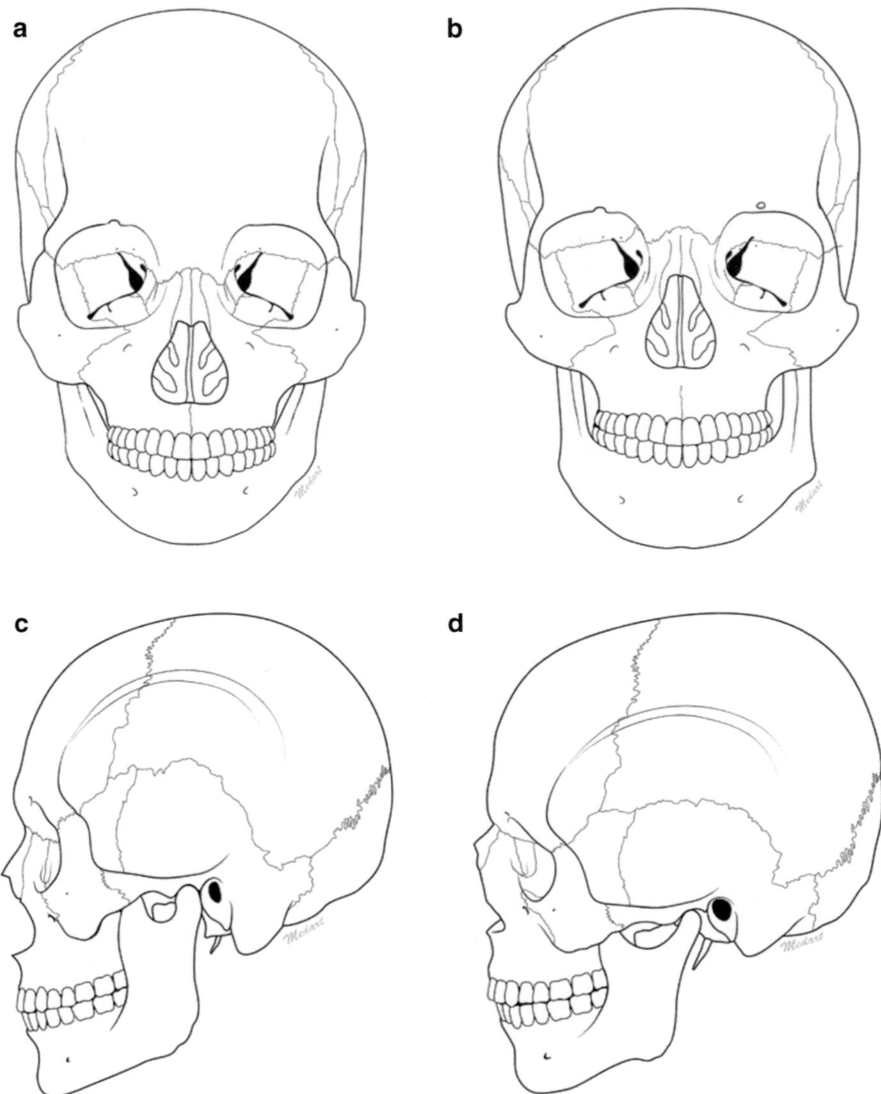

Fig. 6.1 "Comparison of Asian (**a**, **c**) and Caucasian (**b**, **d**) skulls. a, b Anterior view. The Asian skull (**a**) is wider overall, with greater bitemporal, bizygomatic, and bigonial width of the temple, zygoma, and mandible, respectively, compared with the Caucasian skull (**b**). (**c**, **d**) Lateral view. The Asian skull (**c**) has a less anterior projection, with a more retruded frontal bone and supraorbital ridge, recessed nasion, infraorbital rim, medial maxilla, the maxillary process of the zygoma, anterior nasal spine, and pogonion of the mandible compared with the Caucasian skull (**d**). (Illustrations courtesy of Prof Kim)." Reproduced with permission from Liew, S., Wu, W.T.L., Chan, H.H. et al. Consensus on Changing Trends, Attitudes, and Concepts of Asian Beauty. Aesth Plast Surg 40, 193–201 (2016). (http://creativecommons.org/licenses/by/4.0/) [5]

Table 6.1 Asian features compared—clinical features to Caucasian

Asian features compared to Caucasian	Clinical features
Increased width: • Bitemporal • Bizygomatic • Bigonal	Result in wider: • Forehead • Midface • Lower face
Retrusion of the following: • Forehead • Orbital rim • Medial maxilla • Pyriform margin	Flat forehead Heavy eyelids Concave central midface, perialar recession and nasolabial fold, perioral retrusion, shadowing on the base of nose, wide nasal width
Low nasal bridge Deficient anterior nasal spine	Nose: flat, short, retruded columella, broad nasal width
Bimaxillary protrusion	The upper and lower jaws are projected forward
Hypoplastic mandible	Retruded chin

Reproduced with permission from Liew, S., Wu, W.T.L., Chan, H.H. et al. Consensus on Changing Trends, Attitudes, and Concepts of Asian Beauty. Aesth Plast Surg 40, 193–201 (2016). (http://creativecommons.org/licenses/by/4.0/) [5]

Sundaram et al. have further delineated three Asian facial morphotypes, providing a nuanced understanding of the diverse facial structures within Asian populations (Fig. 6.2) [12]. This classification aids clinicians in customizing cosmetic procedures, including thread lifting, to harmonize with the unique anatomical and aesthetic preferences inherent to Asian individuals, ensuring culturally sensitive and effective treatment outcomes.

In East Asian aesthetics, there is a notable preference for enhancing the anterior facial projection to achieve a balanced and harmonious overall facial appearance. This enhancement is particularly sought after in the younger demographic, where genetic predispositions such as masseter hypertrophy and a square jawline—traits less favored aesthetically—are addressed. Additionally, among the aging population, interventions aim to diminish aging signs, augment anterior projection, and refine jawline contouring [13].

Specific facial features are believed to bring good fortune or luck, while others might suggest the opposite, reflecting deep-seated cultural beliefs about the link between physical appearance and life outcomes [14, 15]. For example, the mandibular angle is critical in female facial shape in Asia, as "a woman who has a wide and square face is thought to bring unhappiness to her husband" [16]. In women, an oval face shape is correlated with "beauty and compliance" and the ability to "juggle job and family". People with oval faces are said to be "logical, emotionally stable, and creative" with "very high self-esteem" but "may lack energy".

Another example is that individuals with an equilateral triangle face (small forehead and large cheekbones) are considered "stubborn, indomitable, neurotic, arrogant, and scared of authority", who "work actively and generally get along well with like-minded people". Women with "small eyes" are considered "moody" [17]. In China, Japan, Korea, and India, facial physiognomy is still extensively acknowledged and practised [4]. This has a direct and indirect impact on the field of aesthetic medicine, shaping both the demand for specific treatments and the variety of services provided.

Facial Subtype	Asian Facial Type I—"Northern"	Asian Facial Type II—"Intermediate"	Asian Facial Type III—"Southern"
Regions where these facial types are typical	Mongolia, some parts of Korea, Northern China	Southern China, Hong Kong, Taiwan	Malaysia, Indonesia, Vietnam, and other Southeast Asian Countries
Image	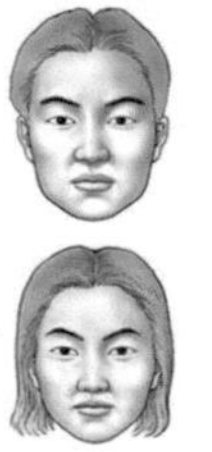	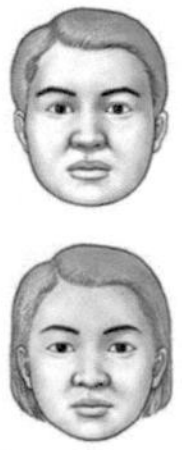	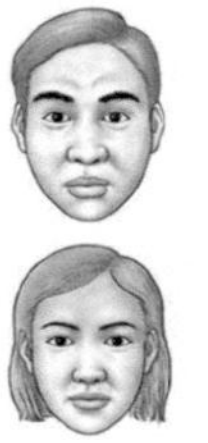
Palpebral fissure	Narrow	Wider than Type I	Widest of the 3 facial types
Supratarsal crease	No	Either present or absent	Present
Medial epicanthal fold	May be present	Usually absent	Absent
Nasal dorsum	Highest and longest of the 3 facial types	May be slightly lower and wider	Flat and short
Nasal ala	Narrow with narrow ellipsoid nostrils	Intermediate in width	Widest of the 3 facial types with wide, round nostrils
Mid face	Medial malar area lends to be flatter than the lateral malar area	Less flattening of the medial malar area than Type I	Medial and Literal malar areas tend to have some convexity
Zygoma	Prominent	Varies in prominence	Not prominent
Mandible	Prominent mandibular angle, giving a square lace or square jaw	Some degree of taper from the maxilla to the mandible can give a narrower appearance to the lower face in comparison to Type I (a round face with small chin and chubby cheeks)	Tapering from maxilla to mandible gives a narrow appearance to the lower face, due to a less prominent bony mandibular angle (oval facial shape)
Skin type	Usually fair	Fair or with intermediate pigmentation	Usually more pigmented than the other 2 facial types
Strategy with Botulinum Toxin Type A	Fitzpatrick skin phototype II–III	Fitzpatrick skin phototype II–IV	Fitzpatrick skin phototype II–IV
General	Avoid eyebrow arching ("Samurai eyebrow"), which is aesthetically displeasing when the face is wide Avoid reduction with botulinum toxin type A of the "charming roll" (pretarsal orbicularis oculi muscle bulge), which widens appearance of the narrow palpebral fissure without supratarsal crease, and hence increases apparent size of the eyes. The "charming roll" is commonly enhanced with filler Reduce width of the face	Avoid eyebrow arching ("Samurai eyebrow"), which is aesthetically displeasing when the face is wide If the palpebral fissure is narrow and without a supratarsal crease, avoid reduction with botulinum toxin type A of the "charming roll" (pretarsal orbicularis oculi muscle bulge). This may be enhanced with filler Reduce facial width, if aesthetically appropriate	Subtle eyebrow arching may be aesthetically appropriate, because the face lends to be narrower than for Type I When an eye-opening effect is desired, increase apparent size of the eyes by slightly lowering the interior ciliary margin to widen appearance of the palpebral fissure with a supratarsal crease. Must be balanced with desire for a "charming roll"
	Reduce prominence of zygoma and mandibular angle to give the face a tapered "V" shape Botulinum toxin to reduce activity of the nasal dilators is not popular, because the base of the nose is relatively narrow	Reduce prominence of the zygoma and mandibular angle, if appropriate, to give the face a tapered "V" shape In general, strategies are intermediate between those for Types I and III	Reduce prominence of base of the nose, which lends to be wide Botulinum toxin to masseter, temporalis, and parotid gland is not popular because the zygoma is smaller and the face is already tapered
Upper face	When injecting frontalis with botulinum toxin, avoid restriction of treatment to the medial portion of the muscle, as this can produce brow arching Botulinum toxin injected into orbicularis oculi at the uppermost point of the lateral canthal rhytids can also provide brow shaping and elevation	When injecting frontalis with botulinum toxin, avoid restriction of treatment to the medial portion of the muscle, as this can produce brow arching Botulinum toxin injected into orbicularis oculi at the uppermost point of the lateral canthal rhytids can also provide brow shaping and elevation.	Botulinum toxin injected into orbicularis oculi at tile uppermost point of the lateral can thai rhytids can also provide brow shaping and elevation Small doses of botulinum toxin to the pars orbitalis of orbicularis oculi superior to the uppermost point of the lateral canthal rhytids may also be appropriate. This injection point is typically at the hairline of the brow
	Avoid botulinum close to inferior ciliary margin, as it may obliterate the "charming roll" Botulinum toxin type A may he injected to temporalis to reduce upper facial width	If "charming roll" is desired, avoid botulinum toxin close to the inferior ciliary margin	When 'charming roll' is not desired, small doses of botulinum toxin can be injected at and/or close to inferior ciliary margin for eye opening
Middle and lower face	Botulinum toxin to masseter is typical to reduce width of the middle and lower face	Botulinum toxin to masseter when reduction of middle and lower facial width is desired	Botulinum toxin to masseter often not indicated
		Botulinum toxin to reduce activity of the nasal dilators only if base of the nose is wide	Botulinum toxin to the nasal dilators, when aesthetically appropriate, to narrow base of the nose
	Botulinum toxin to parotid, if considered appropriate. Further studies are needed to determine long-term safety of this treatment	Botulinum toxin to parotid, if considered appropriate. Further studies are needed to determine long-term safety of this treatment.	Botulinum toxin to parotid typically not indicated

Individual patients, including patients of part-Asian ancestry, may manifest characteristics of different morphotypes in the upper, middle, and lower one-thirds of the face.

Fig. 6.2 New classification of three Asian facial morphotypes and recommendations for appropriate treatment strategies with Botulinum Toxin Type A. Reproduced with permissions from Sundaram, Hema; Huang, Po-Han; Hsu, Nai-Jen; Huh, Chang Hun; Wu, Woffles T.L.; Wu, Yan; Cassuto, Daniel; Kerscher, Martina J.; Seo, Kyle Koo-Il; Pan-Asian Aesthetics Toxin Consensus Group Plastic and Reconstructive Surgery – Global Open 4(12):e872, December 2016

In East Asia, where deep-seated beliefs in facial physiognomy and the nuances of facial morphology intertwine with cultural ideals of beauty, the aspiration to look both beautiful and distinguished takes on heightened importance. This region, home to some of the most densely populated nations on the planet, is experiencing a surge in wealth and prosperity. This economic growth has rendered aesthetic enhancements more desirable and widely accessible to a growing middle class. In societies that place a premium on aesthetic refinement and beauty, the appeal of cosmetic procedures is naturally magnified. Among the array of non-surgical aesthetic options, thread lifting has gained exceptional popularity. This technique caters to East Asian preferences for enhancing specific facial features and achieving a harmonious balance, in line with Asian beauty standards yet adaptable to the individual's unique features. Thread lifting, known for its minimal invasiveness and quick recovery, aligns with the contemporary lifestyle and aesthetic goals of East Asian societies, making it a sought-after procedure.

Thread lifting can effectively improve tissue laxity with a shorter recovery time and less visible scarring [18–20]. The barb suspension for tissue repositioning, lifting, and anterior projection of Asian faces has been reported as an effective technique [21].

The most favourable anatomic characteristics for absorbable thread lifting are said to be [1]:

- Low body mass index
- Minimal fullness to the soft tissues
- Strong underlying bony projections to support the elevated tissue
- Good skin quality

Obesity and thick soft tissues result in poor outcomes [1].

In contrast to the West, East Asians view high cheekbones (a pronounced malar eminence) as masculine and unattractive in women. Rounded cheeks, known as "apple cheeks", without zygomatic prominence, are favoured. Currently, threads are frequently introduced obliquely in instances of midface and mandibular jowl lifts, with rejuvenation vectors oriented toward the temple. Threads unavoidably pass through the malar eminence, emphasising the cheekbones. While this unforeseen consequence may benefit Caucasians, it is undesirable in East Asians and results in dissatisfied patients [22]. Consideration of skin characteristics, such as a predisposition to post-inflammatory hyperpigmentation and keloid formation in Asians, is also essential in treatment planning.

Aesthetic practitioners are tasked with integrating anthropometric, anatomical, and cultural considerations into their treatment planning for facial re-contouring or rejuvenation, ensuring tailored and culturally sensitive approaches to meet the diverse needs of patients from various ethnic backgrounds.

Conclusion

In conclusion, the unique aesthetic preferences and cultural nuances set this region apart from Western standards of beauty. The preference for rounded "apple cheeks" without zygomatic prominence, in contrast to the high cheekbones favoured in the

West, exemplifies the distinct ideals that must be taken into account during treatment planning for East Asian patients.

Furthermore, the importance of understanding and adapting to regional differences in facial anatomy and treatment outcomes should be considered to enable a customised approach based on cultural and anthropometric factors. Additionally, considering skin differences, such as pre-dispositions to post-inflammatory hyperpigmentation and keloid formation, is crucial to delivering safe and effective treatments tailored to individual patient needs.

As aesthetic practitioners, it is essential to recognise and respect the anthropometric, anatomical, and cultural differences between various ethnicities when planning facial re-contouring or rejuvenation treatments. By cultivating a deep understanding of diverse aesthetic ideals and adapting treatment protocols accordingly, practitioners can ensure they provide personalised and satisfactory outcomes for patients across all cultural backgrounds. Ultimately, embracing this inclusive approach to aesthetic medicine will enable practitioners to deliver high-quality, culturally sensitive care that respects and celebrates the unique beauty of each individual.

References

1. Suh DH, et al. Outcomes of polydioxanone knotless thread lifting for facial rejuvenation. Dermatol Surg. 2015;41(6):720–5.
2. Samizadeh S. The ideals of facial beauty among Chinese aesthetic practitioners: results from a large National Survey. Aesthet Plast Surg. 2018;43:1–13.
3. Samizadeh S, Wu W. Ideals of facial beauty amongst the Chinese population: results from a large national survey. Aesthet Plast Surg. 2018;43:1–11.
4. Samizadeh S. Chinese facial physiognomy and modern day aesthetic practice. J Cosmet Dermatol. 2019;19:161–6.
5. Liew S, et al. Consensus on changing trends, attitudes, and concepts of Asian beauty. Aesthet Plast Surg. 2016;40(2):193–201.
6. Wu WT, et al. Consensus on current injectable treatment strategies in the Asian face. Aesthet Plast Surg. 2016;40(2):202–14.
7. Kim H-J, et al. Clinical anatomy of the face for filler and botulinum toxin injection. Springer; 2016.
8. Naini FB, Naini FB. Clinical diagnostic records, natural head position and craniofacial anthropometry. In: Facial aesthetics. Wiley; 2011. p. 71–85.
9. Liu Y, et al. A 3-dimensional anthropometric evaluation of facial morphology among Chinese and Greek population. J Craniofac Surgery. 2013;24(4):e353–8.
10. Le TT, et al. Proportionality in Asian and north American Caucasian faces using neoclassical facial canons as criteria. Aesthet Plast Surg. 2002;26(1):64–9.
11. Choe KS, et al. The Korean American Woman's face: anthropometric measurements and quantitative analysis of facial aesthetics. Arch Facial Plast Surg. 2004;6(4):244–52.
12. Sundaram H, et al. Aesthetic applications of botulinum toxin a in Asians: an international, multidisciplinary, pan-Asian consensus. Plast Reconstr Surg Glob Open. 2016;4(12):e872.
13. Wanitphakdeedecha R, et al. Absorbable barbed threads for lower facial soft-tissue repositioning in Asians. Dermatol Ther. 2021;11(4):1395–408.
14. McGrath C, Liu K, Lam C. Physiognomy and teeth: an ethnographic study among young and middle-aged Hong Kong adults. Br Dent J. 2002;192(9):522–5.

15. Kim N-H, et al. The use of botulinum toxin type a in aesthetic mandibular contouring. Plast Reconstr Surg. 2005;115(3):919–30.
16. Kim SK, Han JJ, Kim JT. Classification and treatment of prominent mandibular angle. Aesthet Plast Surg. 2001;25(5):382–7.
17. Liu Y, et al. A physiognomy based method for facial feature extraction and recognition. J Vis Lang Comput. 2017;43:103–9.
18. Villa MT, et al. Barbed sutures: a review of the literature. Plast Reconstr Surg. 2008;121(3):102e–8e.
19. Atiyeh BS, et al. Barbed sutures "lunch time" lifting: evidence-based efficacy. J Cosmet Dermatol. 2010;9(2):132–41.
20. Park TH, Seo SW, Whang KW. Facial rejuvenation with fine-barbed threads: the simple Miz lift. Aesthet Plast Surg. 2014;38(1):69–74.
21. Hau K. Malar Reshaping (MR) technique for Anterior Projection in Asian faces using bidirectional barb thread suspension surgery. In: 24th world congress of dermatology milan. 2019.
22. Kang SH, Byun EJ, Kim HS. Vertical lifting: a new optimal thread lifting technique for Asians. Dermatol Surg. 2017;43(10):1263–70.

Psychology in Aesthetic Clinic

7

Souphiyeh Samizadeh

Abstract

In aesthetic medicine, practitioners are presented with a broad spectrum of patients, each with unique motivations ranging from a pursuit of aesthetic enhancement to, in some cases, a need for psychiatric intervention. Recognizing this, it is crucial for aesthetic clinics to incorporate mental health screenings into their initial patient evaluations. This should include a thorough review of the patient's psychiatric history and current mental state, aimed at understanding their motivations for seeking cosmetic procedures. By identifying the psychological underpinnings of a patient's desire for aesthetic improvement, healthcare professionals can ensure treatments align with the patient's best interests, thereby elevating patient-centered care and improving outcomes. The necessity of mental health evaluations extends across the spectrum of aesthetic interventions, from minimally invasive techniques to more extensive surgical procedures. By integrating pre-treatment psychiatric assessments, clinics not only enhance the standard of care but also uphold ethical treatment practices. This approach ensures that the provision of cosmetic services is conducted with a keen awareness of the patient's mental wellbeing, thereby fostering a responsible and ethical framework within the field of aesthetic medicine.

S. Samizadeh (✉)
King's College London, London, UK

University College London, London, UK

Great British Academy of Aesthetic Medicine, London, UK
e-mail: info@baamed.co.uk

© Springer Nature Switzerland AG 2024
S. Samizadeh (ed.), *Thread Lifting Techniques for Facial Rejuvenation and Recontouring*, https://doi.org/10.1007/978-3-031-47954-0_7

Keywords

Psychology · BDD · Mental health · Aesthetic practice · Cosmetic clinic · Mental health screening · Body dysmorphic disorder

In aesthetic medicine, the significance of understanding patients' psychological motivations cannot be overstated. Recognizing that cosmetic interventions can lead to significant improvements in self-esteem, quality of life, and social functionality, it is equally important to identify patients who might face less favorable outcomes due to pre-existing psychological disorders, emotional health challenges, and particular social circumstances. This complexity underscores the necessity for comprehensive psychological evaluations as part of the pre-operative assessment process. Such evaluations are critical in ensuring that interventions are not only aligned with patients' physical aspirations but are also considerate of their mental health and well-being, thereby optimizing the therapeutic potential of cosmetic procedures.

Screening for mental health, encompassing psychiatric history and present mental state, is therefore indispensable during the initial consultation in aesthetic practices. This assessment is vital for both patient safety and practitioner insight. An in-depth dialogue should be initiated to understand the motivations and aspirations driving the pursuit of cosmetic procedures. Additionally, it is essential to discuss all possible outcomes and alternative strategies or solutions including their risks and benefits [1]. This process aids in the identification and safeguarding of vulnerable individuals and is a cornerstone of obtaining informed consent.

Evidence suggests that individuals opting for cosmetic enhancements are at a heightened risk of psychiatric disorders (Table 7.1) [2]. This predisposition significantly increases the likelihood of post-procedural dissatisfaction, adjustment difficulties, social withdrawal, exacerbation of existing mental health conditions, and a heightened risk of self-harm.

Psychological and psychosocial factors, including self-consciousness related to appearance, dissatisfaction with body image, life stressors, and social anxiety, significantly motivate the decision to undergo cosmetic surgery [1, 3]. Notable correlations exist between these psychosocial factors and the inclination towards cosmetic interventions, including [1, 4]:

- Exposure to intimate partner violence
- Engagement in dieting behaviors
- Experiences of verbal abuse in women
- Smoking habits
- Usage of medication for sleep or anxiety
- Holding private medical insurance
- Alcohol consumption
- Elevated stress levels
- Compromised mental health

Conversely, cosmetic interventions have been associated with improvements in self-esteem, quality of life, and social functioning for many individuals [1]. These

Table 7.1 Mental disorders are commonly observed in aesthetic surgery clinics

Primary mental disorders
Psychiatric disorders
- Affective/bipolar disorder (F30–F39)
- Factitious disorders/Munchausen syndrome (F68.1)
- Schizophrenia/body dysmorphic delusion (F20–F29)
- Intentional self-harm (suicide) (X60–X84)

Social phobia (anxiety disorders F40)
Somatoform disorders (F45)
- Hypochondriasis (F45.2)
- Body dysmorphic disorder (F45.2)
- Somatisation disorder (multiple complaints of physical illness) (F45.0)

Personality disorder (F60)
- Emotionally unstable personality disorder (borderline disorder) (F60.3)
- Narcissistic personality disorder (F60.8)
- Obsessive-compulsive personality disorder (F60.5)

Secondary mental disorders and comorbidities
Reactions to severe stress (F43)
- Acute stress reaction (F43.0)
- Post-traumatic stress disorder (F43.1)
- Adjustment disorder (F43.2)

Comorbidities
- Anxiety disorder/social phobia (F40)
- Depressive disorder (F30–39)

Reproduced with permission from Harth W. Psychosomatic Disturbances and Cosmetic Surgery. European Dermatology. 2010;5 [8]

improvements underscore the potential benefits of carefully considered aesthetic procedures.

However, it is important to recognize that not all outcomes are universally positive. Research has identified specific factors that may predict less favorable results post-cosmetic surgery, including [1, 5–7]:

- Disorders with a psychological component:
  - Clinical depression
  - Body dysmorphic disorder
- Non-clinically diagnosed disorders associated with negative emotional health status:
  - Low self-esteem
  - Anxiety
  - Depressed mood
- Social parameters:
  - Age
  - Relationship status
- Personality types

In light of these considerations, the consultation process must be meticulously structured to address a comprehensive range of topics. These include a thorough exploration of the patient's concerns, the duration and intensity of these concerns, the timeline of contemplation regarding cosmetic intervention, and the factors leading to the decision to proceed with a consultation. Additionally, a detailed history of past cosmetic procedures, including the number of surgeries, practitioners, and the level of satisfaction with these interventions, should be reviewed. Understanding the patient's social context—specifically, how their decisions are perceived by family and friends, as well as any history of legal issues or altercations with previous providers—is equally critical. Identifying red flags during this initial consultation, as summarized in key guidelines and tables, is essential for ensuring patient safety and optimizing the likelihood of successful outcomes. This comprehensive approach bridges the gap between recognizing potential risks and effectively planning and conducting cosmetic interventions, ensuring that both patient welfare and procedural success are prioritized. In summary: [5]

1. Detail the primary complaint fully.
2. Duration and extent of the issue.
3. Length of time considering cosmetic intervention.
4. Reasons for scheduling the current consultation.
5. History of cosmetic interventions:
    (a) Number and nature of previous procedures
    (b) Number of previous practitioners
    (c) Level of satisfaction with past interventions and practitioners.
6. Perception of outcomes by the patient, family, and friends (cosmetic and psychosocial).
7. Any legal disputes or conflicts with previous providers.

Consultation red flags are summarized in Table 7.2.

Table 7.2 Alarm signals/red flags

- Aggression, lack of insight, hostility, impulsivity, self-manipulation
- Idealisation of the surgeon
- Life crisis, suicidal tendencies
- Pessimism, affective disorders, and anxiety disorders
- Regression and child-like behaviour
- Attribution of guilt or charges (towards other therapists)
- Secondary gain due to disease (especially attention by others)
- Somatisation of mental problems (multiple complaints of illness)
- Carelessness (side effects), denial of reality
- Disturbed compliance, lack of independence
- Disturbed coping with the disease
- Treatment for the sake of another person
- Deep disturbance of self-valuing/self-image, self-valuing problems
- Over-attribution: exaggeration of the physical defect
- Over-identification with the defect
- Unclear motivation
- Unclear previous surgeries
- Too high expectations on treatment

Reproduced with permission from Harth W. Psychosomatic Disturbances and Cosmetic Surgery. European Dermatology. 2010;5 [8]

Body Dysmorphic Disorder

Body Dysmorphic Disorder (BDD) is a significant concern within the field of medical aesthetics, with studies indicating that between 7–15% of individuals seeking cosmetic procedures suffer from BDD. Notably, a 2021 study in the *Journal of Craniofacial Surgery* found BDD prevalence of approximately 10.8% among patients undergoing maxillofacial surgery [5, 9, 10].

Body dysmorphic disorder (BDD) is classified as a psychiatric condition characterized by an intense preoccupation with perceived flaws in one's physical appearance, often perceived as deformities, which can lead to significant distress, functional impairment, and disability. Frequently, these perceived flaws are either nonexistent or minor and not noticeable to others, yet the individual's concern is disproportionately severe [11].

A 2005 study involving 200 subjects highlighted that the majority sought and received nonpsychiatric care, primarily from dermatologists and surgeons, rather than psychiatric intervention. Notably, 12.0% of the participants had been prescribed isotretinoin, with a high prevalence of suicidal ideation (83.3%) and attempts (25.0%) reported. Dermatological treatments, specifically topical agents, along with rhinoplasty, liposuction, and breast augmentation, were the most sought-after procedures, reflecting broader national trends in cosmetic surgery. Additionally, minimally invasive, paraprofessional, and dental treatments were also commonly pursued [11]. This aligns with previous findings, emphasizing the preference for cosmetic solutions over psychiatric help among individuals with BDD [12–14].

Despite the potential for some subjective improvement, cosmetic interventions have not been shown to effectively address the symptoms of BDD [11, 15]. This disconnect highlights a critical issue: individuals with BDD, who often have minimal or non-existent deformities, are at a high risk of poor post-procedure outcomes due to the disorder's nature. BDD is associated with several comorbidities, including the following [5, 16–18]:

- Depression
- Mania
- Social phobias
- Substance abuse
- Alcohol abuse
- Generalised anxiety disorder
- Obsessive-compulsive disorder
- Suicidal tendencies
- Post-traumatic stress disorder
- Narcissism

Reassurance seeking is another prevalent behavior observed in individuals with BDD [19]. BDD is classified within the category of obsessive-compulsive-related disorders in the Diagnostic and Statistical Manual of Mental Disorders, Fifth Edition (DSM-5) [1] (Table 7.3).

Table 7.3 Diagnostic criteria of body dysmorphic disorder (BDD) [23]

Preoccupation with one or more perceived defects or flaws in physical appearance that are not observable or appear slight to others	At some point during the course of the disorder, the individual has performed repetitive behaviours (e.g. mirror checking, excessive grooming, skin picking, reassurance seeking) or mental acts (e.g. comparing his or her appearance with that of others) in response to appearance concerns	The preoccupation causes clinically significant distress or impairment in social, occupational or other important areas of functioning	The appearance preoccupation is not better explained by concern with body fat or weight in an individual whose symptoms meet diagnostic criteria for an eating disorder
• The common focus is on skin, hair and nose • Acne, wrinkles, paleness, size and shape of the nose, hair thinning or excessive hair growth • First one body part and later may add another body part	• The most common feature is mirror gazing • In a survey on mirror use in BDD patients, the mean duration of an extended mirror session was for 73 min as compared to 21 min in controls [22] • Skin picking: A series of 123 patients with BDD reported skin picking; in 27% [23] • Other behaviours include excessive grooming and camouflaging (extensive hair styling, ritualized make up applications, touching of perceived defects, frequent change of clothing and use of hats)	• Impairment can include missing school or work, avoidance of relationship or intimacy, becoming housebound or psychiatrically hospitalized • Increased severity of symptoms associated with poorer functioning in all areas of activities of daily living	• Those patients with muscle dysmorphia type specifier may excessively diet and exercise • These patients must be distinguished from patients with eating disorders such as anorexia nervosa or bulimia nervosa

Reproduced with permission from Jafferany M, Salimi S, Mkhoyan R, Kalashnikova N, Sadoughifar R, Jorgaqi E. Psychological aspects of aesthetic and cosmetic surgery: Clinical and therapeutic implications. Dermatologic Therapy. 2020;33(4):e13727

The DSM-5 outlines specific diagnostic criteria for BDD, detailed in Table 7.3. These include [17, 20]:

A. Preoccupation with one or more perceived defects or flaws in physical appearance that are not observable or appear slight to others.
B. Repetitive behaviors (e.g., mirror checking, excessive grooming, skin picking, reassurance seeking) or mental acts (e.g., comparing one's appearance with that of others) in response to appearance concerns.
C. The preoccupation causes clinically significant distress or impairment in social, occupational, or other areas of functioning.
D. The appearance preoccupation is not better explained by concerns with body fat or weight in an individual whose symptoms meet diagnostic criteria for an v disorder.

This disorder's severity can range from good or fair insight (where the individual recognizes that BDD beliefs are not true or may not be true) to absent insight/delusional beliefs (where the individual is entirely convinced that the BDD beliefs are true), further complicating treatment and management. Specify the level of insight regarding beliefs about BDD:

(a) Good or Fair Insight: The individual acknowledges that their beliefs related to BDD may be unfounded, recognizing that these beliefs are either definitely or probably not true, or they might entertain some doubt about their accuracy.
(b) Poor Insight: The individual somewhat believes in the veracity of their BDD-related beliefs, considering them to likely be true despite evidence to the contrary. This level of insight indicates that the individual acknowledges the possibility that their concerns might not be entirely justified or accurate, yet they still lean towards believing their perceptions are true. Essentially, it reflects a state of ambivalence where the person is caught between recognizing their belief may be exaggerated or unfounded and feeling convinced by their perception of a physical defect.
(c) Absent Insight/Delusional Beliefs: The individual is fully convinced of the reality of their BDD-related beliefs, without acknowledging any possibility of these beliefs being unfounded, reflecting a delusional conviction.

The majority of individuals diagnosed with BDD engage in various compulsive habits and repetitive behaviors that are both time-consuming and ritualistic. These activities often include frequent checks in mirrors, reflections in car bumpers, or any reflective objects like the back of spoons, alongside excessive grooming, makeup application, or tanning. They might also involve constant comparisons with others and seeking reassurance from people around them, despite seldom finding solace in these reassurances [19, 21, 22].

Table 7.3 can be used as a guide. Cosmetic physicians can use the following during the consultation: [5].

Table 7.4 BDD signs, symptoms, and demographics by BDD severity

Mild/moderate	Severe	Both
No significant impairment in global functioning	Avoidant behaviour	Frequent mirror checking
Localised appearance concerns	Impairment in global functioning	Constant comparison with others
Realistic psychosocial concerns	Young	Need for reassurance with regard to perceived flaws
	Significantly depressed	Seeking unnecessary dermatological treatments or cosmetic procedures
	Significantly anxious	Referential thinking: thinking that others are equally disturbed with the defects
	Extremely preoccupied with defect	Camouflaging behaviour
	Debilitating compulsive behaviours (i.e. mirror checking or self-mutilation/do-it-yourself surgery)	Abnormal or demanding behaviour toward surgeon or staff
	Delusional beliefs about appearance	
	Social isolation	
	Unemployment	
	Unrealistic expectations regarding cosmetic outcome	
	Expectation that cosmetic procedure will be solution to problems in other areas of life	

Reproduced with permission from Higgins, S. and Wysong, A., 2018. Cosmetic surgery and body dysmorphic disorder—an update. International journal of women's dermatology, 4(1), pp. 43–48 [24]

- The daily duration spent worrying about the perceived flaw.
- The level of distress the flaw causes to the individual.
- The behavioral consequences stemming from this distress, such as avoiding social situations.

Should a patient display an intense preoccupation with their appearance, coupled with substantial distress or functional impairment, the presence of BDD should be considered [5]. Moreover, research has highlighted a link between cosmetic surgery and an increased risk of developing mental health conditions [1]. Detailed insights into the signs, symptoms, and demographics associated with varying degrees of BDD severity are provided in Table 7.4.

While much of the research on BDD focuses on the context of cosmetic surgery, the importance of assessing and screening for BDD in non-surgical cosmetic environments cannot be overstated. A study involving 154 women seeking minor cosmetic procedures revealed that 25% showed potential signs of BDD, alongside heightened psychological distress and more unrealistic expectations, particularly related to improving social or romantic relationships [25].

Symptoms of BDD manifest similarly across genders, albeit with distinct concerns. Men may exhibit preoccupations predominantly with muscle size (muscle dysmorphia), focusing excessively on certain body parts like genitalia and hairline, often resorting to substance misuse. Women, conversely, are more likely to obsess over weight, breast size, buttocks, thighs, toes, and body hair, with a tendency to engage in frequent comparisons and extensive mirror gazing [26, 27].

Reassuring individuals with BDD about their appearance or the unnecessity of the requested treatment often proves futile and is usually met with skepticism. Simply refusing treatment or referring them to another practitioner does not address the underlying issue. Likewise, preventative or minimal therapies typically offer little benefit, with many patients regarding previous cosmetic interventions as ineffective or worsening their condition [19, 21, 22].

Studies indicate that outcomes of cosmetic interventions in individuals with BDD are often deemed suboptimal, leading to discontent, legal actions, aggression towards the surgeon, dissatisfaction, depression, and in severe cases, suicide [21, 28–30].

Even when a minor cosmetic concern is addressed to the patient's satisfaction, a new perceived flaw often becomes the focus, potentially leading to a cycle of multiple surgeries [21, 30, 31].

Managing a patient with BDD in a medical aesthetics setting is quite challenging, particularly in the absence of typical indicators.

Treatment is most effective when behavioural and pharmaceutical interventions are combined. The Dufresne Body Dysmorphic Disorder Questionnaire can be an effective screening tool in the cosmetic environment and outpatient setting [32].

For comprehensive management guidelines tailored to cosmetic surgeons and dermatologists, the work of Phillips, K.A., and Dufresne, R.G. on Body Dysmorphic Disorder offers invaluable insights [19].

Personality Disorders

Personality disorders should be considered during the consultation. The DSM-IV-TR™ defines personality disorder [33].

> "An enduring pattern of inner experience and behaviours that deviates markedly from the expectations of the individual's culture, is pervasive and inflexible, has an onset in adolescence or early adulthood is stable over time, and leads to distress or impairment."

Narcissistic personality disorder, borderline personality disorder, histrionic disorder, antisocial personality disorder, and other disorders in the same category are frequently described as "dramatic, excitable, erratic, or volatile" [34].

Obsessive-Compulsive Personality

In the general population, obsessive-compulsive personality disorder is the most prevalent personality disorder [35]. It is characterised by extreme perfectionism and inflexibility [8]. Other traits include: [35]

- Obsession with specifics and details
- Excessive dedication to work and productivity
- Over-conscientiousness
- Incapacity to discard useless items
- Inability to delegate
- Miserliness
- Rigidity
- Stubbornness

These individuals may have occupational challenges and anxiety, mainly when presented with unfamiliar situations requiring flexibility/compromise or adaptability.

Narcissistic Personality Disorder

Narcissistic personality disorder (NPD) is notably prevalent among individuals seeking cosmetic surgery. Characterized by an exaggerated sense of self-importance and grandiosity, a continuous need for admiration, heightened sensitivity to the opinions of others, and a pronounced lack of empathy, NPD significantly influences the dynamics within cosmetic surgery settings. While this condition affects less than 1% of the general population, its prevalence increases to between 2 and 16% within clinical settings. Notably, among cosmetic surgery patients, the incidence of NPD can rise to as much as 25%, highlighting the importance of careful psychological assessment in this group [23, 33, 36, 37]. Many of these individuals keep returning to the same clinician despite dissatisfaction with the treatment outcome [37].

According to the diagnostic guidelines, individuals must meet five or more of the following criteria, as outlined in Table 7.5:

- Grandiose sense of self-importance: this includes overestimating achievements and talents, expecting to be recognized as superior without commensurate achievements.
- Preoccupied with illusions of boundless success, strength, intelligence, attractiveness, and/or ideal love: the individual dwells on thoughts of limitless success, power, intelligence, attractiveness, or perfect romance.
- Believes in being unique and "special". The person believes that they are unique and can only be understood by, or should associate with, other special or high-status people or institutions.
- Need for Excessive Admiration: there is a constant requirement for excessive admiration and attention.
- Sense of entitlement
  - Unreasonable expectations
  - Expecting favourable treatment
  - Expecting automatic compliance with their expectations.

Table 7.5 Diagnostic criteria for narcissistic personality disorder

Environment	Genetics	Neurobiology
Mismatches in parent-child relationships with either excessive adoration or excessive criticism that is poorly attuned to the child's experience	Inherited characteristics	The connection between the brain and behaviour and thinking
Has grandiose sense of self-importance (e.g. exaggerates achievements, expects to be recognized as superior without completing the achievements)		
Is preoccupied with fantasies of success power, brilliance, beauty, or perfect love		
Believes that they are special and only "special" and can only be understood by or should associate with other special people (or institutions)		
Requires excessive admiration		
Has a sense of entitlement, such as an unreasonable expectation of favourable treatment or compliance with his (or her expectations)		
Is exploitative and takes advantage of others to achieve their own ends		
Lacks empathy and is unwilling to identify with the needs of others		
Is often envious of others or believes that others are envious of them		
Shows arrogant, haughty behaviours and attitudes		

Reproduced with permission from Jafferany M, Salimi S, Mkhoyan R, Kalashnikova N, Sadoughifar R, Jorgaqi E. Psychological aspects of aesthetic and cosmetic surgery: Clinical and therapeutic implications. Dermatologic Therapy. 2020;33(4):e13727 [23]

- Interpersonally exploitative: the individual takes advantage of others to achieve their own ends.
- Lacks empathy: there is an absence of empathy for the feelings and needs of others.
- Envy of Others or Belief That Others Are Envious of Them: the person often feels jealous of others or believes that others are jealous of them.
- Arrogant and Haughty Behaviors or Attitudes: they display arrogant, haughty behaviors or attitudes.

Histrionic Personality Disorder

A constant pattern of extreme emotion and craving for attention prevails in histrionic personality disorder (also known as dramatic personality disorder) [8]. People with this disorder tend to be flirtatious, overly seductive and inappropriately sexual with the majority of the people they meet, regardless of their sexual attraction, enchanting, charming, manipulative, impulsive, suggestible, and easily manipulated by people they admire, and they are lively. When not the focus of attention, they feel unappreciated or neglected [34].

A histrionic personality disorder is characterised with a persistent and universal pattern of constant attention-seeking behaviours and emotional dysregulation, as

Table 7.6 Diagnostic criteria for histrionic personality disorder

Environment	Genetics	Neurobiology
Mismatches in parent-child relationships with either excessive adoration or excessive criticism that is poorly attuned to the child's experience	Inherited characteristics	The connection between the brain and behaviour and thinking
Uncomfortable when not the centre of attention		
Seductive or provocative behaviour		
Shifting and shallow emotions		
Uses appearance to draw attention		
Impressionistic and vague speech		
Dramatic or exaggerated emotions		
Suggestible		
Considers relationships more intimate than they are		

Reproduced with permission from Jafferany M, Salimi S, Mkhoyan R, Kalashnikova N, Sadoughifar R, Jorgaqi E. Psychological aspects of aesthetic and cosmetic surgery: Clinical and therapeutic implications. Dermatologic Therapy. 2020;33(4):e13727 [23]

indicated by particular symptoms and should have at least five of the following criteria (Table 7.6) [34]:

- Discomfort occurs when the person is not the focus of attention
- Seductive or provocative behaviour
- Emotions that fluctuate are shallow and are fleeting
- Attracts attention via appearance
- Speech that is impressionistic and imprecise
- Emotions that are dramatic or excessive
- Easily influenced by others
- Believes relationships are more intimate than they actually are

These individuals rely heavily on suppression and dissociation as defensive strategies [34]. Furthermore, they frequently have unrealistic expectations of the procedure and also of themselves [38].

Dependent, anxious-reluctant, paranoid, schizoid personality disorders, and emotionally unstable personality disorder (borderline disorder) should not be forgotten [8]. As detailed by Mio Nakamura and John Koo, (Table 7.7) provides a summary of the personality disorders most relevant to aesthetic providers, as well as practical tips for approaching patients with each disorder.

Additional questions for evaluating psychological issues were offered by Grossbart et al. which are shown in (Table 7.8) [40]

Personality Type: A Difficult Patient?

Mio Nakamura and John Koo have discussed the differences between difficult personalities and personality disorders in the clinical context. Understanding this difference is paramount. Fundamentally, personality encompasses the unique patterns

Table 7.7 Summary of personality disorders most relevant to the aesthetic provider and practical tips for approaching patients with each personality disorder as outlined by Mio Nakamura and John Koo

Personality disorder	Clinical presentation	Clinical relevance and implications	Approach
Borderline	• Instability in interpersonal relationships, self-image, and affect • Marked impulsivity • Intense fear of rejection and abandonment • Splitting Self-destructive behaviours	• Presenting complaint is usually due to "need to fill emptiness" • Rejection of requested services or perceived undertreatment is taken as abandonment, causing strong negative emotions	• Do not give in to patient's strong emotionality • Avoid unnecessary treatments/procedures • Provide other options rather than complete rejection • Regular follow-up appointments • Be aware of splitting and potential self-harming behaviour
Histrionic	• Dramatic and excessive emotionality • Attention-seeking, provocative, seductive behaviour • Perceives relationships to be more intimate than they are • Easily influenced by others	• Difficulty in medical decision-making due to impulsivity • Repeated visits due to minor defects causing anxiety • Dissatisfaction when not receiving enough attention	• Assistant or chaperone should be present at all times • Involve patient in decision-making but provide guidance, reassurance, and support • Avoid unnecessary treatment/procedures • Do not let patient's seductive behaviour cloud judgment • Give appropriate attention and compliments focusing on patient as a person • Respond firmly to inappropriate seduction
Obsessive compulsive	• Preoccupation with orderliness, perfectionism, and control • Fear of losing control • Excessive attention to detail • Focus on facts and knowledge to replace or subdue emotions	• Anxiety due to fear of losing control • Knowledge and information gives sense of control over illness • Feeling of loss of control leads to anxiety, depression, and anger	• Professional, structured encounters • Set realistic expectations, be explicit about unattainable outcomes, and document discussion • Detailed explanations and plans (written information and guide to appropriate resources) • Regular follow-up appointments
Narcissistic	• Grandiosity • Uncomfortable in vulnerable or inferior position • Need for admiration • Lack of empathy • Demanding and entitled	• Underlying emptiness, low self-esteem, or insecurities • Need for admiration and power	• Do not take patient's behaviours personally • Focus on an attitude of respect • Engage patient at a medical level (discuss in medical terminology, discuss journal article, etc.) • Allow patient to have a sense of power by engaging in medical decision-making • Discuss details and risks of procedure and document discussion in medical records

Reproduced with permission from Nakamura M, Koo J. Personality disorders and the "difficult" dermatology patient: Maximizing patient satisfaction. Clinics in Dermatology. 2017;35(3):312–8 [39]

Table 7.8 Additional questions useful for exploring psychosocial issues [37, 40]

1. What makes now feel like the right time for surgery rather than a month or a year ago or a month or a year in the future? (Do not stop with purely practical answers like "I have a vacation coming up" or "I just got a bonus check". Continue, "OK but is there anything else?")
2. \zWhat are three wishes about the impact on your life of a successful outcome? Please answer on a pure fantasy level—don't be realistic
3. What are three realistic expectations of the impact that successful surgery will have on your life? Can you imagine any possible disadvantages to a successful surgical outcome?
4. How do you expect key people in your life will respond differently to you after the surgery? How about strangers?
5. Does your (target body part) remind you of anyone you know? Have met? Family members? Whose eyes or whose thighs do you have?
6. Have you noticed that your readiness to have the surgery varies from day to day or week to week? Is the desire greater with certain events, moods, or reactions of others?
7. Have you noticed any unexpected emotional reactions from surgical personnel, the office, or from talking about the surgery?
8. Have you ever had any indications that others see you differently than you see yourself?
9. Do you ever have trouble following health or beauty guidelines that you agree with?
10. What percentage of peoples' first impression of you do you believe your (largest body part) accounts for? What percentage after they get to know you?

of thinking, feeling, and behaving that distinguish an individual. It represents the intrinsic framework through which a person interprets the world, processes experiences, and consistently acts across various situations, relationships, and environments, including reactions to new situations and stress.

Personalities are believed to be long-lasting, stable, and difficult to change. The Five-Factor Model is the most frequently applied system of personality traits. The five broad characteristics include:

- Openness
- Conscientiousness
- Extraversion
- Agreeableness
- Neuroticism

These broad traits can be further dissected into more specific facets, allowing for a deeper analysis of an individual's personality.

The impact of personality on healthcare interactions is profound. It influences how patients articulate their health concerns, interact with medical staff, respond to proposed treatment plans, endure procedures, and manage pain or discomfort [39, 41].

Clinicians can significantly enhance their communication strategies, consultation approach, and overall patient care by comprehensively understanding patient personalities. Although challenging initially, adapting care to align with patients' personality styles fosters greater satisfaction with the healthcare experience. A concordance in beliefs and values between clinicians and patients enhances trust and treatment adherence [39, 42].

Distinguishing personality types from personality disorders is crucial. Personality disorders are characterized by pervasive, maladaptive patterns of thought and behavior that markedly deviate from cultural expectations, potentially causing distress or impairment to the individual and those around them. Interactions with patients having personality disorders can be particularly complex, often leading to dissatisfaction despite the clinician's efforts. A one-size-fits-all approach typically falls short with such patients, underscoring the need for tailored strategies in managing their care [39].

Expectations

Unrealistic expectations about aesthetic procedures are closely linked to suboptimal psychosocial outcomes [5]. Establishing realistic expectations is paramount for the success of any aesthetic procedure. Often, patients may simplify their understanding, expecting the procedure to be painless, straightforward, without any post-treatment visible signs, and requiring no recovery period. Misleading advertisements from product companies, practices, practitioners, and distorted portrayals on social media exacerbate these unrealistic expectations. Thorough discussions encompassing all treatment options, procedural expectations, potential sequelae, and side effects/complications, along with the presentation of before-and-after pictures (including immediate post-procedure images), are vital in fostering realistic patient expectations. It is also crucial to recognize that expectations can be influenced by cultural and racial factors, as perceptions of body image are intertwined with these contexts [23].

Assessment of the patient's expectations regarding the procedure, the anticipated outcome, reactions from others, and potential life changes is essential [5, 43]. A clear distinction should be made between internal motivations, such as enhancing body image, versus external expectations, such as affecting relationships or employment opportunities. A dominance of external motivations can be a poor prognostic indicator, suggesting a higher likelihood of dissatisfaction with the outcome, thus warranting careful consideration before proceeding with the cosmetic intervention [5, 44].

In the case of thread lifting procedures, while significant improvements are achievable, expectations of surgical or flawless results may be unrealistic. Additional treatments might be necessary to achieve and enhance the desired outcome.

Identifying and addressing potential mental health issues, as well as managing unreasonable and unrealistic expectations, are critical steps in preventing harm and potential legal issues [45]. This comprehensive approach emphasizes the importance of aligning patient expectations with realistic outcomes, thereby ensuring patient satisfaction and safeguarding against adverse effects.

Conclusion

This chapter has aimed to illuminate the critical intersection between psychological well-being and aesthetic interventions, emphasizing the importance of patient-centered care and the safeguarding of vulnerable individuals within the aesthetic clinic setting. While the array of psychological concerns discussed here is not exhaustive, it provides a foundational understanding that should prompt educational dialogues between patients and practitioners, and, where necessary, the initiation of referrals to mental health professionals. Recognizing and addressing underlying psychological issues in individuals seeking cosmetic procedures is not solely about refining the practitioner's skills; it is fundamentally about ensuring the well-being and safety of patients. This approach empowers clinicians to make judicious decisions regarding treatment plans, advocating for the execution of procedures only when they align with the best interests of the patient and highlight the need for psychiatric evaluation when indicated.

Optimizing patient care in aesthetic medicine requires a paradigm that extends beyond technical proficiency to embrace comprehensive communication strategies, a structured consultation process, and sensitive, informed interview techniques. This vigilance towards potential psychiatric disorders is pivotal in providing holistic care. By prioritizing patient-centered approaches and remaining attentive to the psychological dimensions of aesthetic medicine, practitioners affirm their commitment to not only enhancing physical appearance but also promoting the overall psychological health of their patients. The cultivation of such an environment within aesthetic clinics is instrumental in safeguarding vulnerable patients, thereby upholding the highest standards of care and ethical responsibility in the field.

References

1. Brunton G, Paraskeva N, Caird J, Bird KS, Kavanagh J, Kwan I, et al. Psychosocial predictors, assessment, and outcomes of cosmetic procedures: a systematic rapid evidence assessment. Aesthet Plast Surg. 2014;38(5):1030–40.
2. Hayashi K, Miyachi H, Nakakita N, Akimoto M, Aoyagi K, Miyaoka H, et al. Importance of a psychiatric approach in cosmetic surgery. Aesthet Surg J. 2007;27(4):396–401.
3. Rumsey N, Harcourt D. The psychology of appearance. McGraw-Hill Education; 2005.
4. Schofield M, Hussain R, Loxton D, Miller Z. Psychosocial and health behavioural covariates of cosmetic surgery: Women's Health Australia Study. J Health Psychol. 2002;7(4):445–57.
5. Honigman RJ, Phillips KA, Castle DJ. A review of psychosocial outcomes for patients seeking cosmetic surgery. Plast Reconstr Surg. 2004;113(4):1229–37.
6. Cook SA, Rosser R, Salmon P. Is cosmetic surgery an effective psychotherapeutic intervention? A systematic review of the evidence. J Plast Reconstr Aesthet Surg. 2006;59(11):1133–51.
7. Picavet V, Gabriëls L, Jorissen M, Hellings PW. Screening tools for body dysmorphic disorder in a cosmetic surgery setting. Laryngoscope. 2011;121(12):2535–41.
8. Harth W. Psychosomatic disturbances and cosmetic surgery. Eur Dermatol. 2010;5(9):736–43.
9. Dey JK, Ishii M, Phillis M, Byrne PJ, Boahene KD, Ishii LE. Body dysmorphic disorder in a facial plastic and reconstructive surgery clinic: measuring prevalence, assessing comorbidities, and validating a feasible screening instrument. JAMA Facial Plast Surg. 2015;17(2):137–43.

10. Kashan DL, Horan MP, Wenzinger E, Kashan RS, Baur DA, Zins JE, et al. Identification of body dysmorphic disorder in patients seeking corrective procedures from oral and maxillofacial surgeons. J Craniofac Surg. 2021;32(3):970–3.
11. Crerand CE, Phillips KA, Menard W, Fay C. Nonpsychiatric medical treatment of body dysmorphic disorder. Psychosomatics. 2005;46(6):549–55.
12. Phillips KA, Grant J, Siniscalchi J, Albertini RS. Surgical and nonpsychiatric medical treatment of patients with body dysmorphic disorder. Psychosomatics. 2001;42(6):504–10.
13. Veale D, Boocock A, Gournay K, Dryden W, Shah F, Willson R, et al. Body dysmorphic disorder: a survey of 50 cases. Br J Psychiatry. 1996;169(2):196–201.
14. Hollander E, Cohen LJ, Simeon D. Body dysmorphic disorder. Psychiatr Ann. 1993;23:359–64.
15. Bowyer L, Krebs G, Mataix-Cols D, Veale D, Monzani B. A critical review of cosmetic treatment outcomes in body dysmorphic disorder. Body Image. 2016;19:1–8.
16. Vindigni V, Pavan C, Semenzin M, Granà S, Gambaro F, Marini M, et al. The importance of recognizing body dysmorphic disorder in cosmetic surgery patients: do our patients need a preoperative psychiatric evaluation? Eur J Plast Surg. 2002;25(6):305–8.
17. Fletcher L. Development of a multiphasic, cryptic screening protocol for body dysmorphic disorder in cosmetic dermatology. J Cosmet Dermatol. 2021;20(4):1254–62.
18. Castle D, Beilharz F, Phillips KA, Brakoulias V, Drummond LM, Hollander E, et al. Body dysmorphic disorder: a treatment synthesis and consensus on behalf of the International College of Obsessive-Compulsive Spectrum Disorders and the Obsessive Compulsive and Related Disorders Network of the European College of Neuropsychopharmacology. Int Clin Psychopharmacol. 2021;36(2):61–75.
19. Phillips KA, Dufresne RG. Body dysmorphic disorder. A guide for dermatologists and cosmetic surgeons. Am J Clin Dermatol. 2000;1(4):235–43.
20. American Psychiatric Association, DSM-5 Task Force. Diagnostic and statistical manual of mental disorders: DSM-5. Washington, DC: APA; 2013.
21. Phillips KA, McElroy SL, Keck PE, Pope HG, Hudson JI. Body dysmorphic disorder: 30 cases of imagined ugliness. Am J Psychiatr. 1993;150:302–8.
22. Phillips KA, Diaz SF. Gender differences in body dysmorphic disorder. J Nerv Ment Dis. 1997;185(9):570–7.
23. Jafferany M, Salimi S, Mkhoyan R, Kalashnikova N, Sadoughifar R, Jorgaqi E. Psychological aspects of aesthetic and cosmetic surgery: clinical and therapeutic implications. Dermatol Ther. 2020;33(4):e13727.
24. Higgins S, Wysong A. Cosmetic surgery and body dysmorphic disorder—an update. Int J Womens Dermatol. 2018;4(1):43–8.
25. Pikoos TD, Rossell SL, Tzimas N, Buzwell S. Is the needle as risky as the knife? The prevalence and risks of body dysmorphic disorder in women undertaking minor cosmetic procedures. Aust N Z J Psychiatry. 2021;55:1191–201.
26. Taqui A, Shaikh M, Gowani S, Shahid F, Khan A, Tayyeb S, Ganatra HA. Body dysmorphic disorder: gender differences and prevalence in a Pakistani medical student population. BMC Psychiatry. 2008;8(1):20.
27. Perugi G, Akiskal HS, Giannotti D, Frare F, Di Vaio S, Cassano GB. Gender-related differences in body dysmorphic disorder (dysmorphophobia). J Nerv Ment Dis. 1997;185(9):578–82.
28. Groenman N, Sauer H. Personality characteristics of the cosmetic surgical insatiable patient. Psychother Psychosom. 1983;40(1–4):241–5.
29. Wright MR. The male aesthetic patient. Arch Otolaryngol Head Neck Surg. 1987;113(7):724–7.
30. Dufresne RG Jr, Phillips KA, Vittorio CC, Wilkel CS. A screening questionnaire for body dysmorphic disorder in a cosmetic dermatologic surgery practice. Dermatol Surg. 2001;27(5):457–62.
31. Fukuda O. Statistical analysis of dysmorphophobia in out-patient clinic. Jpn J Plast Reconstr Surg. 1977;20:569–77.
32. Wilson JB, Arpey CJ. Body dysmorphic disorder: suggestions for detection and treatment in a surgical dermatology practice. Dermatol Surg. 2004;30(11):1391–9.

33. Cooper J. Diagnostic and statistical manual of mental disorders (4th edn, text revision) (DSM–IV–TR) Washington, DC: American Psychiatric Association 2000. 943 pp.£ 39.99 (hb). Br J Psychiatry. 2001;179(1):85.
34. French JH, Shrestha S. Histrionic personality disorder. Treasure Island (FL): StatPearls Publishing; 2020.
35. Diedrich A, Voderholzer U. Obsessive–compulsive personality disorder: a current review. Curr Psychiatry Rep. 2015;17(2):2.
36. Napoleon A. The presentation of personalities in plastic surgery. Ann Plast Surg. 1993;31(3):193–208.
37. Malick F, Howard J, Koo J. Understanding the psychology of the cosmetic patients. Dermatol Ther. 2008;21(1):47–53.
38. Ritvo EC, Melnick I, Marcus GR, Glick ID. Psychiatric conditions in cosmetic surgery patients. Facial Plast Surg. 2006;22(03):194–7.
39. Nakamura M, Koo J. Personality disorders and the "difficult" dermatology patient: maximizing patient satisfaction. Clin Dermatol. 2017;35(3):312–8.
40. Grossbart TA, Sarwer DB. Psychosocial issues and their relevance to the cosmetic surgery patient. Semin Cutan Med Surg. 2003;22(2):136–47.
41. Fortin AH, Dwamena FC, Frankel RM, Smith RC. Smith's patient centered interviewing: an evidence-based method. McGraw Hill Professional; 2012.
42. Krupat E, Bell RA, Kravitz RL, Thom D, Azari R. When physicians and patients think alike: patient-centered beliefs and their impact on satisfaction and trust. J Fam Pract. 2001;50(12):1057–63.
43. Pruzinsky T. Psychological factors in cosmetic plastic surgery: recent developments in patient care. Plast Surg Nurs. 1993;13(2):64–71.
44. Sarwer DB, Didie ER. Body image in cosmetic surgical and dermatological practice. In: Disorders of body image. Stroud: Wrighton Biomedical Publishing; 2002. p. 37–53.
45. Klassen AF, Cano SJ, Alderman A, East C, Badia L, Baker SB, et al. Self-report scales to measure expectations and appearance-related psychosocial distress in patients seeking cosmetic treatments. Aesthet Surg J. 2016;36(9):1068–78.

Part II

Threads in Focus: Types and Materials

Thread Types and Materials

8

Souphiyeh Samizadeh and Sorousheh Samizadeh

Abstract

Synthetic polymers have long been a cornerstone in the fields of tissue engineering, surgical interventions, and pharmacological applications, offering unparalleled versatility and innovation in medical treatments. Their appeal lies in the ability to customize mechanical properties and degradation rates, alongside the capacity to introduce functional groups tailored to specific medical needs. Moreover, their biodegradable and bioresorbable nature makes them particularly suited for integration and eventual absorption within biological systems. Among these polymers, poly(glycolic acid) (PGA), poly(lactic acid) (PLA), and poly(caprolactone) (PCL) are prominent for their widespread use as fundamental components in the manufacturing of sutures and suture anchors. These materials have revolutionized surgical practices, facilitating not only traditional surgical procedures but also pioneering minimally invasive techniques for aesthetic rejuvenation. This chapter discusses the diverse types and materials of threads utilized in lifting procedures, underscoring the technological advancements and material sciences that have propelled the use of polymer sutures to the forefront of surgical innovation.

S. Samizadeh (✉)
King's College London, London, UK

University College London, London, UK

Great British Academy of Aesthetic Medicine, London, UK
e-mail: info@baamed.co.uk

S. Samizadeh
University College London, London, UK

© Springer Nature Switzerland AG 2024
S. Samizadeh (ed.), *Thread Lifting Techniques for Facial Rejuvenation and Recontouring*, https://doi.org/10.1007/978-3-031-47954-0_8

Keywords

Thread lift · Thread lifting · Thread lift method · Thread lift technique · Thread lift procedure · Polydioxanone threads · Facial rejuvenation

Synthetic polymers have been integral to tissue engineering, surgical procedures, and pharmacology for a long time. Degradable medical devices are frequently composed of polymers, which are chains of repeating monomers that might be natural or manufactured. These materials are appealing for medical applications as their mechanical characteristics and degradation profiles can be tailored, the potential to design functional groups for specific medical applications, and their biodegradable and bioresorbable properties [1]. Biodegradable polymers can easily form solid, stable, and porous structures with excellent mechanical properties.They can undergo controlled degradation through various methods, such as particle leaching and phase separation [2]. Additionally, synthetic biodegradable polymers have been crucial in tissue engineering as scaffolds, guiding specific cell growth and differentiation [3].

Sutures, in particular, must exhibit optimal biomechanical properties to ensure their effectiveness and durability in various applications. These characteristics include excellent tensile strength, dimensional stability, absence of memory, and flexibility to avoid tissue injury [4].

The 1960s saw the introduction of synthetic absorbable polymeric surgical devices [4]. Use of these polymers in the medical field includes orthopaedics (fixation devices, bone screws, pins, spinal cages, scaffolds, prosthesis), scaffold (bone/tendon regeneration), soft tissue implants, vascular grafts, drug delivery, encapsulation, sustained release of bioactive compounds, tumour targeting, sutures, and expansion into new fields [5–11]. Bioresorbable materials are frequently used in bone fixation and repair procedures. They eliminate the need for a second operation to remove the implant after healing the bone [12]. Poly(glycolic acid), poly(lactic acid), and poly(caprolactone) are among the most popular and common polymers used as the main components of common sutures and suture anchors (Fig. 8.1) [1]. The use of some of these polymers has attracted the attention of the medical aesthetic community as sutures for non-surgical/minimally invasive dentofacial rejuvenation.

Various suture (thread) materials are available for the suture/thread lifting procedure. Initially, permanent threads made from materials such as silicon, gold, titanium, and polypropylene were used (Fig. 8.2). These threads, which required insertion through an incision and general anaesthesia, did not bring widespread popularity among surgeons and practitioners [13]. The development of biodegradable polymers was a fundamental leap in wound closure and surgical procedures. The choice of suture material is critical, as its properties significantly impact both the procedure's effectiveness and the healing process. These properties are multifaceted and interconnected, including [14]:

- Physical Properties: This encompasses the suture's strength, stiffness, viscoelasticity, friction coefficient, compliance, size, and shape (monofilament or multifilament). Additionally, it covers the suture's ability to absorb and transport fluids, which can affect wound healing.

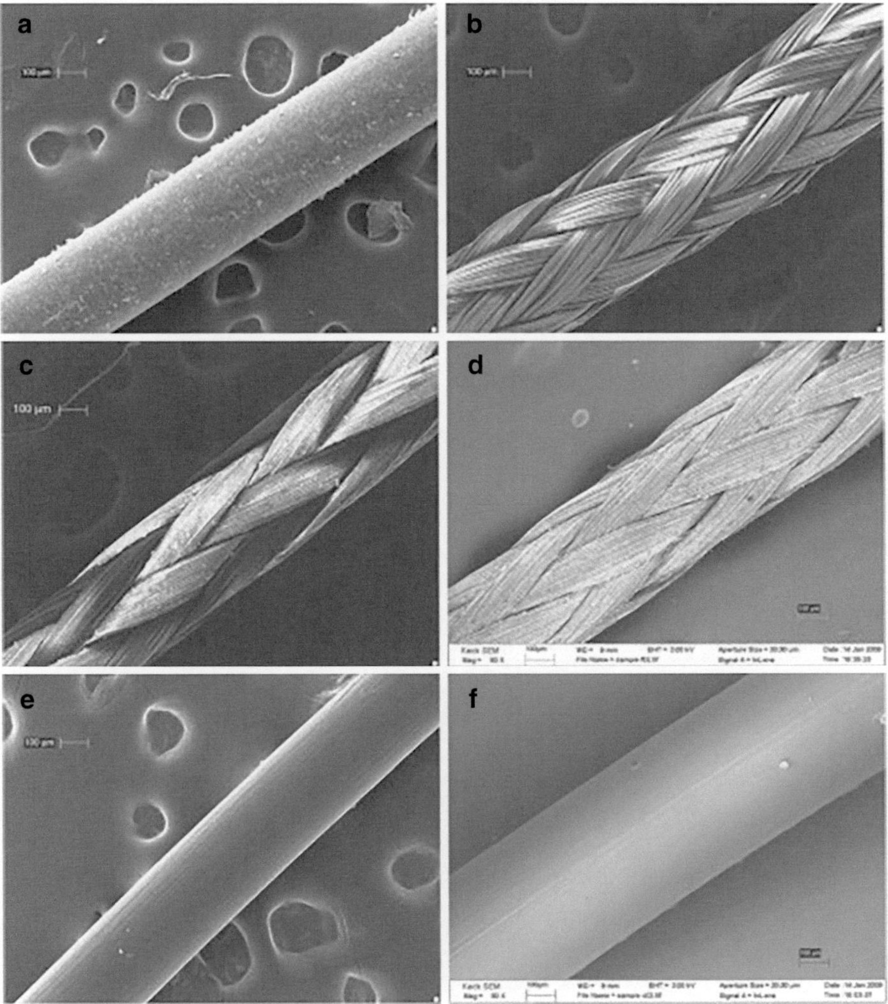

Fig. 8.1 Scanning electron images of some commercial absorbable sutures (**a**) Chromic catgut: polyglycolic acid family; (**b**) Dexon: poly(glycolide/L-lactide) copolymer or polyglactin 910 family; (**c**) Vicryl; (**d**) Vicryl Plus: poly-*p*-dioxanone family; (**e**) PDSII; (**f**) MonoPlus: poly(glycolide/trimethylene carbonate) copolymer or polyglyconate family; (**g**) Maxon: poly(glycolide/ε-caprolactone) copolymer or poliglecaprone 25 family; (**h**) Monocryl: poly(glycolide/trimethylene carbonate/dioxanone) or Glycomer 631 family; (**i**) Biosyn: poly(glycolide/trimethylene carbonate/ε-caprolactone) copolymer or glyconate family; (**j**) Monosyn: poly(glycolide/trimethylene carbonate/lactide/e-caprolactone) copolymer or polyglytone 6211 family; and (**k**) Caprosyn. [Reproduced with permission from Chu, C.C., 2013. Types and properties of surgical sutures. In biotextiles as medical implants (pp. 231–273). Woodhead Publishing]

- Mechanical Properties: Key considerations include tensile strength (both when knotted and unknotted), modulus of elasticity (indicative of stiffness), elongation at break, and overall toughness of the suture material.
- Handling properties: This aspect evaluates how easy the sutures are to use during procedures, affecting the efficiency and outcome of the surgery.

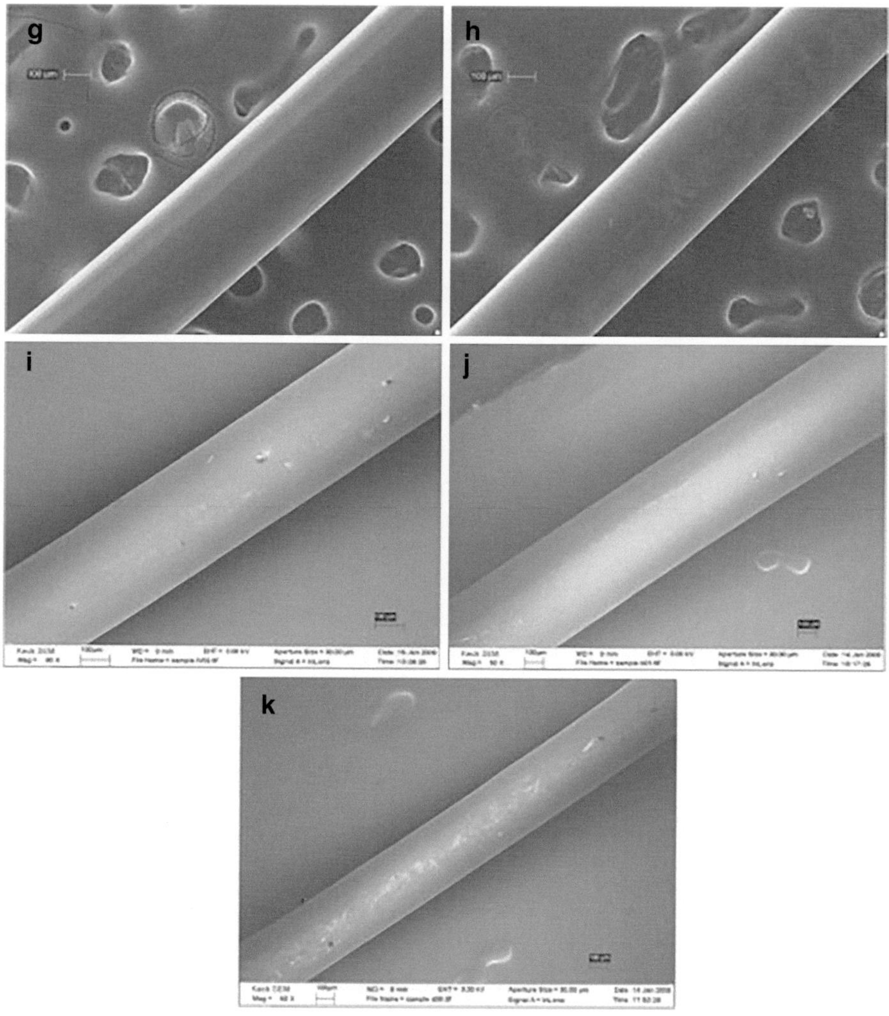

Fig. 8.1 (continued)

- Biological Properties: Biocompatibility is vital, as it measures the suture's impact on surrounding tissues and vice versa. The chemical composition of the sutures and their degradation products can influence the extent of tissue reaction, essential for minimizing complications
- Biodegradation Properties: The rate and manner in which sutures break down in the body are crucial for timed healing and minimizing the need for removal procedures.

It is noteworthy that the physical configuration of the suture, such as its stiffness, can precipitate varying degrees of tissue response, underscoring the importance of material selection predicated upon specific procedural requirements and anticipated outcomes [14].

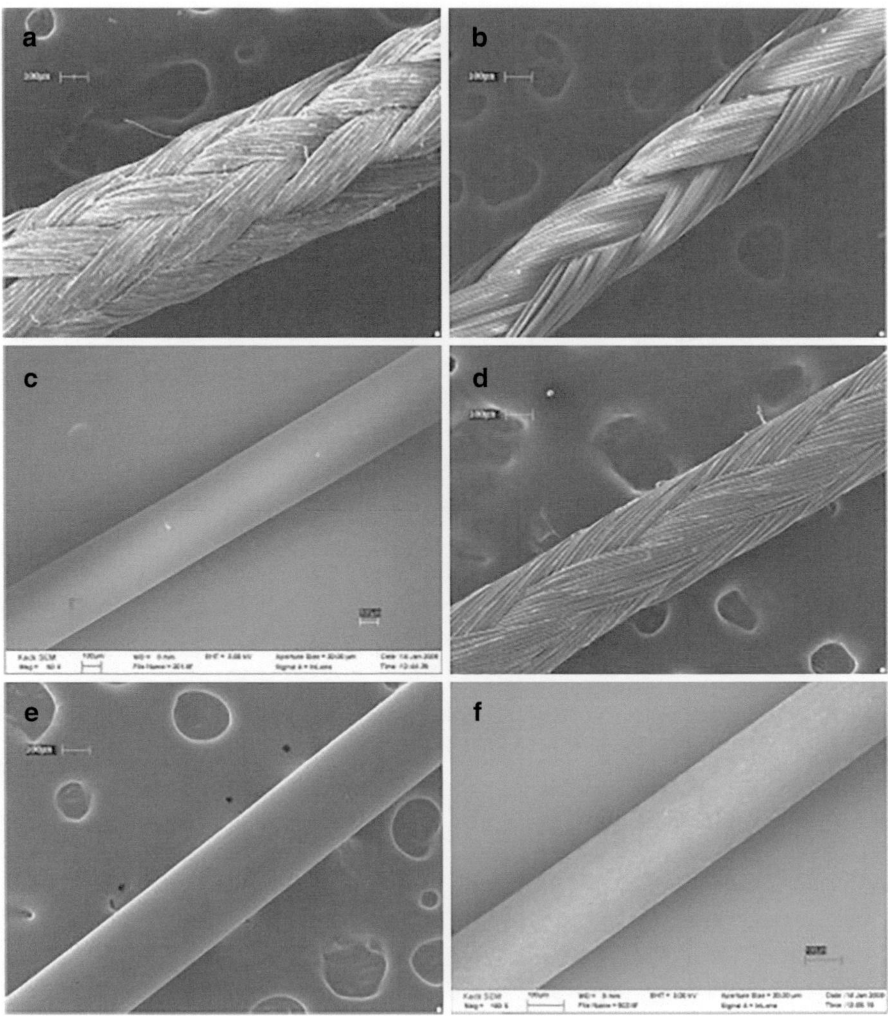

Fig. 8.2 Scanning electron images of some commercial non-absorbable sutures (**a**) Silk: polyester family; (**b**) Mersilene; (**c**) Novafil: polyamide family; (**d**) Nurolon; (**e**) Ethilon; (**f**) Dermalon; (**g**) Supramid: polypropylene family; (**h**) Prolene: polyvinylidene fluoride family; (**i**) Pronova: oly (ether ester) family; (**j**) Dyloc: poly(tetrafluoroethylene) family; (**k**) Gore-Tex; (**l**) Stainless steel. [Reproduced with permission from Chu, C.C., 2013. Types and properties of surgical sutures. In biotextiles as medical implants (pp. 231–273). Woodhead Publishing]

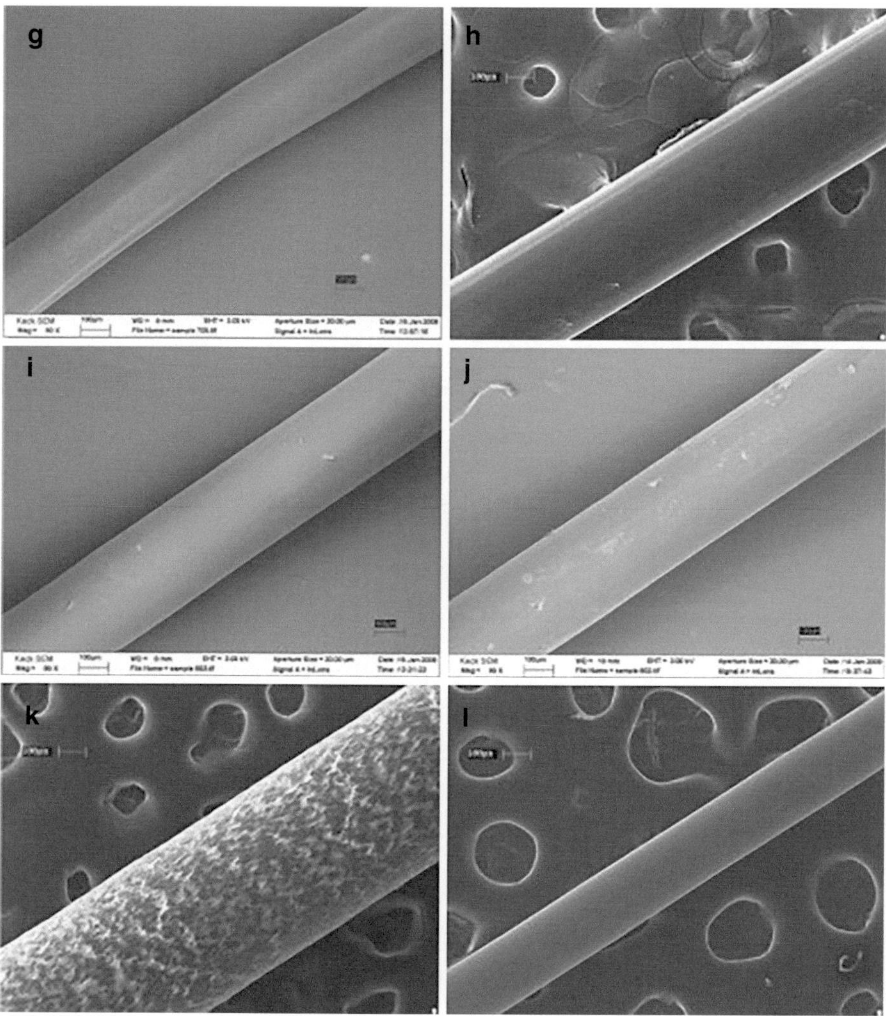

Fig. 8.2 (continued)

Threads utilized in facial rejuvenation procedures can be systematically categorized based on several criteria, including their longevity (absorbable vs. non-
absorbable), composition (e.g., polydioxanone, poly-L-lactic acid), and a variety
of other distinctive features. These features encompass surface characteristics,
thread length (with a demarcation at 90 mm differentiating long from short threads),
and configurations ranging from single to multiple strands, straight to coiled formations, and those pre-attached to needles or cannulae [15, 16]. In terms of the
physical configuration, the sutures can be classified into: monofilament, multifilament, twisted, and braided types, as shown in Fig. 8.1. The taxonomy of threads,
particularly those designated for facial rejuvenation, is continuously evolving, with

manufacturers tirelessly innovating both the threads themselves and the associated techniques to enhance facial and bodily rejuvenation through this modality. The field of tissue engineering and biomaterials research has seen exponential growth, driving advancements in this area.

Upon the implantation of these threads, a biophysical process is initiated, leading to the stimulation of neocollagenesis and the formation of new elastic fibers. This biological response, characterized by an augmented volume of collagen and elastin, coupled with elevated hyaluronic acid production and subsequent water retention, culminates in the fibrosis process. The resultant effect is a discernibly rejuvenated skin appearance, attributed to the improved structural integrity and hydration of the dermal and subdermal tissue [17].

Thread Materials and Longevity

Table 8.1 provides a comprehensive overview of various thread materials, delineating their longevity as observed in both in vivo and in vitro settings.

Polydioxanone (PDO)(Fig. 8.3), are synthetic, biodegradable polymers with an extensive application history and a well-established safety profile. Introduced in the 1980s for intradermal suturing, PDO threads are known for their biocompatibility and are absorbed through hydrolysis approximately six months after placement. When utilized in their smooth form, PDO threads facilitate biostimulation,

Table 8.1 Various thread materials, highlighting their respective longevity.

	Material		Longevity (months)
Thread materials and longevity	Polydioxanone (PDO)		6
	Poly-L-lactic acid (PLLA)		12
	Poly-caprolactone (PCL)		24
	Poly(L-lactide-*co*-caprolactone) (PLCL)		
	Polypropylene (non-absorbable)		Non-absorbable Permanent
	Combination	Polyester (polyethylene terephthalate—PET) and silicone (solid and from medical grade)	Non-absorbable Permanent
		Polylactic acid-caprolactone (PLACL)	18+
		Polylactic-*co*-glycolic acid (PLGA)	24
		Poly(lactic acid/caprolactone acid) hyaluronic acid P(LA/CL) HA	24
	Silicone Polyester coated with silicone		Non-absorbable Permanent

Fig. 8.3 *p*-Dioxanone to polydioxanone (PDO)

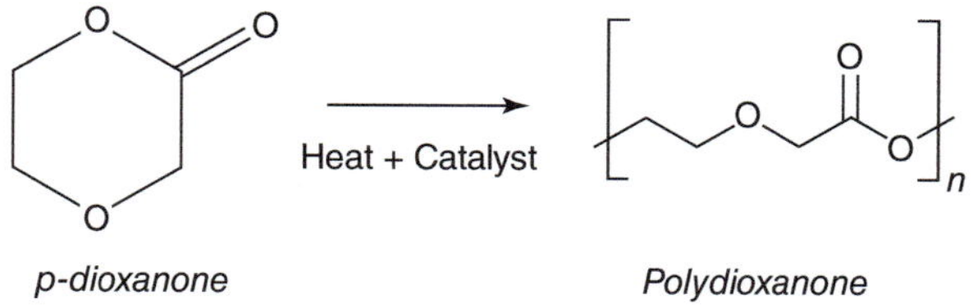

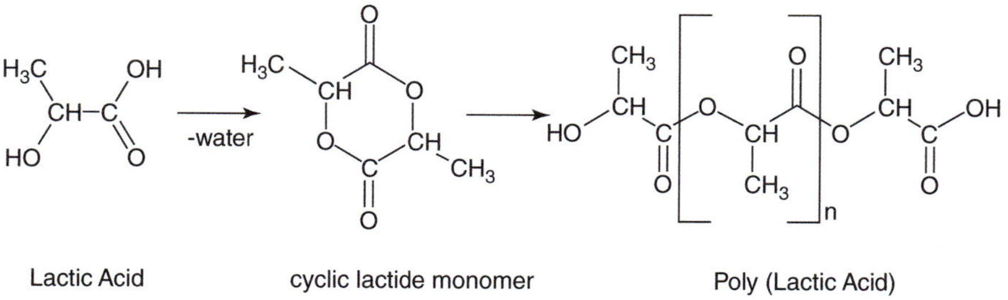

Fig. 8.4 Lactic acid to polylactic acid

effectively treating static rhytids by acting as "solid fillers." Moreover, the incorporation of specific surface modifications, such as barbs and cogs, significantly augments their load-bearing capacity, rendering them highly effective as suspension sutures. The application of PDO threads has proven successful in various aesthetic interventions, including the correction of ptotic soft tissues, mild lipolysis, reducing and eliminating rhytids, and deep facial folds [18].

Poly-L-lactic acid (PLLA) is a biodegradable and absorbable polymer extensively employed in the fabrication of medical implants and resorbable materials, including those based on PLLA and PLGA (Fig. 8.4) [5, 6]. Both polylactic acid and polyglycolic acid polymers, along with their copolymers, are recognized for their bioabsorbable properties. Their widespread use is attributed to their chemical components, which bear a resemblance to those found in bone tissue, and their elastic modulus, closely mirroring that of natural bone [8, 19–21]. Through the process of hydrolytic de-esterification, PLLA is broken down into lactic acid monomers. These monomers subsequently participate in the Krebs cycle and are ultimately expelled from the body as carbon dioxide and water through pulmonary excretion [22–24]. In aesthetic medicine, PLLA is used as an injectable filling agent for volumisation, soft tissue augmentation, and as a thread material for thread lifting procedures. Post-implantation, PLLA incites a foreign body reaction that triggers a cellular inflammatory response. This inflammatory response stimulates neocollagenesis and promotes the production of type I and III collagen. Over a period of approximately 24 months, the implanted PLLA material gradually decomposes and is replaced by newly formed collagen [25]. This induced neocollagenesis, combined with strategic tissue repositioning, is instrumental in the rejuvenation and improving face and body contours. It provides a critical mechanism for substantially improving aesthetic outcomes.

Polylactic-*co*-glycolic acid (PLGA) is a copolymer of polylactic acid (PLA) and polyglycolic acid (PGA) (Fig. 8.5). It is biodegradable and biocompatible. This versatile material is extensively utilized across a myriad of medical and dental fields, ranging from bone regeneration to various branches of dentistry, including

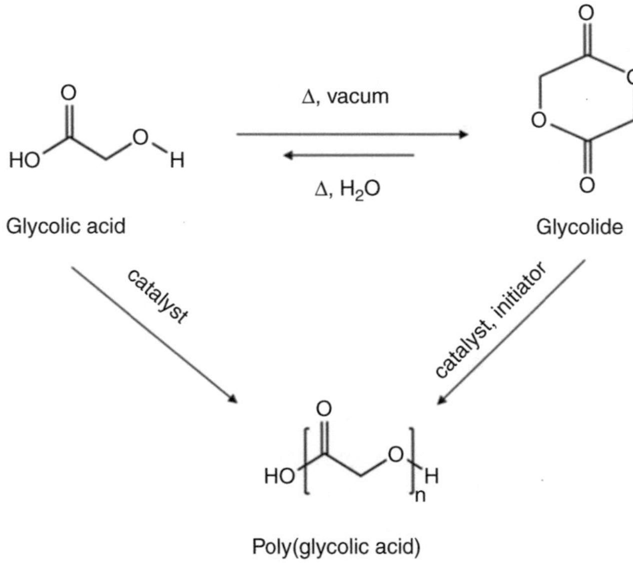

Fig. 8.5 Glycolic acid to polyglycolic acid

Fig. 8.6 Caprolactone to polycaprolactone

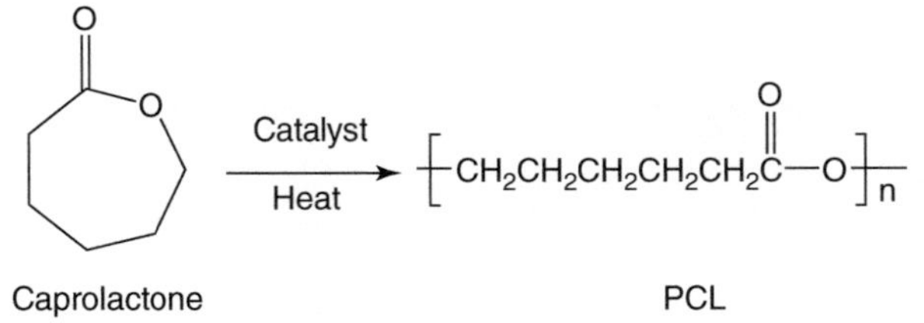

endodontics, periodontology, and implantology. PLGA's applications are broad and diverse, encompassing biomedical research, the fabrication of implants and grafts, the creation of prosthetic devices, the production of sutures and stents, and the development of scaffolds for tissue engineering. Additionally, it is employed in the generation of micro and nanoparticles for targeted therapeutic and diagnostic applications. Some examples include biomedical research, implants, grafts, prosthetic devices, sutures, stents, and scaffolding for tissue engineering applications, as well as micro and nanoparticles [26, 27]. In aesthetic medicine, PLGA is used in the creation of sutures for thread lifting, offering a biocompatible and biodegradable solution for non-surgical rejuvenation and the lifting of ptotic soft tissues.

Polycaprolactone (PCL) is also used as an injectable filling agent and thread material (Fig. 8.6), attributable to its biocompatibility and inherent biodegradability, enabling it to decompose into water and carbon dioxide. This polymer has been utilized in clinical and biomedical applications for over seven decades, facilitating a broad range of uses that span from surgical sutures to the fabrication of three-dimensional printed organs and tissue replacements. Moreover, PCL is integral in the development of 3D scaffolds aimed at enhancing repair and regeneration processes across various tissues, including bone and skin [28]. Poly(L-lactide-*co*-caprolactone)

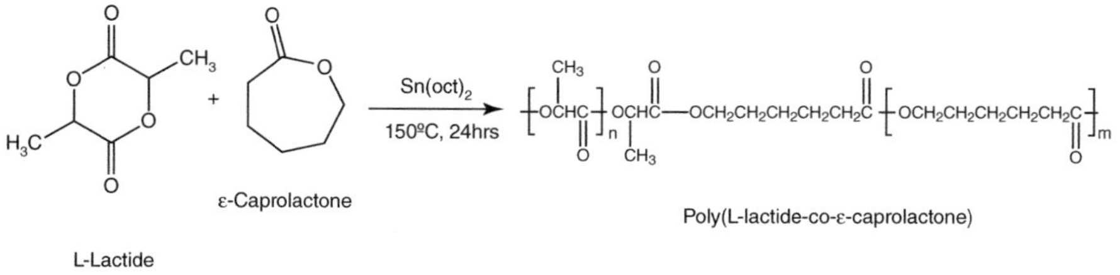

Fig. 8.7 Synthesis of poly(L-lactide-*co*-ε-caprolactone) (PLCL) copolymer

(PLCL) is a polymer obtained by the process of ring-opening polymerisation of L-lactide (cyclic dimer of L-lactic acid) and ε-caprolactone as monomers (Figs. 8.6 and 8.7) and is a promising biomaterial. PLCL has been extensively applied in the construction of tissue engineering scaffolds designed to elucidate the role of mechanical stimulation in facilitating tissue regeneration. Its utility extends to more prolonged applications, encompassing long-term controlled-release drug delivery systems and biodegradable nerve conduits for axonal regeneration, which necessitate an extended degradation timeline to accommodate the gradual process of tissue repair and regeneration [2, 29, 30]. Post-insertion, PLCL undergoes metabolic breakdown into lactic acid and 6-hydroxycaproic acid [31].

Polypropylene

Polypropylene is a non-polar, partially crystalline thermoplastic, non-absorbable polymer. Synthetic polypropylene has been used widely in the medical field. Its applications vary from medical equipment (syringes, storage, transport, electric cables) to synthetic, non-absorbable isotactic polypropylene used for hernia and pelvic organ repair operations in urinary incontinence, oesophageal, and gastrointestinal operations [44, 45]. Moreover, polypropylene monofilament threads have been extensively employed as sutures due to their durability and resistance to biological degradation, making them a staple in various surgical applications [46].

Thread Degradation

During the biodegradation and absorption process of sutures, the pivotal characteristics to monitor are the patterns of strength and mass loss, alongside the biocompatibility of the degradation products. Notably, the reduction in tensile strength often precedes mass loss. The biocompatibility of the degradation byproducts of all currently utilized absorbable sutures typically presents no significant concerns, as these sutures are composed of well-established biocompatible polymers such as glycolide, lactide, and their copolymers. The key factor influencing biocompatibility is the concentration of degradation products within the surrounding tissues, which necessitates efficient removal and metabolism by these tissues. This metabolic capacity is closely linked to the tissue's vascularization, which facilitates the

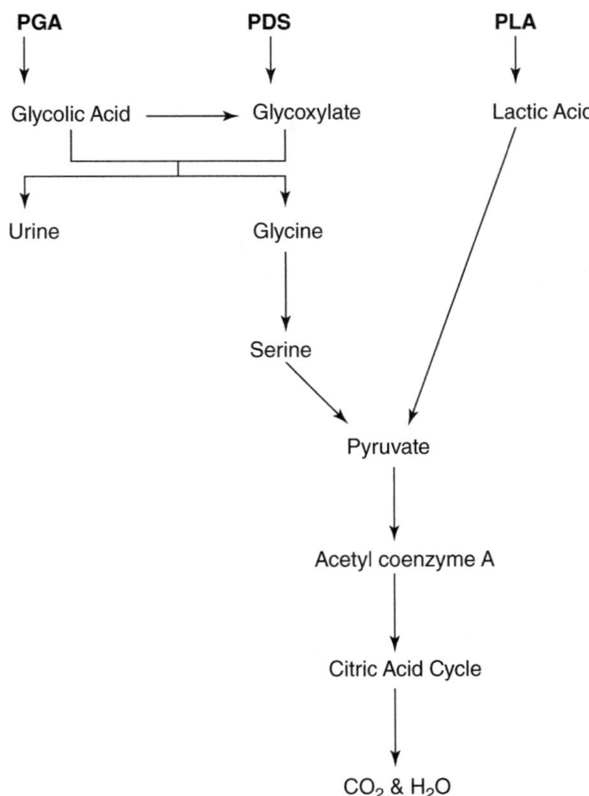

Fig. 8.8 Biodegradation of bioabsorbable polymers. PGA (polyglycolic acid), PLA (polylactic acid), and PDS (polydioxanone)

elimination of degradation products at a rate matching their production from the suture material [14].

In vivo, certain soluble polymers may trigger allergic reactions [32–34]. The degradation of aliphatic polyesters like PGA, PLA, and PCL primarily occurs through non-enzymatic, random hydrolytic scission of ester linkages, with the rate of degradation varying according to the hydrophilicity of the monomeric units—PGA degrades rapidly, PLA more slowly, and PCL very slowly. Enzymatic processes may play a partial role in the degradation of PCL [3, 35, 36]. Water preferentially affects amorphous regions over crystalline ones due to their higher permeability, leading to faster degradation in copolymers compared to homopolymers due to increased water infiltration and reduced crystallinity [3].

The extracellular water in the human physiological medium facilitates hydrolytic degradation processes (Fig. 8.8) [37]. PLGA and PLLA undergo hydrolytic degradation, targeting their ester bonds and resulting in the formation of lactic and glycolic acids [38]. The degradation of PLGA polymer chains occurs uniformly throughout their matrix [38, 39]. The produced glycolic acid lowers the local pH, which can lead to inflammation in surrounding tissues; it is eventually expelled from the body through the urinary system [27, 39].

Upon exposure to air, soluble threads such as PDO begin hydrolysing due to moisture absorption, necessitating moisture-proof packaging, typically in aluminium-coated bags. This hydrolysis process renders the thread increasingly fragile, compromising its structural integrity and mechanical lifting capability, as it may break before complete absorption [32].

Non-absorbable threads/sutures, including both natural (e.g., surgical steel, silk, cotton, linen) and synthetic variants (e.g., nylon, polypropylene, polybutester), are distinguished by their durability, resistance to premature breakage, and minimal inflammatory reaction risk [4, 40–43].

Thread Surface Characteristics

The physical configuration of sutures/threads plays a crucial role, significantly influencing a range of biological effects, including their interaction with the body's tissues and susceptibility to bacterial colonizationts [14]. The design and structural attributes of sutures dictate their performance and functionality, impacting both clinical outcomes and the potential for infection.

Sutures/Threads can be differentiated based on their surface characteristics and physical properties. The categorization includes (Table 8.2, Fig. 8.9):

- Monofilament (Mono): These sutures possess smooth surfaces, minimizing tissue trauma.
- Spring/Twin Thread: This category encompasses monofilament threads that are either braided or twined together, enhancing tensile strength and flexibility.
- Barbed/Cog/Spicules/Teeth: These sutures feature protruding elements designed to anchor securely within soft tissues. The design variations—unidirectional, bidirectional, or multidirectional—further refine their application by providing adjustable tension and distribution along the suture line.

Various modifications, such as cogs, cones, "teeth," spicules, and barbs, have been developed to enhance thread anchoring within soft tissues. These modifications are known by different names, varying by the manufacturing company, production method, and the specific design of the modification. Initially, barbed threads were created by making incisions along the thread, which could lead to weak points and potential breakage. Recent advancements have seen a shift towards molded threads, which offer improved tensile strength and maintain structural integrity more

Table 8.2 Thread surface characteristics

Thread surface characteristics	Smooth	Single threads per needle/cannula (monofilament thread)
		Multiple threads per needle/cannula
		Screw/spring/coiled
		Braided
		Mesh
	Barbs/cogs	Unidirectional
		Bidirectional/zig zag
		Multidirectional
	Cones	

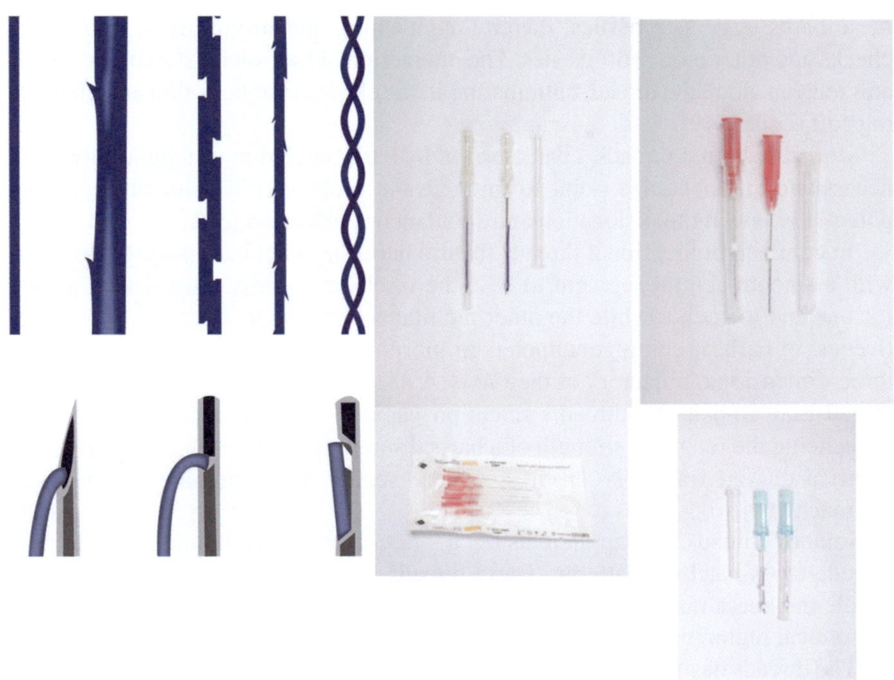

Fig. 8.9 A schematic figure of examples of some of the different types of threads, including smooth, unidirectional, bidirectional, screw/spring/coiled and needle/cannula tips, monofilament, and multifilament, including thread packaging and threads

effectively. The enhanced "holding power" of molded cogs, for instance, has been documented to be superior, providing a more reliable and durable solution for tissue engagement [47]. Additionally, threads may undergo surface treatment or coating with substances such as silicone, hyaluronic acid, or calcium hydroxyapatite to improve biocompatibility, facilitate tissue integration, and promote therapeutic effects. These advancements underscore the continuous evolution and optimization of suture materials to meet the specific requirements of various medical and surgical applications.

Smooth monofilament threads are predominantly used for biostimulation, leading to enhancement in cutaneous tissue firmness, reduction of pore size and fine rhytids, and augmentation of the papillary dermis thickness. Threads with varied surface modifications are used for the repositioning of soft tissue, thereby facilitating a "lifting" and "volumising" effect, while screw/spring-type threads contribute to volumetric enhancement in the designated area.

Threads embedded with barbs operate analogously to cogs and hooks, grasping, engaging, elevating, and suspending soft tissues. As a result, bidirectional and multidirectional threads demonstrate inherent 'self-retaining' characteristics [48]. The deployment of these barbs, expanding in an umbrella-like fashion, establishes a structural support system that effectively elevates ptotic tissues. Beneath the skin, these barbs aggregate tissues, thereby augmenting and lifting areas such as the cheeks and other ptotic soft tissues. The interaction of barbs with skin tissue generates tension along the thread, culminating in the elevation of both skin and underlying soft tissues [49].

Monodirectional threads, characterized by barbs angled in a singular direction, necessitate an anchorage point to mitigate the propensity for thread migration, potentially leading to dislocation and spontaneous extrusion [50].

In contrast, bidirectional threads feature barbs oriented in opposing directions with a smooth central segment to ease the insertion process. This design allows for one end to anchor while the other facilitates tissue approximation. The effectiveness of barbs is contingent upon their morphology, spatial distribution, and the three-dimensional trajectory of their axis. A needle diameter exceeding that of the thread may impair the thread's retention capacity [51]. The paramount factor influencing the retention strength of a barbed suture is its three-dimensional alignment; a curved trajectory ensures a more secure hold compared to a linear approach [10].

Smooth threads are applied using a "free-floating" technique, which may include cross-hatching patterns. These threads vary in diameter and length, with needle thickness ranging from 18 to 31 gauge, and length tailored to the specific anatomical region under treatment [52].

The threads designed for medical and aesthetic procedures are usually mounted on needles or cannulas, which vary in gauge from 18 to 31, accommodating a range of procedural requirements. These implements are characterized by their diverse lengths and diameters, tailored to specific applications to ensure precision and efficacy in treatment delivery. The configuration of the threads—whether monofilament or multifilament—paired with the needle or cannula, is crucial for optimizing procedure outcomes and patient comfort. Importantly, the threads are designed to be partially housed within the cannula and extend into its lumen, facilitating seamless insertion and placement within the target tissue area.

Threads According to Their Function

Threads used in medical aesthetics can serve dual functions: as suspension devices to mechanically lift and reposition tissues, and as regenerative bio-stimulatory agents to promote tissue healing and rejuvenation. Their operation is grounded in distinct mechanisms (Table 8.3):

Table 8.3 Classification of Threads by Function

Action	
	Bio-stimulation: Stimulates collagen production and tissue regeneration, improving skin elasticity, firmness, and thickness.
	Suspension: Mechanically lifts and repositions soft tissues for aesthetic enhancement.

1. Suspension: Achieved through a mechanical effect, suspension involves the distribution of gravitational forces across a thread to adjacent areas. This method can have long-lasting effects, especially if the threads are non-biodegradable and precisely placed, facilitating sustained tissue elevation and support [32, 53].
2. Bio-stimulation: The presence of the thread as a foreign object in the tissue instigates fibrosis in the surrounding areas. This response occurs regardless of the thread's material composition and contributes to the formation of subcutaneous fibrous tissue, enhancing the structural integrity and appearance of the skin [32, 53].

Monofilament threads are typically inserted into the superficial hypodermis or deep dermis to induce skin tightening and rejuvenation. The immediate tensile effect of these threads is visible upon implantation. Conversely, suspension threads achieve traction through their unique surface features or by anchoring to stable structures, such as the periosteum [54]. Threads can be anchored in place by various methods, such as stabilising onto the facial fascia, including deep temporal fascia or using bi/multidirectional threads for enhanced efficacy.

The bio-stimulatory impact of threads is an area of ongoing research. Initial bio-stimulation may occur due to needle or cannula trauma during insertion, leading to vasodilation and hyperemia, even in the absence of threads. The subsequent inflammatory response triggered by thread insertion contributes to the bio-stimulatory effect. True bio-stimulation should result in enrichment and an increase in type III collagen and connective tissue. Furthermore, enhanced action against free radicals, improved skin elasticity, firmness, and thickness are expected [54]. Furthermore, post-insertion fibrosis is a commonly reported phenomenon, underscoring the threads' capacity to produce significant structural changes within the treated tissues [55]. A review of studies indicates that threads utilized for bio-stimulation elicit satisfactory outcomes in terms of patient contentment over a medium-term period [54].

Thread insertion technique is critical for maximizing the benefits of both suspension and bio-stimulation. The thread is introduced against the direction of the barb's bevel to prevent premature engagement with the tissue. Once positioned, pulling the thread in the reverse direction engages the barbs with the fatty, fibrous adipose tissues, effectively transferring force, anchoring the thread, and facilitating the desired lifting effect on the overlying skin [50, 56].

Thread Size

Suture sizes are classified according to two primary standards: the United States Pharmacopeia (USP) and the European Pharmacopeia (EP), with the USP being more commonly used:

- USP (United States Pharmacopeia)
- EP (European Pharmacopeia)

The size designation involves a combination of two Arabic numerals, starting with zero (e.g., 2/0), where the numeral before the slash indicates the thread's gauge. The guiding principle is straightforward: a higher preceding number indicates a finer gauge of the suture material. For sizes exceeding zero, such as 1/0 (referred to simply as "1"), 2, 3, etc., the numerical value directly correlates to the suture's thickness. It's important to note that this sizing convention is distinct from the material composition of the suture [14]. This system allows for a standardized approach to suture selection, facilitating the choice of the appropriate suture size for various medical procedures based on the specific needs and requirements of the surgical site.

Larger diameter threads offer enhanced biomechanical strength but may increase the risk of dimpling at the insertion site. The formation of collagen around the threads and their specific design features, such as cogs or barbs, intensifies their effects [48, 49, 57–61].

Tissue Reaction to Threads

The tissue's reaction to suture placement is a dynamic process that unfolds in several stages, indicative of the body's natural healing and immune response mechanisms [14]:

- Day 1–3: The initial phase is marked by the infiltration of polymorphonuclear leukocytes, signaling the body's immediate response to the foreign material.
- Day 3–4: The acute response phase is characterized by the infiltration of lymphocytes and monocytes, key players in the immune system's reaction to injury or foreign bodies.
- Day 4–7: This period sees the presence of macrophages and fibroblasts, crucial for phagocytosis and the beginning of the healing process through tissue repair and regeneration.
- Day 7–10: The final stage involves the maturation of fibrous connective tissue alongside chronic inflammation, indicative of the body's ongoing efforts to integrate or encapsulate the suture material.

Within the first week post-implantation, the differential in tissue reactivity between synthetic absorbable and non-absorbable sutures is minimal. Nonetheless, synthetic absorbable sutures may elicit a slightly heightened inflammatory response, which subsides as the suture material is metabolized and absorbed by the body. In contrast, non-absorbable sutures typically provoke a mild, chronic inflammatory response that culminates in the formation of a thin fibrous tissue capsule around the suture by the 28th day, a mechanism that secures the suture in place while minimizing tissue irritation [14].

Choice of Threads

Selecting the appropriate threads involves consideration of their application and the targeted area. Making an informed choice requires a thorough understanding of various thread properties and their clinical indications. Key factors include:

1. Patient-specific factors and meticulous patient selection.
2. Choice of thread, encompassing thread material.
3. The planning of vectors and anchorage points for optimal lift and tissue engagement.
4. Careful post-operative management.

Incorporating biochemical factors in enforcing the physicomechanical lift will help practitioners achieve better results [62].

Conclusion

The history and application of threads in both medicine and aesthetic medicine is marked by a multitude of considerations that dictate the selection of optimal suture for tissue repair. Factors influencing this decision range from the physical properties of the suture, such as diameter, to the physiological characteristics of the target tissue, encompassing fascia, tendon, or bone. Moreover, attributes of the fixation process itself, including its rigidity and elasticity—as observed in fracture fixation or tendon repair—contribute to this decision. The repair's position, whether superficial or deep, also plays a pivotal role, as do the factors of biocompatibility or biodegradability of the suture [4].

In a parallel fashion, sutures used for thread lifting must be subjected to a thorough evaluation before their use in treatment. Threads specifically engineered for facial rejuvenation and lifting warrant a comprehensive appraisal both in the laboratory and clinically. The evaluation should encapsulate a myriad of factors: biocompatibility, longevity, complication potential, and possible side effects [61]. The efficacy of these threads is profoundly influenced by their composition, interaction, and design. For clinicians to make informed decisions, they must acquire a comprehensive understanding of the anatomy and material science pertaining to the threads they employ. This should be tempered with the recognition that there is no universal material perfectly suited to all circumstances. Therefore, a careful weighing of the merits and demerits of each material is indispensable in determining the most suitable choice for a specific application and patient.

In conclusion, the historical and contemporary use of threads in medicine and aesthetic medicine illustrates the necessity of a multidimensional evaluation process for selecting appropriate materials. As the field continues to evolve, so too must our understanding and application of these valuable tools in the pursuit of optimal patient outcomes.

References

1. Martins JA, et al. Polydioxanone implants: a systematic review on safety and performance in patients. J Biomater Appl. 2020;34(7):902–16.
2. Kim SI, et al. Preparation of enhanced hydrophobic poly(L-lactide-*co*-ε-caprolactone) films surface and its blood compatibility. Appl Surf Sci. 2013;276:586–91.
3. Jeong SI, et al. In vivo biocompatibility and degradation behavior of elastic poly(L-lactide-*co*-ε-caprolactone) scaffolds. Biomaterials. 2004;25(28):5939–46.
4. Choi Y, et al. Biomechanical properties and biocompatibility of a non-absorbable elastic thread. J Funct Biomater. 2019;10(4):51.
5. Pihlajamaki H, et al. Absorbable pins of self-reinforced poly-L-lactic acid for fixation of fractures and osteotomies. J Bone Jt Surg Br. 1992;74(6):853–7.
6. Inui A, et al. Potency of double-layered poly-L-lactic acid scaffold in tissue engineering of tendon tissue. Int Orthop. 2010;34(8):1327–32.
7. Lee DW, et al. Comparison of poly-L-lactic acid and poly-L-lactic acid/hydroxyapatite bioabsorbable screws for tibial fixation in ACL reconstruction: clinical and magnetic resonance imaging results. Clin Orthop Surg. 2017;9(3):270–9.
8. Liu S, et al. Current applications of poly(lactic acid) composites in tissue engineering and drug delivery. Compos Part B Eng. 2020;199:108238.
9. Da Silva D, et al. Biocompatibility, biodegradation and excretion of polylactic acid (PLA) in medical implants and theranostic systems. Chem Eng J. 2018;340:9–14.
10. Shebi A, Lisa S. Pectin mediated synthesis of nano hydroxyapatite-decorated poly(lactic acid) honeycomb membranes for tissue engineering. Carbohydr Polym. 2018;201:39–47.
11. Al Tawil E, et al. Microarchitecture of poly(lactic acid) membranes with an interconnected network of macropores and micropores influences cell behavior. Eur Polym J. 2018;105:370–88.
12. Wan P, et al. Fabrication and evaluation of bioresorbable PLLA/magnesium and PLLA/magnesium fluoride hybrid composites for orthopedic implants. Compos Sci Technol. 2014;98:36–43.
13. Cui H. Aesthetic thread rejuvenation in Asians. In: Sulamanidze, editor. Several viewpoints on thread rejuvenation. Peking University Medical Press; 2019.
14. Chu CC. 10—Types and properties of surgical sutures. In: King MW, Gupta BS, Guidoin R, editors. Biotextiles as medical implants. Woodhead Publishing; 2013. p. 231–73.
15. Ruff G. Technique and uses for absorbable barbed sutures. Aesthet Surg J. 2006;26(5):620–8.
16. Paul MD. Barbed sutures for aesthetic facial plastic surgery: indications and techniques. Clin Plast Surg. 2008;35(3):451–61.
17. Lee CG, et al. Histological evaluation of bioresorbable threads in rats. Korean J Clin Lab Sci. 2018;50(3):217–24.
18. Suárez-Vega DV, et al. In vitro degradation of polydioxanone lifting threads in hyaluronic acid. J Cutan Aesthet Surg. 2019;12(2):145–8.
19. Damadzadeh B, et al. Effect of ceramic filler content on the mechanical and thermal behaviour of poly-L-lactic acid and poly-L-lactic-*co*-glycolic acid composites for medical applications. J Mater Sci Mater Med. 2010;21(9):2523–31.
20. Vasenius J, et al. Absorbable self-reinforced polyglycolide (SR-PGA) screws for the fixation of fractures and osteotomies: strength and strength retention in vitro and in vivo. Clin Mater. 1994;17(3):119–23.
21. Vert M, et al. Something new in the field of PLA/GA bioresorbable polymers? J Control Release. 1998;53(1–3):85–92.
22. Kulkarni R, et al. Polylactic acid for surgical implants. Washington, DC: Walter Reed Army Medical Center; 1966.
23. Hollinger JO. Preliminary report on the osteogenic potential of a biodegradable copolymer of polyactide (PLA) and polyglycolide (PGA). J Biomed Mater Res. 1983;17(1):71–82.
24. Mäkelä P, et al. Strength retention properties of self-reinforced poly-L-lactide (SR-PLLA) sutures compared with polyglyconate (MaxonR) and polydioxanone (PDS) sutures. An in vitro study. Biomaterials. 2002;23(12):2587–92.

25. Bohnert K, et al. Randomized, controlled, multicentered, double-blind investigation of injectable poly-L-lactic acid for improving skin quality. Dermatol Surg. 2019;45(5):718–24.
26. Makadia HK, Siegel SJ. Poly lactic-*co*-glycolic acid (PLGA) as biodegradable controlled drug delivery carrier. Polymers. 2011;3(3):1377–97.
27. Budak K, Sogut O, Aydemir Sezer U. A review on synthesis and biomedical applications of polyglycolic acid. J Polym Res. 2020;27(8):208.
28. Christen M-O, Vercesi F. Polycaprolactone: how a well-known and futuristic polymer has become an innovative collagen-stimulator in esthetics. Clin Cosmet Investig Dermatol. 2020;13:31–48.
29. Wong V. The science of absorbable poly(L-lactide-*co*-ε-caprolactone) threads for soft tissue repositioning of the face: an evidence-based evaluation of their physical properties and clinical application. Clin Cosmet Investig Dermatol. 2021;14:45–54.
30. Jelonek K, et al. Novel poly(L-lactide-*co*-ε-caprolactone) matrices obtained with the use of Zr[Acac]$_4$ as nontoxic initiator for long-term release of immunosuppressive drugs. Biomed Res Int. 2013;2013:607351.
31. Ramot Y, et al. Long-term local and systemic safety of poly(L-lactide-*co*-ε-caprolactone) after subcutaneous and intra-articular implantation in rats. Toxicol Pathol. 2015;43(8):1127–40.
32. Fukaya M. Two mechanisms of rejuvenation using thread lifting. Plast Reconstr Surg Glob Open. 2018;6(12):e2068.
33. Della Torre F, Della Torre E, Di Berardino F. Side effects from polydioxanone. Eur Ann Allergy Clin Immunol. 2005;37(2):47–8.
34. Guardiani E, Davison SP. Angioedema after treatment with injectable poly-L-lactic acid (sculptra). Plast Reconstr Surg. 2012;129(1):187e–9e.
35. Gan Z, et al. Enzymatic degradation of poly(ε-caprolactone)/poly(DL-lactide) blends in phosphate buffer solution. Polymer. 1999;40(10):2859–62.
36. Nakayama A, et al. Hydrolytic degradation of poly(L-lactide-*co*-ε-caprolactone). In: Advanced biomaterials in biomedical engineering and drug delivery systems. Tokyo: Springer Japan; 1996.
37. Sabino MA, et al. Study of the hydrolytic degradation of polydioxanone PPDX. Polym Degrad Stab. 2000;69(2):209–16.
38. Loo JSC, Ooi CP, Boey FYC. Degradation of poly(lactide-*co*-glycolide) (PLGA) and poly(L-lactide) (PLLA) by electron beam radiation. Biomaterials. 2005;26(12):1359–67.
39. Azimi B, et al. Poly(lactide-*co*-glycolide) fiber: an overview. J Eng Fibers Fabrics. 2014;9(1):155892501400900107.
40. Al-Mubarak L, Al-Haddab M. Cutaneous wound closure materials: an overview and update. J Cutan Aesthet Surg. 2013;6(4):178–88.
41. Pillai CKS, Sharma CP. Absorbable polymeric surgical sutures: chemistry, production, properties, biodegradability, and performance. J Biomater Appl. 2010;25(4):291–366.
42. Luck RP, et al. Cosmetic outcomes of absorbable versus nonabsorbable sutures in pediatric facial lacerations. Pediatr Emerg Care. 2008;24(3):137–42.
43. Moon H-J, Chang D, Lee W. Short-term treatment outcomes of facial rejuvenation using the mint lift fine. Plast Reconstr Surg Glob Open. 2020;8(4):e2775.
44. Gavrila DE, et al. Advanced polypropylene and composites with polypropylene with applications in modern medicine. In: Composite materials. IntechOpen; 2020.
45. Orringer M, et al. Polypropylene suture in esophageal and gastrointestinal operations. Surg Gynecol Obstet. 1977;144(1):67–70.
46. Razumov M, et al. Polypropylene suture material with anti-inflammatory action. Iran Polym J. 2018;27(9):629–34.
47. Kim B, Oh S, Jung W. Type of absorbable thread products. In: The art and science of thread lifting. Springer; 2019. p. 73–7.
48. Wu WT. Barbed sutures in facial rejuvenation. Aesthet Surg J. 2004;24(6):582–7.
49. Kalra R. Use of barbed threads in facial rejuvenation. Indian J Plast Surg. 2008;41(Suppl):S93–S100.

50. Fundaro SP, et al. Expert consensus on soft-tissue repositioning using absorbable barbed suspension double-needle threads in Asian and Caucasian patients. J Cutan Aesthet Surg. 2021;14(1):1–13.
51. Cui H. Aesthethic thread rejuvenation in Asians. In: Ruff GL, editor. Several viewpoints on thread rejuvenation. Peking University Medical Press; 2019.
52. Cobo R. Use of polydioxanone threads as an alternative in nonsurgical procedures in facial rejuvenation. Facial Plast Surg. 2020;36(04):447–52.
53. Fukaya M. Long-term effect of the insoluble thread-lifting technique. Clin Cosmet Investig Dermatol. 2017;10:483–91.
54. Alcolea JM, Trelles M. Biostimulation threads: scientific evidence and systematic review of their efficacy and safety. Union of Aesthetic Medicine-UIME; 2016. p. 26.
55. Amuso D, et al. Histological evaluation of a biorevitalisation treatment with PDO wires. Union of Aesthetic Medicine-UIME; 2015. p. 111.
56. Villa MT, et al. Barbed sutures: a review of the literature. Plast Reconstr Surg. 2008;121(3):102e–8e.
57. Bisaccia E, et al. Midface lift using a minimally invasive technique and a novel absorbable suture. Dermatol Surg. 2009;35(7):1073–8.
58. Matarasso A, Rosen AD. New and emerging uses of barbed suture technology in plastic surgery. Aesthet Surg J. 2013;33(3_Supplement):90S–5S.
59. Beer K. Delayed complications from thread-lifting: report of a case, discussion of treatment options, and consideration of implications for future technology. Dermatol Surg. 2008;34(8):1120–3.
60. Kim J, et al. Investigation on the cutaneous change induced by face-lifting monodirectional barbed polydioxanone thread. Dermatol Surg. 2017;43(1):74–80.
61. DeLorenzi CL. Barbed sutures: rationale and technique. Aesthet Surg J. 2006;26(2):223–9.
62. Song JK, et al. Favorable crisscrossing pattern with polydioxanone: barbed thread lifting in constructing fibrous architecture. Aesthet Surg J. 2021;41(7):NP875–86.

Polydioxanone (PDO) Threads

9

Souphiyeh Samizadeh and Sourosheh Samizadeh

Abstract

Polydioxanone (PDO) is a synthetic, bioabsorbable monofilament suture renowned for its colorless, crystalline properties. Derived from paradioxanone, PDO is available in various forms, lengths, and surface characteristics, making it versatile for medical applications. PDO threads have been utilized for many years across different medical applications and specialities. Particularly, PDO threads have garnered significant interest in aesthetic medicine for their role in thread-lifting procedures, which aim to stimulate and reposition ptotic soft tissues, resulting in rejuvenation. The placement of PDO threads initiates a biostimulatory response, promoting tissue regeneration and improving skin texture, elasticity, and overall quality. This chapter explores the characteristics of PDO threads and their diverse applications within the field of aesthetic medicine.

Keywords

Thread lift · Thread lifting · Thread lift method · Thread lift technique · Thread lift procedure · Polydioxanone · Polydioxanone threads · PDO threads · Facial rejuvenation

S. Samizadeh (✉)
King's College London, London, UK

University College London, London, UK

Great British Academy of Aesthetic Medicine, London, UK
e-mail: info@baamed.co.uk

S. Samizadeh
University College London, London, UK

© Springer Nature Switzerland AG 2024
S. Samizadeh (ed.), *Thread Lifting Techniques for Facial Rejuvenation and Recontouring*, https://doi.org/10.1007/978-3-031-47954-0_9

Polydioxanone (PDO) Threads

Polydioxanone PDO threads have become popular in the field of aesthetic medicine. PDO threads are available in a range of sizes, forms, surface characteristics, and application devices, each tailored for targeted facial and body rejuvenation procedures. The strategic placement of PDO threads for rejuvenation has been reported to linked to repositioning soft tissues, enhancing skin texture, complexion improvement, and improving skin elasticity [1]. Despite their widespread use, it is important to note that much of the existing clinical and histological research on PDO threads is derived from animal studies, indicating a need for further investigation in human subjects.

PDO threads are composed of a synthetic, colorless, crystalline, bioabsorbable monofilament made from the polymer paradioxanone, a substance derived from the monomer of the same name. Introduced in 1981 as a groundbreaking absorbable suture, they were initially designed for wound closure applications, particularly in high-tension areas or where prolonged dermal support is necessary. Over the years, their application has expanded beyond cardiac surgery and laparotomies to include esophageal stents and a variety of cosmetic procedures. The physical properties of PDO—such as its glide characteristics and minimal tissue reactivity—minimize the risk of wound infection and facilitate ease of passage through tissues [2–6].

The structural integrity of PDO sutures is noteworthy, with an initial tensile strength retention of 74% after the first two weeks post-implantation, decreasing to 50% by the fourth week, and eventually to 25% after six weeks. This durability underlines their suitability for applications requiring sustained support and wounds under high tension [2, 3].

As a thermoplastic polymer, PDO exhibits a high degree of hydrophilicity, leading to its gradual bioabsorption and hydrolytic degradation over time. Typically, the absorption process is partially complete around 90 days after placement, with total absorption occurring within 6-7 months. This process not only eliminates the material from the body without residue but also stimulates the production of a new dermal matrix, enhancing the overall quality and appearance of the skin (Fig. 9.1) [1, 2, 7–10].

Suture threads made of PDO have been shown to be effective in elevation of ptotic soft tissue, lipomatosis, bio-stimulation and collagen stimulation, reduction of lines and wrinkles, and reduction of deep folds on the face and body [7]. Following the insertion of the threads, a fibrotic response occurs with the surrounding biomaterial [11, 12]. The fibrotic tissue that forms around PDO threads as a result of the body's healing response is often referred to as "fibrotic pathways".

Fig. 9.1 Biochemical degradation pathway for PDO

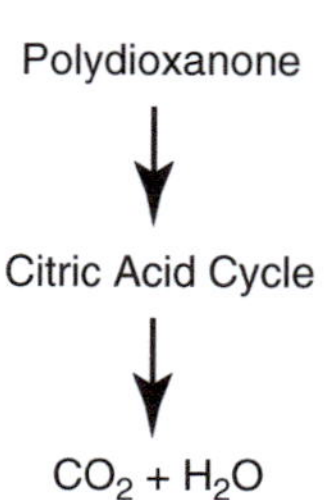

These pathways consist of newly formed collagen and other connective tissue components that organize around the threads. This fibrotic encapsulation not only supports the mechanical lifting effect provided by the threads but also serves as a scaffold for tissue remodeling and regeneration. As the PDO threads stimulate collagen production, the fibrotic pathways become integral to maintaining the structural integrity and aesthetic improvements achieved through the treatment. [13]. Importantly, the duration of this "lifting effect" is governed by the rate of biodegradation and hydrolysis of the threads.

Within the initial 12 months post-implementation, the biostimulatory action of PDO threads promotes neocollagenesis and fibrillogenesis, alongside the contraction of the fibrosed dermis, culminating in a noticeable tightening and rejuvenation of the skin [14, 15].

PDO threads are available in various configurations, each designed to address specific aesthetic goals: (Fig. 9.2) [16].

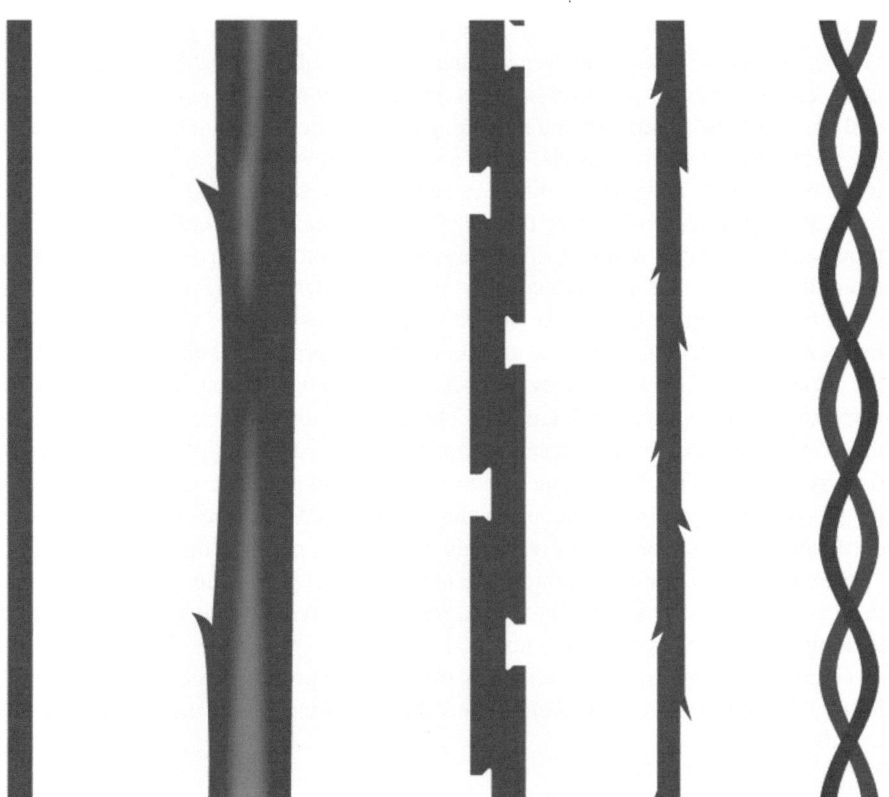

Fig. 9.2 Examples of knotless PDO thread devices demonstrate different thread surface characteristics

- Smooth monofilament threads offer a uniform structure for subtle rejuvenation.
- Spiral or screw threads are designed to provide volume and lift through their helical structure.
- Multiple monofilament threads combine several strands for enhanced structural support.
- Barbed sutures, which have tiny projections, offer tissue repositioning by mechanically anchoring to the tissue.

PDO threads are encapsulated within either a cannula or a needle, facilitating their insertion into the tissue. These threads, available in both smooth and barbed varieties, are designed in a V-shaped configuration. This design involves one half of the thread being enclosed within the needle or cannula, while the other half extends outside, secured by a specialized fixing sponge (Fig. 9.3) [16]. All threads are manufactured in an array of diameters and lengths to accommodate different treatment areas and objectives. Correspondingly, the gauge of the needles, indicative of their thickness, spans from 18 to 31 gauge. This variation in size allows practitioners to select the most appropriate needle and thread combination based on the specific anatomical region being addressed [16].

PDO threads are typically placed subdermally and in the subcutaneous layer of the skin, which is beneath the dermis. This placement allows for the threads to effectively engage with the skin's structural components, stimulating collagen production and providing the desired lift and tightening effects. The subcutaneous layer, consisting of fat and connective tissues, offers a suitable environment for the PDO threads to anchor securely and promote tissue integration and regeneration. By targeting this layer, PDO threads can leverage the body's natural healing and collagen production processes to achieve aesthetic improvements. Smooth, spiral, screw, or multiple monofilament threads are strategically placed subdermally (Fig. 9.4) [16]. The smooth threads, in particular, are placed using a "free-floating" method that establishes a cross-hatching, mesh, or net-like structure, primarily aimed at stimulating the production of new collagen [16]. All these patterns elicit a bio-stimulatory response, encouraging neocollagenesis. The introduction of smooth threads beneath the skin surface leads to a noticeable firming effect, contributing to tissue regeneration, skin brightening, and enhancements in skin texture, elasticity, and overall quality [1, 16]. The precise mechanisms through which PDO threads instigate these dermatological transformations remain an area of ongoing investigation.

Screw, spiral, or multiple monofilament threads increase volume in the implantation area due to neocollagenesis around the threads, resulting in enhanced volume and improved skin elasticity and texture [16].

Cog/barbed threads, characterized by their surface protuberances, are engineered for targeted soft tissue engagement and can be categorized based on their directional features into [16]:

- Unidirectional: Barbs are aligned in a single direction.
- Bidirectional: Barbs extend in two opposite directions from the midpoint.
- Multidirectional: Barbs are oriented in multiple directions along the thread

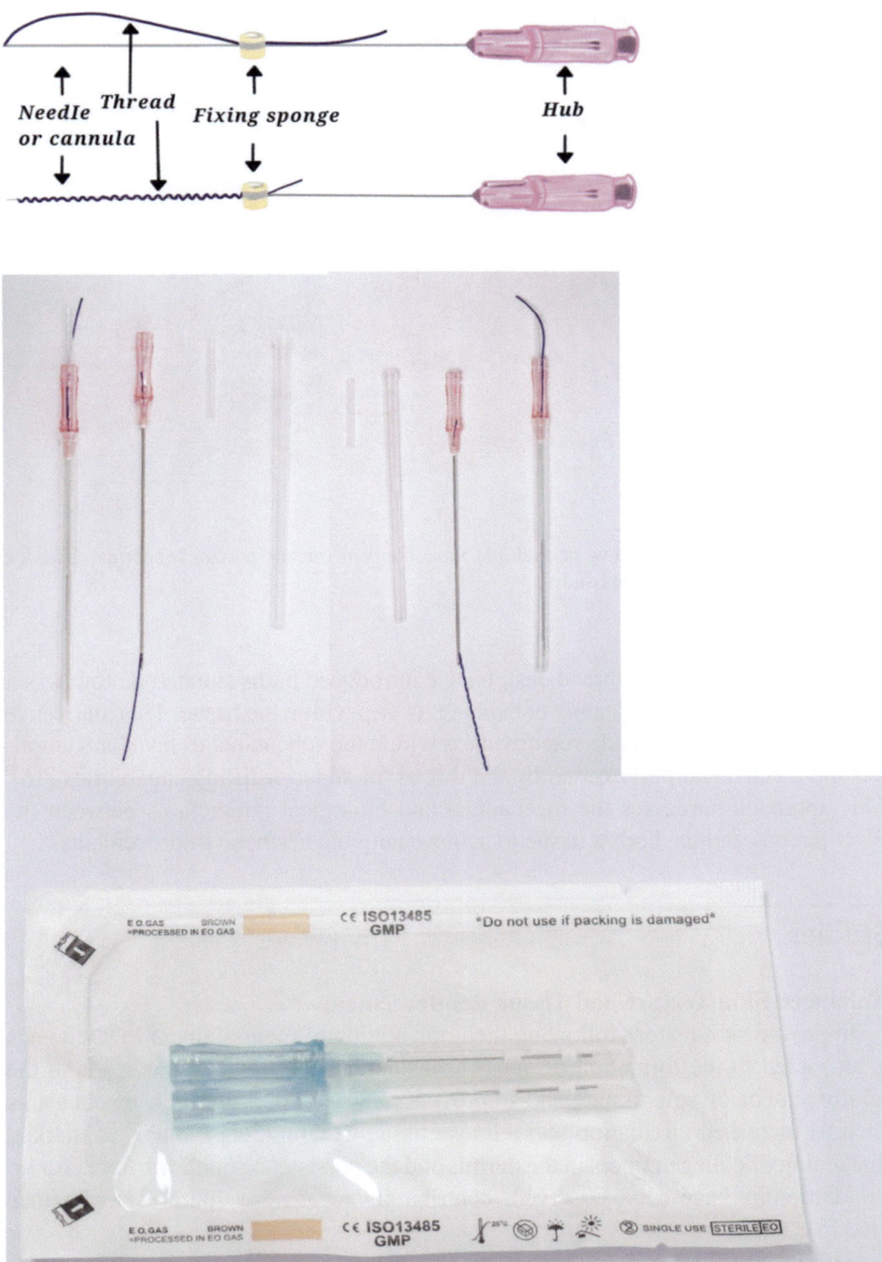

Fig. 9.3 Polydioxanone (PDO) threads are intricately designed for precise insertion and placement within the tissue. Each thread is attached to a hub that serves as the connecting point to the needle or cannula. The PDO thread is threaded through this hub and extends out through the tip of the needle or cannula. This arrangement results in half of the thread being exposed outside the needle or cannula. To ensure stability and secure placement during the insertion process, this exposed portion of the thread is anchored with a small sponge attached to the external part of the needle or cannula. This design feature ensures that the PDO thread can be accurately positioned within the target area for optimal lifting and tissue engagement [10, 16]

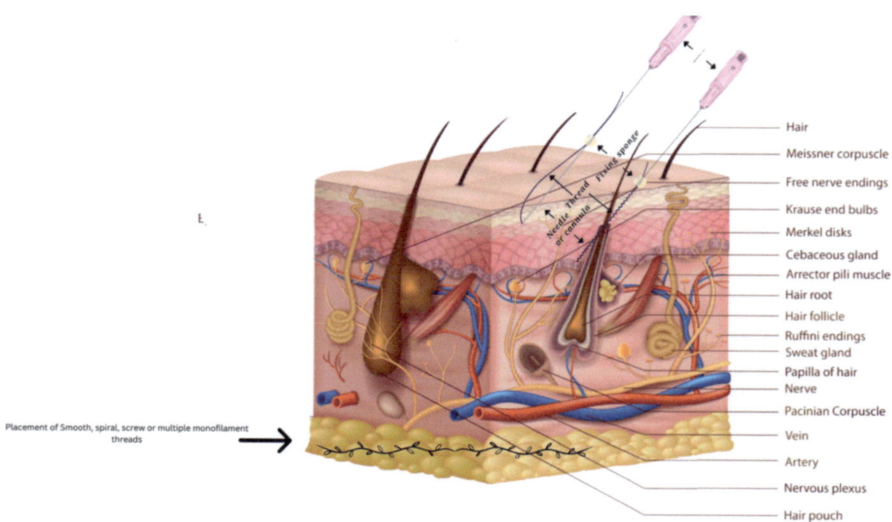

Fig. 9.4 Smooth, spiral, screw, or multiple monofilament threads remain subdermal after the needle is inserted and then removed

Recent advancements in thread design have introduced barbs situated on four to six sides of the thread, significantly enhancing its grip within the tissue. This innovative feature increases the thread's retentiveness within the subcutaneous layer and amplifies the mechanical pull exerted by the thread for superior lifting capabilities [16]. This approach harnesses the mechanical and biological interactions between the PDO threads and the body's tissue to achieve tangible aesthetic improvements.

Studies

Enhanced Skin Texture and Tissue Reinforcement

Improved skin texture following the implantation of monofilament PDO threads is attributed to the formation of new fibrous connective tissues. This leads to the reinforcement of soft tissues and improved facial contours through mechanisms such as increased circulation and adipose tissue denaturation. Notably, a marked thickening of collagen fibers in the dermis and the persistence of elastic fibers for up to 12 months have been observed, contributing to a more youthful appearance [10, 15].

Animal Studies: Insights into PDO Thread Effects

White Yucatan pygmy pigs Study: An investigation using White Yucatan pygmy pigs, which have skin closely resembling human skin, explored the effects of a 9-cm USP 4.0 PDO thread. Reported tissue changes included neocollagenesis, fibrous merging, fat reduction, tissue contracture, and an improved vascular environment. Threads maintained their shape for 12 weeks, with fragmentation by 24 weeks and complete dissolution by 48 weeks, indicating that the aesthetic effects of PDO threads can last up to a year [17].

Guinea Pig Study: In a detailed study involving the placement of monofilament, unidirectional PDO threads into the dorsal skin of 12 guinea pigs, significant tissue changes were observed, shedding light on the histological impact of PDO threads. The threads were implanted into the panniculus carnosus layer. Tissue samples were systematically harvested at intervals of 1, 3, and 7 months post-implantation to assess the histologic changes induced by the PDO threads. Early examinations, particularly at 1 and 3 months, revealed the threads to be encased within a fibrous sheath, indicating a protective tissue response. Notably, the capsular structure around the threads was markedly thicker at 1 month, suggesting an initial robust reaction to the foreign material. Over time, the presence of the threads stimulated an accumulation of inflammatory cells and fibroblasts, especially noticeable in the core region around the suture material, illustrating the body's response to facilitate integration and healing. By the 7-month mark, the threads became less distinguishable, indicative of their biodegradation and assimilation into the surrounding tissue. Concurrently, the formation of granulation tissue, rich in fibroblasts and multinucleated giant cells, was evident at the sites of thread insertion. Despite these significant internal changes, the overlying epidermis remained notably unaffected. The deeper dermal layers, however, showed denser collagen composition compared to untreated skin, a testament to the threads' ability to stimulate collagen production and reorganization. These histological changes culminated in the replacement of the initial fibrous sheaths with mature connective tissue, highlighting a transition from an acute response to a more stabilized tissue integration. The findings underscore the PDO threads' capacity to provoke fibrous encapsulation, inflammation, and subsequent collagen and TGF-beta elevation, mechanisms that collectively contribute to tissue realignment and the observed "lifting effect." This enhanced understanding of tissue responses to PDO threads at the microscopic level reinforces their potential for cosmetic applications, emphasizing the need for ongoing research to optimize their use in aesthetic medicine [18].

Rat Studies: An animal study focusing on rats demonstrated significant findings related to the biophysical interaction and tissue response to cog PDO threads. Four weeks after implantation beneath the skin, the presence of myofibroblasts around the threads was noted, indicating a role in fibrous tissue contracture. This process is pivotal for the structural stability and mechanical strength of the treated area. Further, a longitudinal study on the dorsal skin of Sprague Dawley rats revealed the persistence of PDO threads for up to eight months. This period allowed for substantial neocollagenesis around the threads, with the extent of collagen formation being directly related to the surface area of the implanted threads. Predominantly, Type 3 collagen was induced, matching or exceeding the collagen production observed with other suture materials like PLLA and PCL. The study underscores the threads' capacity to support and enhance the dermal matrix through collagen synthesis, a cornerstone for rejuvenation and structural integrity. [19, 20].

Design and Placement Influence

The design and pattern of thread placement were highlighted as critical factors for achieving optimal outcomes. A specific study reported that PDO threads with larger barbs, when arranged in crisscross patterns, significantly foster fibrous capsulation. This structural arrangement creates effective zones for lifting and tension suspension, exemplifying the importance of technique alongside material properties in clinical applications [21].

Stent-shaped Scaffold Device Study

Another intriguing approach was the examination of a stent-shaped hollow scaffold device, braided with multiple PDO filaments, implanted into the subcutaneous layer (animal study). This innovative design was intended to generate a space conducive to collagen accumulation both internally and externally around the implant. Conducted on rat and mini-pig models, the study observed a gradual transition from Type I to Type III collagen within the accumulated matrix, pointing to the threads' role in facilitating an adaptable and durable collagenous environment conducive to tissue rejuvenation and structural support. [8].

Human Study

A histological examination was conducted on five patients treated with five different brands of PDO threads, with follow-up periods at 6, 12, and 18 months post-implantation. The findings highlighted fibrosis persisting up to 12 months, alongside the production of Type I collagen. Notably, there was an absence of Type III collagen production, suggesting a differential tissue response in humans compared to animal models [15]. This study is crucial in understanding the long-term effects and tissue integration of PDO threads in clinical practice, providing a foundational basis for further research and optimization of treatment protocols. Furthermore, the study elucidated several key physiological processes triggered by the PDO threads, including:

- Granulation tissue formation
- Neovascularisation, collagen matrix formation
- Merging of the new and old collagen tissues
- Biodegradation takes place when fluids penetrate the suture material and break its molecules [22]

Degradation

The degradation of PDO sutures is a critical aspect of their functionality and safety profile in medical applications. These sutures exhibit a total loss of resistance approximately 63 days post-implantation, with degradation primarily occurring through hydrolytic excision within the amorphous regions of the suture material [23–25]. The process of excision is initiated as early as 15 days after placement, leading to significant alterations in the suture's interfibrillar architecture. Over time, these structural changes precipitate the rupture of the suture threads. The inevitable loss of mechanical properties observed with the PDO sutures is a direct consequence of this degradation process [25]. This predictable biodegradation timeline is essential for the designed temporary support and subsequent absorption, aligning with the tissue healing process to minimize long-term foreign body reactions.

Following the degradation dynamics of PDO sutures, the role of hyaluronic acid (HA) in this process merits special attention. HA is known to catalyze the biodegradation of PDO threads by initiating hydrolysis within 24 hours of thread contact. The inherent hydrophilicity of PDO threads makes them particularly susceptible to the catalytic action of uncross-linked HA, facilitating their hydrolytic breakdown. In practical applications, the strategic insertion of PDO threads in conjunction with HA is utilized to expedite the suture's biodegradation process, This interaction notably diminishes the chemical resistance of the threads, a phenomenon especially advantageous for superficially placed threads where rapid biodegradation is desired. Thus, the combination of PDO with non-crosslinked HA not only accelerates the degradation timeline but also aligns with clinical objectives for minimizing the duration of foreign material presence within the body [7, 21].

- Increased Fibrous Encapsulation: The crisscross placement pattern resulted in a threefold increase in fibrous capsulation around the barbed areas compared to barb-free areas, indicating a heightened local tissue response.
- Enhanced Fibrotic Area Density: In the crisscross pattern, the width and density of fibrotic areas were fivefold greater, suggesting a more robust framework for tissue support and lift.
- Crucial Factors for Enhanced Lift: The study highlighted two critical factors for optimizing lift effects:
  - Utilization of threads with larger PDO barbs
  - Adoption of a crisscross placement pattern
- Biological Architecture and Stability: The crisscross placement facilitates the formation of a grid of fibrous capsules, echoing the architecture of internal support structures. This arrangement allows for tension dispersion following biotensegrity principles, akin to the organization of biological structures like muscles, bones, fascia, ligaments, tendons, and cell membranes. This biomechanical synergy enhances the stability and longevity of the lift.
- Longevity and Structural Integrity: The strategic formation of a dense grid of fibrous capsules, mimicking biotensegrity principles found in natural biological structures, contributed to the superior stability and extended longevity of the lifting effect.
- Clinical Outcomes: Employing these techniques in over 300 cases led to immediate improvements in soft tissue lifting, significantly reduced malar widening, decreased post-operative discomfort, and markedly prolonged effect duration.

This research underscores the significance of incorporating biochemical enhancements and adopting a crisscross thread placement pattern in barbed thread lifting. By aligning with the principles of biotensegrity and optimizing thread characteristics, practitioners can achieve more effective, stable, and lasting lifting outcomes [21].

Conclusion

In conclusion, PDO threads have emerged as a popular and innovative tool in the field of cosmetic medicine, providing new possibilities for facial and body rejuvenation. With their diverse types and applications, these threads have been associated with numerous benefits, including soft tissue repositioning, enhanced skin texture, complexion improvement, and increased skin elasticity. Despite the promising results observed thus far, it is crucial to emphasise the need for further clinical and histological research to better understand the mechanisms, long-term effects, and potential complications of PDO thread usage. By conducting rigorous studies and expanding the evidence base, clinicians and practitioners will be better equipped to optimise treatment outcomes and ensure the safety and efficacy of PDO thread-based interventions. As the field of cosmetic medicine continues to evolve, PDO threads stand as a testament to the importance of ongoing research, innovation, and the pursuit of excellence in patient care.

References

1. Unal M, et al. Experiences of barbed polydioxanone (PDO) cog thread for facial rejuvenation and our technique to prevent thread migration. J Dermatol Treat. 2021;32(2):227–30.
2. Dart AJ, Dart CM. 6.636—Suture material: conventional and stimuli responsive. In: Ducheyne P, editor. Comprehensive biomaterials. Oxford: Elsevier; 2011. p. 573–87.
3. Weitzul S, Taylor RS. Suturing technique and other closure materials. In: Surgery of the skin. Elsevier Inc.; 2005. p. 225–44.
4. Ray J, et al. Polydioxanone (PDS), a novel monofilament synthetic absorbable suture. Surg Gynecol Obstet. 1981;153(4):497–507.
5. Bartholomew R. PDS (polydioxanone suture): a new synthetic absorbable suture in cataract surgery. Ophthalmologica. 1981;183(2):81–5.
6. Martins JA, et al. Polydioxanone implants: a systematic review on safety and performance in patients. J Biomater Appl. 2020;34(7):902–16.
7. Suárez-Vega DV, et al. In vitro degradation of polydioxanone lifting threads in hyaluronic acid. J Cutan Aesthet Surg. 2019;12(2):145–8.
8. Kim H, et al. Novel polydioxanone multifilament scaffold device for tissue regeneration. Dermatol Surg. 2016;42(1):63–7.
9. Molea G, et al. Comparative study on biocompatibility and absorption times of three absorbable monofilament suture materials (polydioxanone, poliglecaprone 25, glycomer 631). Br J Plast Surg. 2000;53(2):137–41.
10. Suh DH, et al. Outcomes of polydioxanone knotless thread lifting for facial rejuvenation. Dermatol Surg. 2015;41(6):720–5.
11. Ali YH. Two years' outcome of thread lifting with absorbable barbed PDO threads: innovative score for objective and subjective assessment. J Cosmet Laser Ther. 2018;20(1):41–9.
12. Ilankovan V. Erratum to: Recent advances in face lift to achieve facial balance. J Maxillofac Oral Surg. 2017;16(1):134.
13. De Masi EC, De Masi FD, De Masi RD. Suspension threads. Facial Plast Surg. 2016;32(6):662–3.
14. Fundaro SP, et al. Expert consensus on soft-tissue repositioning using absorbable barbed suspension double-needle threads in Asian and Caucasian patients. J Cutan Aesthet Surg. 2021;14(1):1–13.
15. Amuso D, et al. Histological evaluation of a biorevitalisation treatment with PDO wires. Union of Aesthetic Medicine-UIME; 2015. p. 111.

16. Cobo R. Use of polydioxanone threads as an alternative in nonsurgical procedures in facial rejuvenation. Facial Plast Surg. 2020;36(04):447–52.
17. Yoon JH, et al. Tissue changes over time after polydioxanone thread insertion: an animal study with pigs. J Cosmet Dermatol. 2019;18(3):885–91.
18. Kim J, et al. Investigation on the cutaneous change induced by face-lifting monodirectional barbed polydioxanone thread. Dermatol Surg. 2017;43(1):74–80.
19. Jang HJ, et al. Effect of cog threads under rat skin. Dermatol Surg. 2005;31(12):1639–43. discussion 1644
20. Lee CG, et al. Histological evaluation of bioresorbable threads in rats. Korean J Clin Lab Sci. 2018;50(3):217–24.
21. Song JK, et al. Favorable crisscrossing pattern with polydioxanone: barbed thread lifting in constructing fibrous architecture. Aesthet Surg J. 2021;41(7):NP875–86.
22. Karimi K, Reivitis A. Lifting the lower face with an absorbable polydioxanone (PDO) thread. J Drugs Dermatol. 2017;16(9):932–4.
23. Ping Ooi C, Cameron RE. The hydrolytic degradation of polydioxanone (PDSII) sutures. Part II: micromechanisms of deformation. J Biomed Mater Res. 2002;63(3):291–8.
24. Medeiros AC, Araújo-Filho I, de Carvalho MDF. Fios de sutura. J Surg Clin Res. 2016;7(2):74–86.
25. Sabino MA, et al. Study of the hydrolytic degradation of polydioxanone PPDX. Polym Degrad Stab. 2000;69(2):209–16.

Poly-ʟ-Lactic Acid Cone Threads: Silhouette Soft Threads

10

Souphiyeh Samizadeh, Sorousheh Samizadeh, and Kyungkook Hong

Abstract

This chapter investigates the application and biological integration of Silhouette Soft threads, composed of poly-ʟ-lactic acid (PLLA) and poly (ʟ-lactic-*co*-glycolic) acid in aesthetic medicine. These biodegradable and biocompatible polymers serve as the foundation for a dual-action technique that combines immediate tissue repositioning with long-term regenerative effects, facilitating facial and body contour enhancements and rejuvenation. Highlighting the transition towards less invasive cosmetic interventions, this analysis underscores the threads' operational principles, focusing on the nuanced interplay between their chemical structure and the biological response they elicit. A detailed exploration into the histological interactions of Silhouette Soft threads with human tissue is presented, aiming to provide a comprehensive understanding of the cellular and extracellular matrix responses critical for achieving desired aesthetic outcomes. Through this scientific lens, the chapter contributes to a broader discourse on the efficacy, safety, and potential applications of thread lifting techniques, offering insights into their strategic utility in aesthetic practices and patient care.

S. Samizadeh (✉)
University College London, London, UK

King's College London, London, UK

Great British Academy of Aesthetic Medicine, London, UK
e-mail: info@baamed.co.uk

S. Samizadeh
University College London, London, UK

K. Hong
Clinque hus-hu, Cheongdam, Seoul, South Korea

© Springer Nature Switzerland AG 2024
S. Samizadeh (ed.), *Thread Lifting Techniques for Facial Rejuvenation and Recontouring*, https://doi.org/10.1007/978-3-031-47954-0_10

Keywords

Thread lift · Thread lifting · Thread lift method · Thread lift technique · Thread lift procedure · Poly-L-lactic acid cone threads · Silhouette threads · Terminology

Poly-L-Lactic Acid (PLLA)

Poly(L-Lactic-*co*-Glycolic) Acid (PLGA)

Silhouette Soft threads are absorbable, sterile, implantable, single-use sutures/threads (absorbable suspension sutures) made up of poly-L-lactic acid (PLLA) and poly(L-lactic-*co*-glycolic) acid (PLGA). These threads are used in multiple pairs for repositioning facial and neck soft tissues for rejuvenation. These threads facilitate soft tissue repositioning through a dual-action mechanism:

1. Immediate repositioning of the soft tissues
   (a) Compression and elevation of the soft tissues
2. Gradual tissue regeneration
   (a) Remodelling the target tissues by stimulating fibroblasts and activating collagen production and volume restoration

Biodegradable and bioresorbable synthetic polymers, including PLLA, have been used in tissue engineering and bioresorbable devices in surgery and pharmacology. Synthetic absorbable polymeric surgical devices were first used in surgery in the 1960s [1].

One of the main applications of resorbable PLLA- and PLGA-based materials is medical implants and implant materials [2, 3]. Examples include fixation devices in orthopaedics (bone screws, pins, spinal cages, prostheses), internal fixation with absorbable self-reinforced poly-L-lactide pins, bone scaffold, scaffold in tendon regeneration, screws for tibial fixation, and soft tissue implants [4–7]. Polylactic acid and polyglycolic acid polymers and their copolymers are recognised and prominent bioabsorbable polymers because they include chemical components similar to those found in bone and have a similar elastic modulus [2, 7–9]. Compared to metallic implants, bioresorbable materials are commonly employed for bone fixation and repair applications, eliminating the need for a second surgery to remove the implant after the bone has healed [3]. Furthermore, they have been used for vascular grafts, drug delivery, encapsulation, sustained release of bioactive compounds, tumour-targeting, as sutures, and in expansion to new fields [7, 10–12].

Polylactic acid is a linear aliphatic biopolymer made from renewable sources such as corn and sugarcane. Polylactic acid exists in three stereochemical forms: poly(L-lactide) (PLLA), poly(D-lactide), and poly(DL-lactide) [7]. By combining different stereo-copolymers, aliphatic polyesters of the PLLA family can be tailored to various mechanical characteristics and degradation profiles [13].

PLLA, a biodegradable, absorbable polymer, is degraded by hydrolytic de-esterification into lactic acid monomers. These monomers enter the carboxylic acid cycle and are excreted by the lungs as carbon dioxide and water [1, 14, 15].

Poly-L-glycolide (PGA) is a highly crystalline polymer. It is biodegradable and biocompatible and is used in biomedical research, including implants and grafts, sutures, prosthetic devices, surgical sealant films, stents, scaffolds for tissue engineering applications, and micro- and nanoparticles [16, 17]. The degradation rate of these synthetic polymers can be modified to suit their application [18]. PGA is a different material from PLGA (PLGA is a copolymer of L-lactide and glycolide, while PGA is a homopolymer of glycolide). The degradation of PLGA is favourable for sustained drug release at desirable doses by implantation without surgical procedures, and its overall physical properties can be modified [16]. The first biodegradable and absorbable polymeric surgical sutures were made of PGA and were introduced in the 1970s [17]. It has been widely used as a favourable suture material with a low melting temperature and remarkable tensile strength [17, 19, 20].

Biodegradation

The breakdown rate of PLGA and PLLA may be controlled by numerous factors, such as pH, molecular weight, temperature, size, additives, processing conditions, and the copolymer ratio for PLGA. PLLA is ultimately decomposed into lactic acid monomers and PLGA into its monomers, lactic acid and glycolic acid. Lactic acid is a typical by-product of muscle activity; it is converted to pyruvic acid and then metabolised by the tricarboxylic acid cycle before being expelled as water and carbon dioxide via respiration (Fig. 10.1). Glycolic acid is eliminated in the urine. Furthermore, glycolic acid reacts to generate glycine. Glycine is utilised to synthesise serine, which is converted to pyruvic acid. Pyruvic acid is expelled in the form of water and carbon dioxide after completing the tricarboxylic acid cycle [21]. The acid by-products of PLGA degradation may generate undesirable foreign body responses and may function as an autocatalyst for PLGA breakdown. While associated with some degree of cellular response, the long history of safe and efficacious use indicates that the products of degradation and resorption are well tolerated by the human body.

The Silhouette range can be seen below (Fig. 10.2, Table 10.1):

- Lift-Permanent Polypropylene
- Soft: Absorbable, PLLA, cones: PLGA
- Instalift: entirely made of PLGA

Silhouette Soft® thread is made of polylactic acid, and the cones are made of lactic acid (82%) and glycolic copolymer (18%).

Each suture comprises two sets of cones that are uniformly spaced and oriented in opposing directions, along with a central monofilament. The cones are separated by knots and can move freely between the retaining knots until the subcutaneous tissue engages them upon implantation. This enables the advancement of the soft tissue

Over time, the body breaks down both PLLA ans PLGA via normal metabolic pathways. Biodegradation and resorption of both these materials is well tolerated by tissue and there is a long history of their safe and efficacious use in implantable medical device applications.

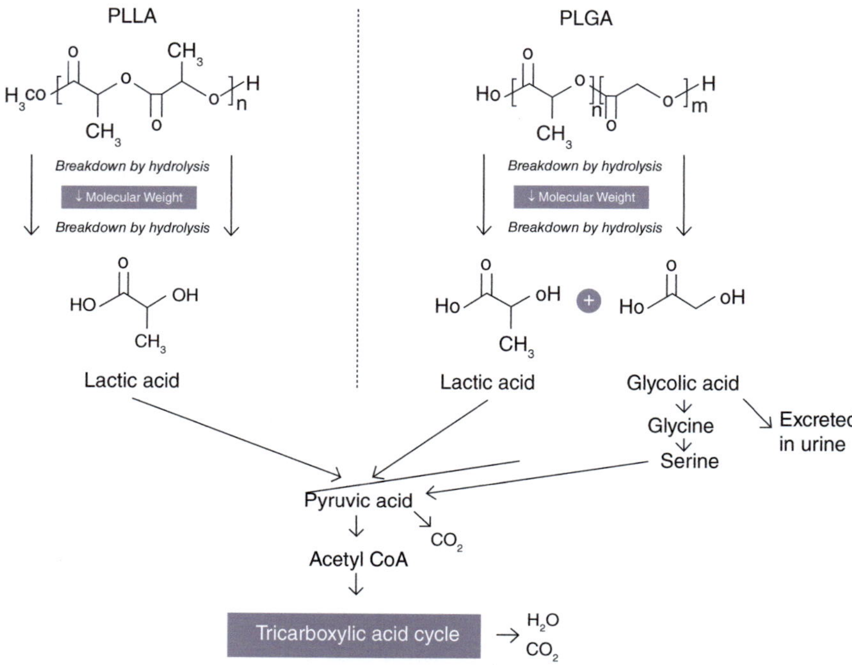

Fig. 10.1 Schematic diagram of the metabolic degradation of PPLA and PLGA

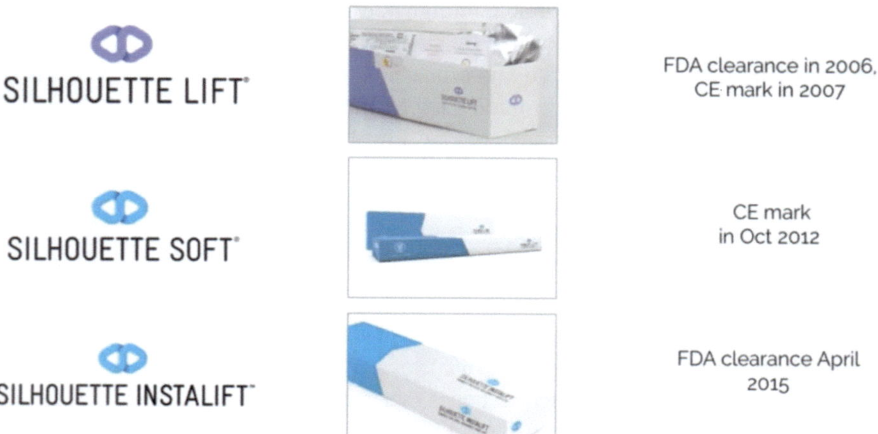

Fig. 10.2 Silhouette Soft range

Table 10.1 Silhouette Soft range

Product	8 cones	12 cones	12-cone short	16 cones
Length	30 cm	27.5 cm	27.5 cm	26.8 cm
Active length[a]	8 cm	14.1 cm	10.4 cm	18 cm
Direction of cones	Bidirectional			
Space between cones	5 mm	8 mm	5 mm	8 mm
Material	PLLA (monofilament) and PLGA (cones)			
Needle	2 needles (23 G) of 12 cm each			

[a]Refers to tensioned device length

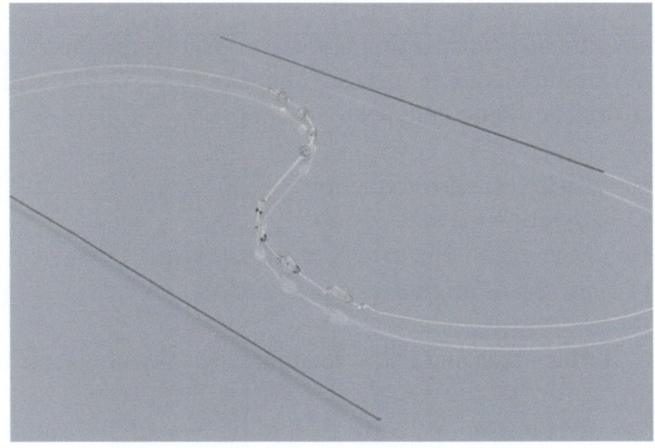

Fig. 10.3 Each suture comprises two groups of evenly spaced cones oriented in opposite directions, along with a central monofilament. The cones are separated by knots and can freely move between them until they become engaged by the subcutaneous tissue post-insertion

over the distal cones and elevation of the soft tissue by the proximal cones (Fig. 10.3). Sutures made of these materials are resorbable, biocompatible, and biodegradable.

Characteristics (Fig. 10.3)

- Monofilaments 100% poly-lactic acid (PLLA)
- Cones in poly-lactic acid (82%) and glycolic polymer (18%) (PLGA)
- Bidirectional cones (face in opposite directions)
- Central monofilament: cones evenly spaced on either side of the cone-free central zone of 2 cm. Freely moving cones don't compromise the device strength
- Each cone is separated by tied knots and is free-floating between them until tissue engagement
- A 12 cm needle is attached to both ends

Silhouette Soft Range

Sutures are available in four different sizes; 8, 12, 12-short, and 16 cones to accommodate a range of facial shapes and sizes and target tissues. The consensus report states that the 8-cone suture is acceptable for almost all face applications [22, 23].

This opinion was formed prior to the introduction of the 12-cone short product variant, which is anticipated to be equally versatile.

Cones (Fig. 10.4)

Why are cones utilized in these sutures? The design serves three primary functions: firstly, it provides resistance against the traction forces of suspension, ensuring the suture's stability and effectiveness. Secondly, it facilitates the repositioning of tissues, allowing for precise adjustments and improvements in facial structure. Lastly, the cones offer strong anchorage within the subcutaneous tissues, securing the lifted position and contributing to the procedure's durability and effectiveness. This combination of features makes Silhouette Soft sutures a reliable option for achieving desired aesthetic outcomes. In summary:

- Resists suspension traction
- Reposition the soft tissues
- Strong anchorage in subcutaneous tissue
- Low risk of migration and extrusion

Surface area and tissue retaining capacity are inextricably linked:

- For example, one barb of molding type of 1–0 suture with 0.4 mm barb usually has a surface area of 0.072 mm^2 (this kind of molding type barbed suture is known to have the largest barbs in the market).
- The actual shape of a cone in Silhouette Soft is pendulum, and its external surface is much wider than same height cone. Hence actual external surface area of a cone is ~8 mm^2. For the purpose of tissue retention, the internal surface area is also relevant, which is ~5.5 mm^2.

This comparison clearly shows that cones offer a substantially larger surface area for anchorage compared to barbs. The implications of this increased surface area are multifaceted:
- Increased surface area, enhances the capacity for secure anchorage.
- It minimizes potential damage to surrounding tissues.

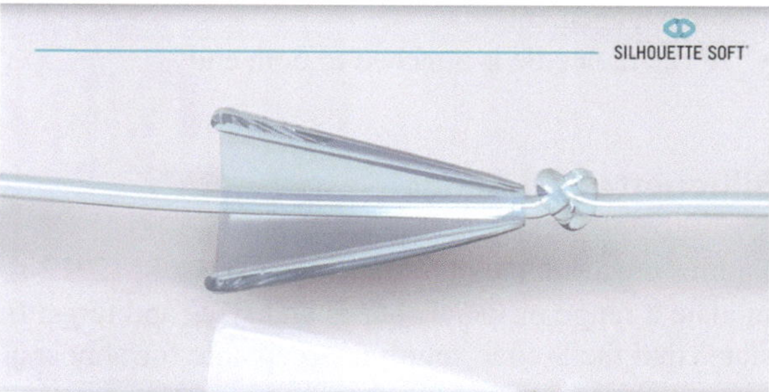

Fig. 10.4 Cones in Silhouette threads and their features. External surface area (i.e. just outside of the cone, not including the "hollow") = 8 mm^2. The total volume displaced by an 8-cone device, as the volume contained within the "hollow" of one cone, is ~1.0 mm^3

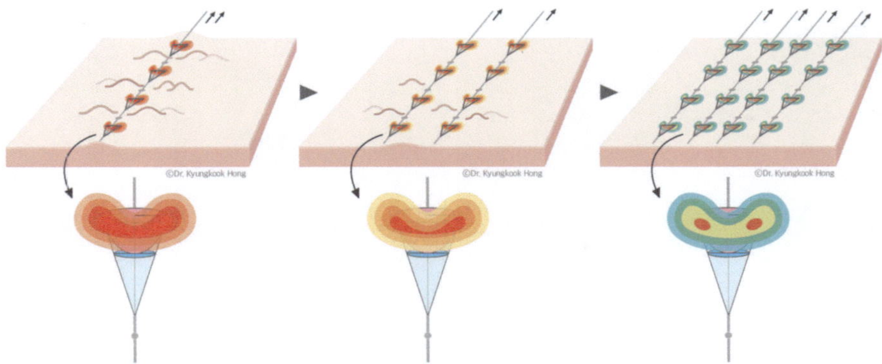

Fig. 10.5 Increasing the number of threads increases the overall anchoring force and the amount of collagen stimulation. Meanwhile, this reduces the traction loading around each cone, contributing to lesser irregularity

- Ensures more effective engagement of repositioned tissues, leading to robust anchoring and suspension. Cones significantly reduce the risk of migration, extrusion, or dislocation/deformation of the device, providing superior resistance against suspension traction.

Cones engage the repositioned tissue, resulting in anchoring and suspension. Cones significantly limit the possibility of migration or extrusion and dislocation/deformation of the device and provide excellent resistance to suspension traction [24, 25]. In comparison to barbs, cones give more volume for anchoring. The number of cones is proportional to the anchoring force (Fig. 10.5). Moreover, cones offer a greater volume for anchorage than barbs, with the anchoring force directly correlating to the number of cones. Increasing cone density not only augments the anchoring force but also reduces tissue deformation. Consequently, a higher number of threads enhances the overall anchoring force and collagen stimulation while decreasing the load on each cone, leading to less tissue irregularity.

Studies

PLLA facilitates neocollagenesis. Utilization of Silhouette Soft, composed of PLLA monofilament and poly (l-lactic-co-glycolic) acid (PLGA) cones, has been demonstrated to initiate the induction of type I collagen. This process effectively doubles the diameter of the PLLA monofilament by 12 months through a mechanism of encapsulation, with this level of collagen deposition enduring up to 24 months. At this juncture, both the suture and cones commence disintegration [26–28].

Punch biopsies were taken 2 mm from the path of the suture PLLA/PLGA monofilament and cones in a study to determine the effect of the PLLA/PLGA on collagenesis. Three to four threads were placed in the midface on each side to improve midface volume loss and reduce the appearance of the nasolabial folds. The author explained that a global improvement in skin quality and facial contours is seen post-treatment.

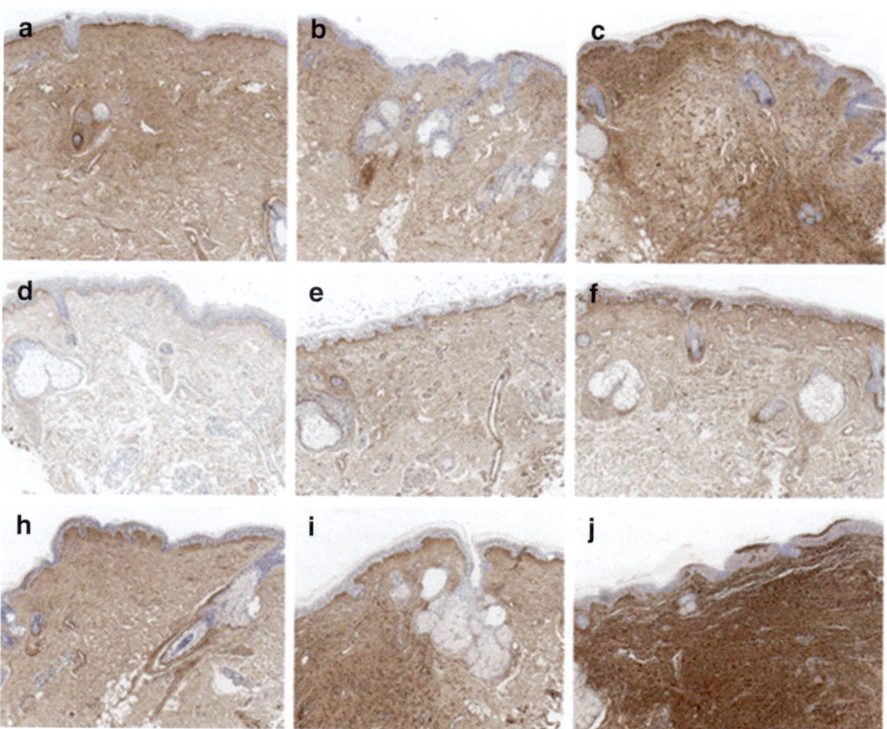

Fig. 10.6 Illustrative examples of staining for collagen type I. Between day 1 (**a, d, g**) and day 90 (**b, e, h**), the deposition of procollagen-1 can be qualitatively appreciated, but this increase is not significant. Between day 1 (**a, d, g**) and day 180 (**c, f, i**), the increase in collagen is significant ($P = 0.0016$). The increase is also significant between day 1 (**a, d, g**) and day 270 ($P = 0.0015$). The increase between days 90 (**b, e, h**) and 180 (**c, f, i**) is also significant ($P = 0.0004$). These changes are consistent with the long-term results and satisfaction observed in clinical practice. [Reproduced with permission from Goldberg, D.J., 2020. Stimulation of collagenases by poly-L-lactic acid (PLLA) and -glycolide polymer (PLGA)-containing absorbable suspension suture and parallel sustained clinical benefit. Journal of Cosmetic Dermatology, 19(5), pp. 1172–1178]

This study aimed to examine the validity that the global improvement seen is not limited to the area adjacent to the suture. The author reported significant changes in collagen from baseline at days 180 and 270 and a substantial increase between day 90 and day 180 (Fig. 10.6) [29]. This trend matched patient satisfaction in clinical practice and was reported by clinical studies using absorbable suspension sutures at 6 and 12 months [23, 29]. Furthermore, collagen deposition paralleled the improvement reported in the appearance of the nasolabial fold by both patients and investigators, with patients noting more significant and longer-lasting improvement [29].

Between January 2007 and December 2009, De Benito et al. implanted the Silhouette Lift device (3–0 polypropylene sutures with absorbable cones) in 316 patients. On average, 8.1 sutures were implanted per patient, and the sutures were fixed to a small polypropylene mesh over the deep temporal fascia. The findings were favourable over an average follow-up duration of 18 months, with high patient satisfaction. Forty-two individuals (13.3%) suffered mild and transient complications. The inflammatory reaction gradually degrades the cones; this ongoing reaction is responsible for the long-lasting effect. In 11 months, 75% of the cone material is reabsorbed, implying that the cones will be wholly reabsorbed after a maximum of 2 years. All patients maintained consistent outcomes over the 18-month follow-up period following implantation [24, 25].

A study by Consiglio and colleagues assessed the biological reactions of Silhouette Sutures in human tissues at different time intervals. Furthermore, they looked to determine the sutures' resistance index in subcutaneous tissue. This was done by placing threads in the lower abdomen of eight patients. Histologic examination was performed on the section of soft tissue containing the sutures at 1 month, 3 months, 6 months, and 1 year following suture placement. A persistent inflammatory response was identified at 1 month, with histiocytes, lymphocytes, and multinucleated giant cells clustered around the cones and knots. Additionally, the suture was effectively encircled at this point by a very modest quantity of scar tissue. Until month 3, when just a small amount of collagen and connective tissue remained, the inflammatory tissue predominated. By month 6, there was a significant decrease in the number of inflammatory cells and an increase in connective tissue deposition. After 6 months, the cone material began to degrade and continued for about 12 months. Fibrous tissue encircled the suspension sutures, most prominently at the knot level. At the 1-year mark, physical examination revealed fracture around the knots in all instances (behind or in front of the knot). Histologic examination in this study showed a steady rise in the scar tissue surrounding the suspension sutures, a decrease in inflammatory cells, and an increase in collagenous tissue. By 12 months, the lactic acid and glycolic acid cones had been completely reabsorbed.

Additionally, this study demonstrated that until 12 months following suture insertion (end of the study), the hyaline fibrous tissue (formed of collagen and elastin fibres) underwent progressive remodelling. The physical analysis indicated that the thread structure weakened after 1 year, resulting in a decrease in traction resistance. The architecture of adipose fascial tissue in the abdomen differs significantly from that in the facial and cervical regions.

However, the basic scarring mechanism is consistent throughout the body. This study concluded that following the insertion of these threads in the subcutaneous tissue, there is a rise in the hypodermis, forming a solid fibrous tissue that seems most evident at the node level, and a steady increase in scar tissue formation. Cones totally resorb by 6 months post-insertion, and over the period of the year, the index of resistance decreases. The authors believe that increased scar tissue results in a more robust and permanent support [30, 31].

Conclusion

Silhouette Soft threads represent an innovative tool in aesthetic medicine, providing a minimally invasive option for facial and neck soft tissue rejuvenation. Constructed from biocompatible and bioresorbable synthetic polymers, poly-l-lactic acid (PLLA) and poly-l-glycolide (PLGA), these threads are deployed as sterile, single-use implants, often referred to as absorbable suspension sutures.

The application of these threads engenders a bifurcated mechanism of action: immediate repositioning of the soft tissues, accomplished through mechanical redistribution, and a subsequent, gradual regeneration of tissue. This immediate tissue repositioning is achieved through strategic positioning of the threads, facilitating the desired restructuring and elevation of ptotic tissues. Concurrently, these sutures stimulate a regenerative process, stimulating fibroblast activity and promoting collagen synthesis, resulting in the restoration of tissue volume over time.

The use of these biodegradable synthetic polymers traces its roots back to the 1960s, establishing a significant historical precedent within medical applications, ranging from surgical procedures to tissue engineering, thus substantiating their safety and efficacy profiles. Over the decades, these synthetic absorbable polymeric surgical devices have experienced constant refinement to meet the evolving needs of medical practice.

In conclusion, Silhouette Soft threads offer an effective, minimally invasive approach to aesthetic rejuvenation, achieving immediate tissue repositioning whilst catalysing a progressive natural tissue regeneration process. However, while these threads are effective for specific signs of ageing, it is crucial to underscore that they represent one tool within a multidisciplinary approach necessary to address the complex, multi-faceted nature of ageing. Complementary treatments should be considered to effectively tackle other signs of ageing not directly addressed by thread lifting. By understanding the precise physicochemical properties of these threads, along with the mechanisms propelling their effects, practitioners can optimize their therapeutic arsenal to deliver safe, efficient, and comprehensive aesthetic interventions. The continual refinement and development of these threads hold significant promise for the future landscape of aesthetic medicine.

Acknowledgments Thanks to Sinclair for providing the Silhouette Soft Safety Profile document and Physicians Guide.

References

1. Kulkarni R, et al. Polylactic acid for surgical implants. Washington, DC: Walter Reed Army Medical Center; 1966.
2. Damadzadeh B, et al. Effect of ceramic filler content on the mechanical and thermal behaviour of poly-L-lactic acid and poly-L-lactic-*co*-glycolic acid composites for medical applications. J Mater Sci Mater Med. 2010;21(9):2523–31.
3. Wan P, et al. Fabrication and evaluation of bioresorbable PLLA/magnesium and PLLA/magnesium fluoride hybrid composites for orthopedic implants. Compos Sci Technol. 2014;98:36–43.
4. Pihlajamaki H, et al. Absorbable pins of self-reinforced poly-L-lactic acid for fixation of fractures and osteotomies. J Bone Jt Surg Br. 1992;74(6):853–7.
5. Inui A, et al. Potency of double-layered poly L-lactic acid scaffold in tissue engineering of tendon tissue. Int Orthop. 2010;34(8):1327–32.
6. Lee DW, et al. Comparison of poly-L-lactic acid and poly-L-lactic acid/hydroxyapatite bioabsorbable screws for tibial fixation in ACL reconstruction: clinical and magnetic resonance imaging results. Clin Orthop Surg. 2017;9(3):270–9.
7. Liu S, et al. Current applications of poly(lactic acid) composites in tissue engineering and drug delivery. Compos Part B Eng. 2020;199:108238.

8. Vasenius J, et al. Absorbable self-reinforced polyglycolide (SR-PGA) screws for the fixation of fractures and osteotomies: strength and strength retention in vitro and in vivo. Clin Mater. 1994;17(3):119–23.
9. Vert M, et al. Something new in the field of PLA/GA bioresorbable polymers? J Control Release. 1998;53(1–3):85–92.
10. Da Silva D, et al. Biocompatibility, biodegradation and excretion of polylactic acid (PLA) in medical implants and theranostic systems. Chem Eng J. 2018;340:9–14.
11. Shebi A, Lisa S. Pectin mediated synthesis of nano hydroxyapatite-decorated poly(lactic acid) honeycomb membranes for tissue engineering. Carbohydr Polym. 2018;201:39–47.
12. Al Tawil E, et al. Microarchitecture of poly(lactic acid) membranes with an interconnected network of macropores and micropores influences cell behavior. Eur Polym J. 2018;105:370–88.
13. Tesfamariam B. Bioresorbable vascular scaffolds: biodegradation, drug delivery and vascular remodeling. Pharmacol Res. 2016;107:163–71.
14. Hollinger JO. Preliminary report on the osteogenic potential of a biodegradable copolymer of polylactide (PLA) and polyglycolide (PGA). J Biomed Mater Res. 1983;17(1):71–82.
15. Mäkelä P, et al. Strength retention properties of self-reinforced poly l-lactide (SR-PLLA) sutures compared with polyglyconate (MaxonR) and polydioxanone (PDS) sutures. An in vitro study. Biomaterials. 2002;23(12):2587–92.
16. Makadia HK, Siegel SJ. Poly(lactic-*co*-glycolic acid) (PLGA) as biodegradable controlled drug delivery carrier. Polymers. 2011;3(3):1377–97.
17. Budak K, Sogut O, Aydemir Sezer U. A review on synthesis and biomedical applications of polyglycolic acid. J Polym Res. 2020;27(8):208.
18. Lim TY, Poh CK, Wang W. Poly(lactic-*co*-glycolic acid) as a controlled release delivery device. J Mater Sci Mater Med. 2009;20(8):1669–75.
19. Maurus PB, Kaeding CC. Bioabsorbable implant material review. Oper Tech Sports Med. 2004;12(3):158–60.
20. Pillai CKS, Sharma CP. Absorbable polymeric surgical sutures: chemistry, production, properties, biodegradability, and performance. J Biomater Appl. 2010;25(4):291–366.
21. Shuwisitkul D. Biodegradable implants with different drug release profiles. 2011.
22. Lorenc ZP, et al. Expert consensus on achieving optimal outcomes with absorbable suspension suture technology for tissue repositioning and facial recontouring. J Drugs Dermatol. 2018;17(6):647–55.
23. Nestor MS. Facial lift and patient satisfaction following treatment with absorbable suspension sutures: 12-month data from a prospective, masked, controlled clinical study. J Clin Aesthet Dermatol. 2019;12(3):18.
24. de Benito J, et al. Facial rejuvenation and improvement of malar projection using sutures with absorbable cones: surgical technique and case series. Aesthet Plast Surg. 2011;35(2):248–53.
25. Loo JSC, Ooi CP, Boey FYC. Degradation of poly(lactide-co-glycolide) (PLGA) and poly(l-lactide) (PLLA) by electron beam radiation. Biomaterials. 2005;26(12):1359–67.
26. Goldberg D, et al. Single-arm study for the characterization of human tissue response to injectable poly-ʟ-lactic acid. Dermatol Surg. 2013;39(6):915–22.
27. Stein P, et al. The biological basis for poly-ʟ-lactic acid-induced augmentation. J Dermatol Sci. 2015;78(1):26–33.
28. Russo P, et al. Histological findings after insertion of PLLA sutures with bi-directional cones in humans: 2 years follow-up. J Plast Path Dermatol. 2018;14(2):121–5.
29. Goldberg DJ. Stimulation of collagenesis by poly-ʟ-lactic acid (PLLA) and -glycolide polymer (PLGA)-containing absorbable suspension suture and parallel sustained clinical benefit. J Cosmet Dermatol. 2020;19(5):1172–8.
30. Consiglio F, et al. Suture with resorbable cones: histology and physico-mechanical features. Aesthet Surg J. 2016;36(3):NP122–7.
31. Azimi B, et al. Poly(lactide-*co*-glycolide) fiber: an overview. J Eng Fibers Fabrics. 2014;9(1):155892501400900107.

P(LA/CL)-ʟ-Polylactide-Σ-Caprolactone Threads—APTOS Threads: APTOS Solution-APTOS Methods and Threads

11

Souphiyeh Samizadeh, Sorousheh Samizadeh, George Sulamanidze, Kajaia Albina, Konstantin Sulamanidze, and Marlen Sulamanidze

Abstract

In the ever-evolving field of aesthetic medicine, the advent of P(LA/CL)-l-Polylactide-Σ-Caprolactone threads, commonly known as APTOS threads, marks a significant innovation in minimally invasive facial and body rejuvenation techniques. This chapter provides an in-depth exploration of the APTOS solution, including its threads, thread material, and histology findings. It explores the unique properties of APTOS threads, which are designed for effective soft tissue lifting and support, offering a promising alternative or adjunct to more invasive surgical procedures. The chapter highlights the biocompatible and biodegradable nature of these threads, their mechanism of action in stimulating collagen production, and the subsequent enhancement of facial and

S. Samizadeh (✉)
King's College London, London, UK

University College London, London, UK

Great British Academy of Aesthetic Medicine, London, UK
e-mail: info@baamed.co.uk

S. Samizadeh
University College London, London, UK

G. Sulamanidze
Clinic of Plastic and Aesthetic Surgery and Cosmetology, Total Charm Clinic, Tbilisi, Georgia
e-mail: aptos@aptos.ge

K. Albina
Department of Clinic of Plastic Surgery and Dermatology, Total Charm Clinic, Tbilisi, Georgia

K. Sulamanidze · M. Sulamanidze
Total Charm Clinic, Tbilisi, Georgia

© Springer Nature Switzerland AG 2024
S. Samizadeh (ed.), *Thread Lifting Techniques for Facial Rejuvenation and Recontouring*, https://doi.org/10.1007/978-3-031-47954-0_11

body contours, and reduction of ptotic tissues. Emphasis is placed on the technical nuances of thread placement, patient selection criteria, and post-procedural care to optimize outcomes and minimize complications. By integrating scientific research with clinical insights, this chapter aims to equip aesthetic practitioners with the knowledge and skills necessary to incorporate APTOS thread lifting into their practice, thereby expanding the scope of aesthetic solutions available to patients seeking facial rejuvenation.

Keywords

Thread lift · Thread lifting · Thread-lift method · Thread-lift technique · Thread-lift procedure · Poly-L-lactic acid cone threads · APTOS solution · APTOS methods and products · Thread lifting · Poly(L-lactide-*co*-*ε*-caprolactone) · Thread with hyaluronic acid · Polypropylene · Non-surgical body and face rejuvenation · Body and face thread lifting · Face thread lifting

Thread lifting serves as an exceptional complement to other non-surgical and minimally invasive procedures aimed at contouring and rejuvenation. This option holds particular appeal for patients reluctant to undergo surgery, those who wish to avoid general anesthesia, and those seeking a comparatively shorter recovery period. While surgical interventions remain the gold standard for certain cases, thread lifting can offer significant benefits in instances of mild to moderate soft tissue ptosis.

However, not all individuals are suitable candidates for thread lifting. Those with autoimmune diseases, blood disorders, ongoing anticoagulant therapy, untreated or uncontrolled inflammatory conditions, a predisposition to keloid or hypertrophic scar formation, pregnant women, individuals with non-absorbable threads or benign and malignant tumors at the target site, and those allergic to the thread materials are advised against this procedure. Patients with cancer undergoing treatment are often advised to postpone non-essential aesthetic procedures until after their cancer treatment has been completed and their health status has been re-evaluated. Ensuring patient safety and achieving optimal outcomes are paramount, and each case should be considered individually, with decisions made in close consultation with the patient's medical team.

Currently, the market offers threads made from materials such as polydioxanone (PDO), poly-L-lactic acid (PLLA), polyglycolic acid (PGA), and polycaprolactone (PCL). Scientists and clinicians continue to explore a variety of polymers, striving to advance the development and refinement of products and techniques. The goal is to enhance both the safety and efficacy of thread lifting, ensuring it remains a viable and effective option for facial rejuvenation and contouring.

APTOS Solutions

Starting in the late 1990s, APTOS company has been manufacturing unique products for plastic and aesthetic surgery and non-surgical/minimally invasive aesthetic medicine. Its contributions are recognized globally, with the company's inventions being utilized in over 85 countries. APTOS also emphasizes the importance of education, offering extensive training programs to physicians to ensure the proficient application of its techniques. Since 1996 plastic surgeons in the Sulamanidze family have been developing new technologies and techniques to minimize complications and optimize outcomes. Currently, APTOS has more than 30 products that can be used with more than 50 APTOS ON LABEL Methods including various facial areas and body concerns. Absorbable PLLA/PCL threads are used to:

- Re-position the soft tissues
- Provide long-lasting biostimulation

The enrichment with hyaluronic acid (HA) has been reported to reduce post-procedure downtime, enhance and accelerate rejuvenation, and provide more significant patient satisfaction [1].

Thread Composition

Polymeric materials play a pivotal role across various sectors, including industry, medicine, drug delivery systems, and technology. Absorbable and non-absorbable polymers are extensively utilized in the production of surgical sutures. Various suture materials, such as polypropylene (PP), polydioxanone (PDO), poly-L-lactic acid (PLLA), polyglycolic acid (PGA), and polycaprolactone (PCL), are employed for repositioning and supporting subcutaneous tissue. PLLA, in particular, has been used in the medical field for nearly 40 years, serving not only as suture material but also in absorbable implants like screws. The application of PLLA induces a foreign tissue reaction, characterized by an increase in macrophages, mast cells, and lymphocytes, a decrease in fibroblastic activity, and a gradual enhancement of neocollagenesis [2, 3].

For over three decades, P(LA/CL)-l-polylactide-Σ-caprolactone has been a staple material in surgical applications. APTOS products utilize three main types of thread materials: Three types of thread materials are used for APTOS products:

- Non-absorbable material: polypropylene
- Two types of absorbable thread materials:
    - L-Polylactide-Σ-caprolactone P(LA/CL), which fully absorbs over approximately 2 years.
    - L-Polylactide-Σ-caprolactone P(LA/CL) enriched with hyaluronic acid (HA), offering the added benefits of enhanced tissue and skin stimulation.

Polypropylene

Polypropylene, a monofilament synthetic suture, stands out among biocompatible, biostable polymers for its broad clinical utility, extending from sutures to implants. Its low tissue reactivity paired with an extremely low friction coefficient renders it exceptionally suitable for use in aesthetics. Distinguished by its resistance to degradation in tissue, polypropylene is the material of choice for applications necessitating prolonged support. The suture's superior tensile strength further underscores its clinical value. Leveraging polypropylene's unique physical and mechanical properties, APTOS has developed a minimally invasive technique for addressing facial asymmetry due to facial paresis. The strategic placement of APTOS threads within the subcutaneous tissue facilitates effective lifting, fixation, and volumization of the impacted areas, offering a refined approach to restoring facial symmetry.

Poly L-Polylactide-Σ-Caprolactone P(LA/CL)

P(LA/CL)-L-polylactide-Σ-caprolactone as a suture material has been used in surgery for over 30 years. The main component of the APTOS absorbable, APTOS P(LA/CL) threads, is L-lactic acid (75%), which provides an additional rejuvenating effect, stimulating the natural revitalization of tissues and slowing down the ageing process. During the biodegradation of the thread, L-lactic acid is released into the surrounding tissues, promoting the formation of elastin and collagen types 1 and 3. PCL is highly effective at stimulating collagen synthesis [4]. An animal study revealed approximately 50% increase in new collagen formation at eight weeks in PCL thread groups, surpassing both PDO and PLLA thread groups [5]. Additionally, PCL threads have shown superiority in collagen regeneration over longer periods compared to PDO and PLLA threads [5].

Σ-Caprolactone, constituting the remaining 25% of the APTOS P(LA/CL) threads, augments connective tissue stimulation, retards biodegradation, prolongs the tissue lifting effect, facilitates lactic acid delivery to tissues, and enhances thread strength relative to pure polylactic acid compositions.

The dual-component polymer blend of PCL/PLA exhibits desirable biomaterial properties due to its thermoplastic and eco-friendly nature, garnering significant interest for its potential in diverse applications. The unique formulation of absorbable PLLA/caprolactone (PCL) threads, further augmented with HA on their surface, presents a compelling option. These biodegradable aliphatic polyesters demonstrate a gradual degradation rate in subcutaneous implant models, maintaining about 40% integrity at 18 months, thereby offering a durability advantage over previous generations of absorbable threads.

Poly-L-Lactic Acid (PLLA)

Poly-l-Lactic Acid (PLLA) is a synthetic polymer derived from L-lactic acid, extensively utilized in medical applications, including suture materials and absorbable screws, for nearly four decades. Its biocompatibility and efficacy have been well-established in numerous studies, highlighting PLLA's safety and effectiveness [6, 7]. In 1999, a PLLA-based filler, initially branded as 'New Fill' in Europe, was introduced, and subsequently approved in the United States as Sculptra L for treating HIV-related lipoatrophy [3]. Subsequent research has thoroughly evaluated PLLA's safety, efficacy, and longevity, demonstrating its utility in treating lipoatrophy associated with aging and its adaptability for off-label soft-tissue contouring purposes. Patients report high satisfaction rates, with effects lasting from one year to up to 36 months following additional treatment sessions [6–14].

PLLA elicits a localized immune response upon administration, characterized by an influx of macrophages, mast cells, and lymphocytes, and a decrease in fibroblast activity, which cumulatively enhances neocollagenesis [2]. MRI scans have confirmed significant increases in subcutaneous thickness one year post-treatment in the majority of cases [15]. Recognized for its versatility, PLLA is used to address bone resorption, fat loss, and skin laxity, consistently improving skin quality following administration [3, 16].

Poly Caprolactone (PCL)

PCL is a biodegradable polymer that degrades to carbon dioxide and water. Characterized by its high flexibility and elasticity, PCL is associated with reduced pain and discomfort compared to Polydioxanone (PDO) and Poly-L-lactic Acid (PLLA) sutures [5].

The durability of PCL is notable, with its chemical structure and bonds being robust and complex, allowing it to remain intact for up to two years before fully dissolving. Moreover, PCL has demonstrated a pronounced capacity for promoting collagen synthesis [4]. In a comparative animal study, PCL thread applications resulted in a 50% increase in new collagen formation at 8 weeks, outperforming both PDO and PLLA threads in terms of both the degree and duration of collagen regeneration [5]. This efficacy underscores PCL's potential in aesthetic and reconstructive procedures, offering sustained improvements in tissue structure and function.

Hyaluronic Acid-Coated Threads

Third Generation APTOS Threads, enriched with HA, offer a dual benefit of simultaneous lifting and skin stimulation. The innovative composition of these threads leads to a marked enhancement in skin quality post-treatment. The incorporation of HA into these threads not only facilitates the lifting and stimulating effects on the skin but also ensures a consistent enhancement of skin texture and health post-procedure [3, 16]. The enrichment with HA has been reported to reduce post-procedure downtime, enhance and accelerate rejuvenation, and provide more significant patient satisfaction [1, 17–19]. This breakthrough in thread technology exemplifies the synergy between mechanical support and biochemical improvement, setting a new standard in minimally invasive aesthetic treatments.

Thread Types

APTOS threads are meticulously designed to cater to a wide range of indications across different facial and body regions. Expert plastic surgeons have not only refined the techniques for their placement but also established extensive training and support frameworks to ensure optimal outcomes. The APTOS product line includes over 30 distinct offerings, compatible with more than 50 on-label techniques. These products feature carefully engineered variations, including adjustments in thread length, needle type and size, as well as barb configurations. Such precision in design allows for tailored applications, enabling targeted enhancements and corrections in specific facial and bodily areas.

APTOS threads are designed for a broad spectrum of applications, tailored to meet specific aesthetic goals across facial and body regions. These threads are systematically classified to address diverse needs:

- HA-Enriched P(LA/CL) Threads for Facial Contouring and Tissue Repositioning: These threads, enhanced with Hyaluronic Acid, are formulated to refine facial contours and stimulate skin revitalization. These include Visage Excellence Method HA, Visage Excellence Method Soft HA, and Nano Excellence Method HA.
- P(LA/CL) Threads for Addressing Age-Related Changes in the Face and Neck: Designed to counteract visible signs of aging. These include Light Lift Needle Method, Light Lift Thread Method, Light Lift Spring Method, and Light Lift Linea Method.
- Threads for the Reduction of Superficial rhytids: Tailored to minimize the appearance of fine lines, the options include the Nano Excellence Method, Nano Spring Method, and Nano Vitis Method.
- Body Contouring and Shaping Threads: Crafted for non-surgical lifting and rejuvenation, the options include Body Excellence Method, Body Needle Method, and Body Wire Method N.
- Specialized Applications: These threads are meticulously engineered for targeted interventions, including rhinoplasty, otoplasty, and enhancements within intimate regions. This customization underscores the adaptability and precision of APTOS technology across a spectrum of aesthetic medical practices.

APTOS Barbs

The efficacy of thread lifting techniques in achieving a lasting lifting effect hinges on the ability to securely maintain tissues in an elevated position through robust fixation mechanisms. Threads designed for aesthetic enhancements encompass both free-floating varieties and those equipped with fixation units such as barbs or cones.

The main fixational unit of APTOS threads is APTOS barbs. The design of APTOS barb, which is crafted using a proprietary cutting technique. The unique specifications of the APTOS barb—encompassing length, cutting edge, density, and directional orientation—facilitate immediate and firm soft tissue engagement. These barbs are engineered with a three-dimensional geometry, optimizing their capacity to mechanically lift and secure sagging tissues.

APTOS threads are classified based on the directional orientation of the barbs into uni-directional, bi-directional, and multi-directional categories. Bi-directional threads employ barbs positioned to exert counteracting forces, akin to a Tug of War, ensuring the thread remains steadfastly in place.

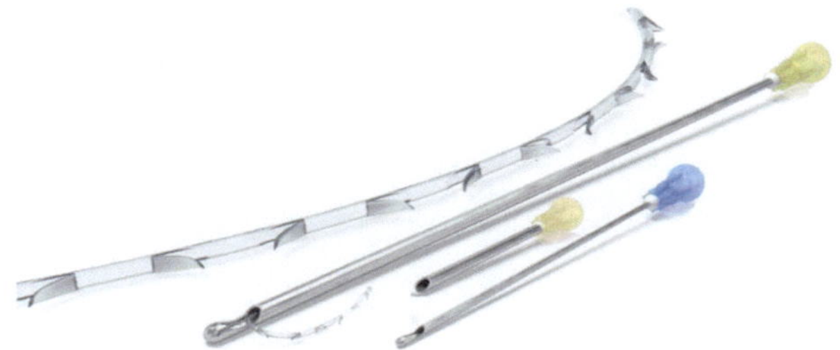

Fig. 11.1 Multi-directional barbed thread with accompanying accessories. (Image credit APTOS)

The configuration of multi-directional barbs (Fig.11.1) ensures equal distribution of tissue tension along the entire length of the thread, and the three-dimensional arrangement of the barbs allows to achieve the most reliable fixation avoiding thread breaking. The three-dimensional barb layout enhances fixation reliability, minimizing the risk of thread breakage. This arrangement means that each pair of barbs operates independently, allowing for immediate tissue fixation. This innovative arrangement guarantees sustained fixation strength, as the failure of a single barb does not compromise the thread's overall stability within the tissue.

Thread Design for Optimal Outcome and Safety

These threads are designed with optimal safety and efficacy (Fig. 11.2).
   Safety of APTOS threads is ensured by:
   - Anatomical Considerations for Enhanced Safety: APTOS threads are strategically implanted within the subcutaneous adipose layer, deliberately avoiding the dermis or muscular layers. This careful placement is crucial to circumvent facial danger zones and mitigate the risk of complications, further emphasizing the procedural safety of APTOS thread treatments.

The efficacy of this device is attributed to several key factors:
1. Thread materials
   - Biocompatibility profile, safety, and tolerability for various biomedical applications.
2. Safety-Enhancing Accessories: The threads come in a comprehensive kit that includes specialized tools designed to augment procedural safety:
   - A lance point needle is provided to create precise entry points.
   - A round-tip cannula (23 G × 80 mm) facilitates the infiltration of anesthetic solution into the subcutaneous tissue, laying the groundwork for a pain-free procedure.
   - Pre-loaded round-tip cannulas enable the gentle insertion of the thread through the subcutaneous layer, ensuring an atraumatic process with minimized risk of damage to major vessels, nerves, or tissues (Fig. 11.1).
     - Anatomical Considerations for Enhanced Safety: APTOS threads are strategically implanted within the subcutaneous adipose layer, deliberately avoiding the dermis or muscular layers. This careful placement is crucial to circumvent facial danger zones and mitigate the risk of complications, further emphasizing the procedural safety of APTOS thread treatments.

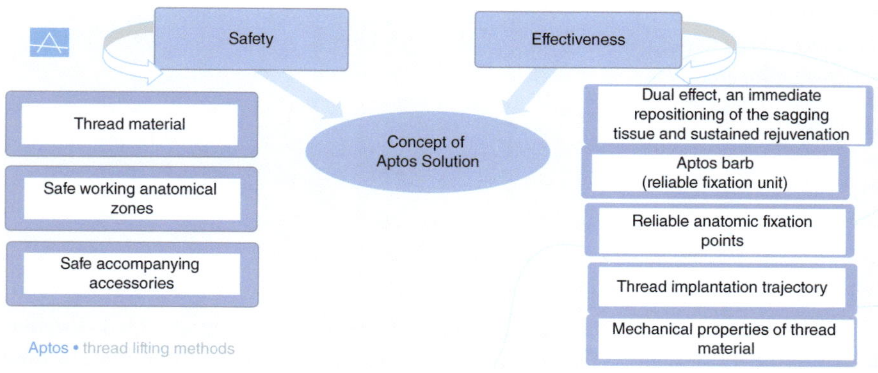

Fig. 11.2 Concept of APTOS solution. (Image credit APTOS)

The efficacy of this device is attributed to several key factors:

1. Minimally Invasive Technique: The procedure for inserting threads is designed to be minimally invasive and atraumatic, significantly shortening the recovery and rehabilitation phase. Consequently, the results become evident within 2–3 weeks post-treatment.
2. Strategic Implantation Pathway: The method for thread implantation is meticulously planned based on the anatomical and physiological understanding of ptosis, ensuring an effective approach to addressing facial sagging.
3. Robust Fixation Mechanisms:
   - The multi-directional arrangement of barbs on the surface of the thread.
   - Anatomic fixation points for threads: ligaments. The use of facial ligaments as fixation points is pivotal for securing the threads. This strategic anchoring allows for the lifted subcutaneous tissue compartments to be maintained in their elevated positions, contributing significantly to the overall aesthetic enhancement.

These features collectively ensure not only the safe application of the threads but also minimize potential adverse effects such as hematomas and swelling, thereby streamlining the post-treatment recovery process.

Histology

The introduction of biomaterials into the body triggers specific cellular responses, including the recruitment of macrophages and the formation of multinucleated foreign body giant cells, which are among the earliest to respond. These cells adhere to the biomaterial surface, instigating fibrosis and leading to the creation of a fibrous capsule encasing the implant. This fibrotic reaction is often accompanied by significant neovascularization. The specific cellular and tissue responses elicited vary with the type of biomaterial implanted [20]. The induced neocollagenesis and neovascularization consequentially alter skin texture, structure, and color [20].

APTOS Company has rigorously investigated the safety and efficacy of APTOS threads through a comprehensive series of foundational studies encompassing sensitization, irritation, biocompatibility, in-vivo and in-vitro degradation, chemical characterization, and biostimulation effects, alongside clinical data on product longevity and efficiency. These studies incorporate objective assessments of the threads' fixation strength and structural integrity post-implantation.

- In a study evaluating the degradation and local tissue response to APTOS P(LA/CL) threads implanted subcutaneously in rabbits, according to ISO 10993-6 standards, these threads were deemed non-irritant at 4 and 26 weeks. However, they were classified as slightly irritant at subsequent intervals—13, 34, 52, 64, and 72 weeks—when compared to a control group using High-Density Polyethylene (HDPE). Both the P(LA/CL) threads and the HDPE controls elicited comparable responses in the subcutaneous tissue of rabbits. Notably, the analysis revealed only minor traumatic changes in muscle fibers, specifically myofiber atrophy, near the sites of P(LA/CL) thread implantation, indicating a relatively mild reaction to the implanted material.

In an animal study published in 2018, tissue reaction on l-lactide-*co*-caprolactone threads was observed at 0, 4, 13, 26, 34, 52, 64, and 72 weeks after implantation in 21 rabbit models. l-Lactide-*co*-caprolactone implantation resulted in an effective inflammation involving macrophages and giant cells, which was proceeded by the gradual creation of fibrous connective tissue surrounding the threads and barbs and the construction of a homogenous fibrous capsule around the thread. The authors believe post-thread degradation, fibrotic tissue, and capsule development are likely to maintain the position of the realigned tissues. Consequently, the persistent fibrotic response along the thread's trajectory, which continues even after the thread has fully dissolved, is believed to be the mechanism behind the lasting thread-lifting effect [20].

Further research involving a cohort of 8 mature pigs (40–50 kg) aimed to assess the cellular inflammatory response, evaluate the thickness of the connective tissue capsule in subcutaneous adipose tissue, and examine the collagen (type I and III) and elastin stimulation following thread implantation. Results from this study indicated that 45 days post-implantation, APTOS P(LA/CL) threads neither caused necrosis nor induced an inflammatory reaction at the implantation sites, demonstrating the threads' biocompatibility and their potential in stimulating collagen and elastin production without adverse tissue responses. (Figs. 11.3 and 11.4).

Research findings indicate that APTOS P(LA/CL) threads augmented with Hyaluronic Acid (HA) significantly boost the production of collagen types I and III, as well as elastin, when compared to threads composed solely of P(LA/CL). Specifically, threads infused with HA exhibit a prolonged and more consistent effect in stimulating elastin production. Additionally, HA-enhanced threads are notably finer than their non-HA counterparts, leading to less connective tissue formation. This property allows for more frequent thread treatments, with intervals of approximately 1.5 to 2 years between sessions. Importantly, the unique composition of these threads minimizes the formation of scar tissue in the treatment area, enabling a smoother recovery and maintaining aesthetic outcomes (Fig. 11.5).

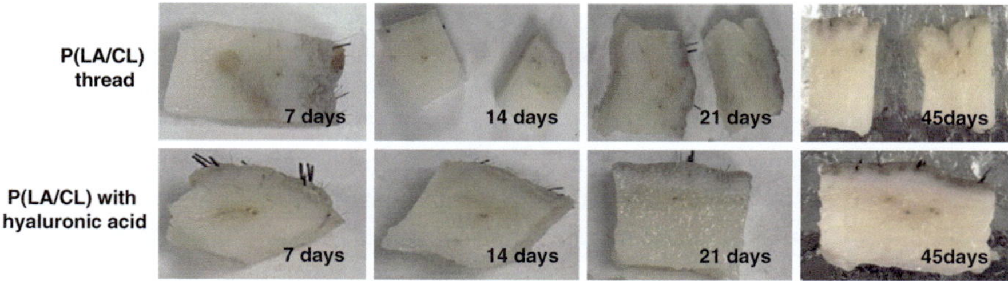

Fig. 11.3 Macroscopic evaluation of implantation sites. (Image credit APTOS)

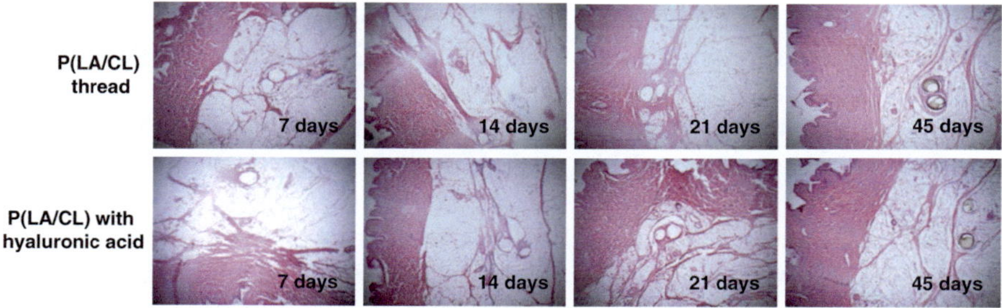

Fig. 11.4 Microscopic evaluation of implantation sites. (Image credit APTOS)

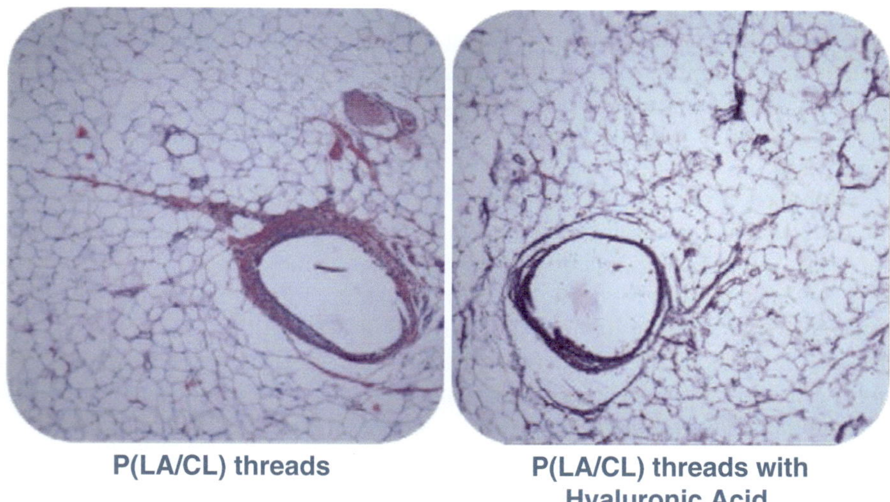

Fig. 11.5 Connective tissue formation. (Image credit APTOS)

In another animal study, 20 white rats, 72 tissue samples were analyzed histologically to assess morphological changes post-implantation of APTOS filaments, in comparison to smooth polypropylene threads. Key findings include [21].

- Collagen synthesis begins more rapidly and persists for an extended period with APTOS filaments, affecting a larger volume of tissue and offering a more robust response than that observed with polypropylene threads.
- The formation of a fibrous capsule around the filament shaft and barbs leads to the development of connective tissue strands extending into both the epidermis and subcutaneous fat layer, integrating with the connective tissue fibers of these areas.
- A notable increase in microvessel density was observed in the vicinity of APTOS filaments compared to areas surrounding polypropylene threads. These microvessels exhibit an open lumen, indicative of the "phenomenon of persistent hyperemia," contrasting with the transient hyperemia seen with polypropylene threads.
- The barbs of APTOS filaments are encased in their distinct connective tissue capsule, which is thicker than that surrounding the main filament shaft, enhancing the filaments' anchorage to adjacent tissues.
- The capsule around the barbs is less mature than that around the filament shaft, suggesting a heightened stimulatory impact on surrounding tissues by the barbs, thereby prolonging collagen production and improving tissue fixation.
- Mast cells, which play a role in vasodilation and HA transport to surrounding tissues, were consistently present near APTOS filaments throughout the observation period, without eliciting a phagocytic response.
- Following APTOS filament implantation, there was a 26% increase in the microvascular network density, significantly enhancing local tissue oxygenation and blood circulation.

Conclusion

Thread-lifting has emerged as a globally recognized technique among minimally invasive cosmetic interventions, reflecting a shift towards procedures that ensure patient comfort and reduced recovery periods. This chapter has undertaken a rigorous analysis of the safety and efficacy of a variety of thread-lifting materials, with a particular emphasis on APTOS threads, which are engineered for targeted facial and body recontouring and rejuvenation. The spectrum of available polymeric threads varies in their capacity to achieve a lifting effect, with a distinct disparity in their ability to induce collagen synthesis. Through the lens of scientific inquiry, it has been determined that P(LA/CL) threads, especially those augmented with Hyaluronic Acid (HA), provide enhanced and enduring biostimulatory effects on elastin and collagen types I and III. The unique design attributes of these threads, including specified density, orientation, and fixation mechanisms, alongside their composition and biodegradation characteristics, significantly influence their performance. The generation of connective tissue post-procedure not only serves as an indicator of these threads and methods' effectiveness but also permits the possibility of repeated treatments, potentially contributing to sustained patient satisfaction over time. The advancement in thread technology, particularly the development of P(LA/CL) and HA-enriched P(LA/CL) variants, coupled with their structural innovations, underscores the significant role of APTOS threads in the evolution of aesthetic medicine. Their capacity to facilitate aesthetic enhancement with minimal procedural downtime, together with their profound effects on critical dermal components, underscores the scientific foundation of thread-lifting as an essential modality in minimally-invasive and non-surgical aesthetic medicine.

References

1. Irina P, Albina K. Single-blind comparative study of the aesthetic outcome of armouring procedures with PLLA/PCL-and HA-enriched absorbable threads. Trichol Cosmetol Open J. 2019;3:15–20.
2. Lowe NJ. Optimizing poly-L-lactic acid use. J Cosmet Laser Ther. 2008;10(1):43–6.
3. Girgin A. The effectiveness of PLLA/PCL aptos thread on skin quality. International Union of Aesthetic Medicine-UIME; 2019. p. 25.
4. Agarwal B, Mishra P. Thread lift in aesthetic and regenerative gynecology. In: Aesthetic and regenerative gynecology. Springer; 2022. p. 153–63.
5. Cho SW, et al. Efficacy study of the new polycaprolactone thread compared with other commercialized threads in a murine model. J Cosmet Dermatol. 2021;20(9):2743–9.
6. Hanke CW, Redbord KP. Safety and efficacy of poly-L-lactic acid in HIV lipoatrophy and lipoatrophy of aging. J Drugs Dermatol. 2007;6(2):123–8.
7. Rotunda AM, Narins RS. Poly-L-lactic acid: a new dimension in soft tissue augmentation. Dermatol Ther. 2006;19(3):151–8.
8. Mest D, Humble G. Duration of correction for human immunodeficiency virus-associated lipoatrophy after retreatment with injectable poly-L-lactic acid. Aesthet Plast Surg. 2009;33(4):654–6.
9. Mest D. Experience with injectable poly-L-lactic acid in clinical practice. Cosmet Dermatol. 2005;18(2):S2.
10. Mest DR, Humble GM. Retreatment with injectable poly-L-lactic acid for HIV-associated facial lipoatrophy: 24-month extension of the Blue Pacific Study. Dermatol Surg. 2009;35(s1):350–9.
11. Schulman MR, Lipper J, Skolnik RA. Correction of chest wall deformity after implant-based breast reconstruction using poly-L-lactic acid (Sculptra). Breast J. 2008;14(1):92–6.
12. Burgess C. The evolution of injectable poly-L-lactic acid from the correction of HIV-related facial lipoatrophy to aging-related facial contour deficiencies. J Drugs Dermatol. 2011;10(9):1001–6.
13. Levy RM, Redbord KP, Hanke CW. Treatment of HIV lipoatrophy and lipoatrophy of aging with poly-L-lactic acid: a prospective 3-year follow-up study. J Am Acad Dermatol. 2008;59(6):923–33.
14. Lam SM, Azizzadeh B, Graivier M. Injectable poly-L-lactic acid (Sculptra): technical considerations in soft-tissue contouring. Plast Reconstr Surg. 2006;118(3 Suppl):55s–63s.

15. van Rozelaar L, et al. Semipermanent filler treatment of HIV-positive patients with facial lipoatrophy: long-term follow-up evaluating MR imaging and quality of life. Aesthet Surg J. 2014;34(1):118–32.
16. Avelar L, Cazerta C. The improvement of the skin quality with the use of PLLA. J Dermat Cosmetol. 2018;2(2):101–2.
17. Nikishin D, Sulamanidze G, Kajaia A. Effectiveness of using poly lactide and caprolactone acid with hyaluronic acid material. Adv Plast Reconstr Surg. 2019;3(2):274–84.
18. Krasiński R, Tchórzewski H, Lewkowicz P. Antioxidant effect of hyaluronan on polymorphonuclear leukocyte-derived reactive oxygen species is dependent on its molecular weight and concentration and mainly involves the extracellular space. Postepy Hig Med Dosw. 2009;63(20):205–12.
19. Röck K, Fischer K, Fischer JW. Hyaluronan used for intradermal injections is incorporated into the pericellular matrix and promotes proliferation in human skin fibroblasts in vitro. Dermatology. 2010;221(3):219–28.
20. Sulamanidze G, et al. The subcutaneous tissue reaction on poly(L-lactide-*co*-caprolactone) based threads. Int J Clin Exp Dermatol. 2018;3:1–9.
21. Adamyan A, et al. Morphological foundations of facelift using APTOS filaments. In: Miniinvasive face and body lifts-closed suture lifts or barbed thread lifts. IntechOpen; 2013.

Thread Lifting: Understanding the Fundamentals

12

Hsieh Chia-Hsien, Peter Hsien-Li Peng, and Souphiyeh Samizadeh

H. Chia-Hsien
Diamond Cosmetic Clinic, Taipei, Taiwan, People's Republic of China

Diamond-Biotechnology Co., Ltd., Taipei, Taiwan, People's Republic of China

P. H.-L. Peng (✉)
P-Skin Professional Clinic and Hair Restoration Center,
Kaohsiung, Taiwan, People's Republic of China

Department of Dermatology, Tri-Service General Hospital, National Defense Medical Center,
Taipei, Taiwan, People's Republic of China

Laser, and Photonics Medicine Society of Taiwan (LMSTW),
Taipei, Taiwan, People's Republic of China

Taiwanese Dermatological Association (TDA), Taipei, Taiwan, People's Republic of China

Taiwanese Society for Dermatological and Aesthetic Surgery (TSDAS),
Taipei, Taiwan, People's Republic of China

Taiwan Society of Hair Restoration Surgery (TSHRS),
Taipei, Taiwan, People's Republic of China

Chinese Across the Strait Association of Plastic and Aesthetic (CASAPA), Beijing, China

ISDS, Darmstadt, Germany

DASIL, Milwaukee, WI, USA

International Medicine Affairs Committee, Kaohsiung City Medical Association,
Kaohsiung, Taiwan, People's Republic of China

S. Samizadeh
University College London-Division of Surgery & Interventional Science, London, UK

King's College London-Dentistry, Oral & Craniofacial Sciences, London, UK

Great British Academy of Aesthetic Medicine, London, UK
e-mail: info@baamed.co.uk

Abstract

Thread lifting, gaining momentum in both East Asia and Western countries, has evolved with technological and technique advancements, offering a refined approach to facial rejuvenation. Initially hampered by limitations, current medical-grade sutures enable effective contouring, rejuvenation, and alignment of soft tissues. Understanding the procedure's fundamentals—differentiating volumization, lifting, and skin tightening techniques—is crucial for achieving favorable outcomes. Ongoing research is vital for improving thread selection, placement strategies, and patient selection, thereby enhancing procedural safety and efficacy. This chapter underscores the importance of a comprehensive grasp of thread lifting principles for optimizing aesthetic results.

Keywords

Thread lifting · Thread lift · Facelift · Nonsurgical facelift · Surgical facelift · Facial rejuvenation · Liquid facelift · Asian beauty

Over the past decade, the global medical aesthetics market has witnessed exponential growth, expanding at an annual rate of approximately 25%. This remarkable surge can be attributed to ongoing technological advancements and innovations in medical materials. Notably, there has been a significant rise in demand for minimally invasive procedures that require fewer visits and entail minimal to no downtime, particularly among both young and elderly patients. The ever-increasing demand for facial lifting procedures has established non-surgical face lifting treatments as the dominant force, accounting for more than 90% of the market. This can be attributed to the popularity of such procedures, as well as individuals' apprehension towards surgical interventions due to associated risks and the need for extended recovery periods.

The pursuit of youthful appearance has long been ingrained in human aspirations. While not everyone seeks procedures such as rhinoplasty, double eyelid surgery, or liposuction, the concerns and distress caused by sagging, drooping facial features, and crepey skin are evident. Common signs of deviating from a youthful appearance manifest as diminished skin firmness, compromised integrity, the emergence and deepening of nasolabial folds, marionette lines becoming more pronounced, and eyelids sagging.

Facial aging encompasses three major aspects: volume loss, alterations in the integrity of both hard and soft tissues, and ptosis of the soft tissues. To effectively address each aspect, numerous treatment options with a shared objective can be employed, including volumization, lifting, and skin tightening.

A plethora of treatment modalities exists for achieving the goals of tightening, lifting, and volumizing. The application of a three-dimensional diagram can effectively illustrate the available options and their distinct mechanisms of action.

Figure 12.1 offers a comprehensive understanding of the distinct roles played by various treatment modalities in addressing facial aging, thereby enabling the customization of individualized treatment plans based on the diagram's insights. It is crucial to recognize that no single modality or treatment can comprehensively address all the mentioned aspects, similar to how we cannot treat multiple medical conditions like heart disease, high blood pressure, and diabetes with a single medication.

As a minimally invasive procedure, thread lifting has gained increasing popularity. This technique involves the subcutaneous passage of sutures to counteract tissue descent and laxity.

The concept of barbed sutures for aesthetic tissue suspension was initially introduced by Georgian author Marlen Sulamanidze in the late 1980s, with thread lifting evolving as a minimally invasive technique utilizing anti-ptosis threads and sutures since the late 1990s [1–4].

The unique concepts of thread lifting hold significant potential for recontouring and rejuvenating various facial and body areas. Key concepts that warrant consideration and understanding include:

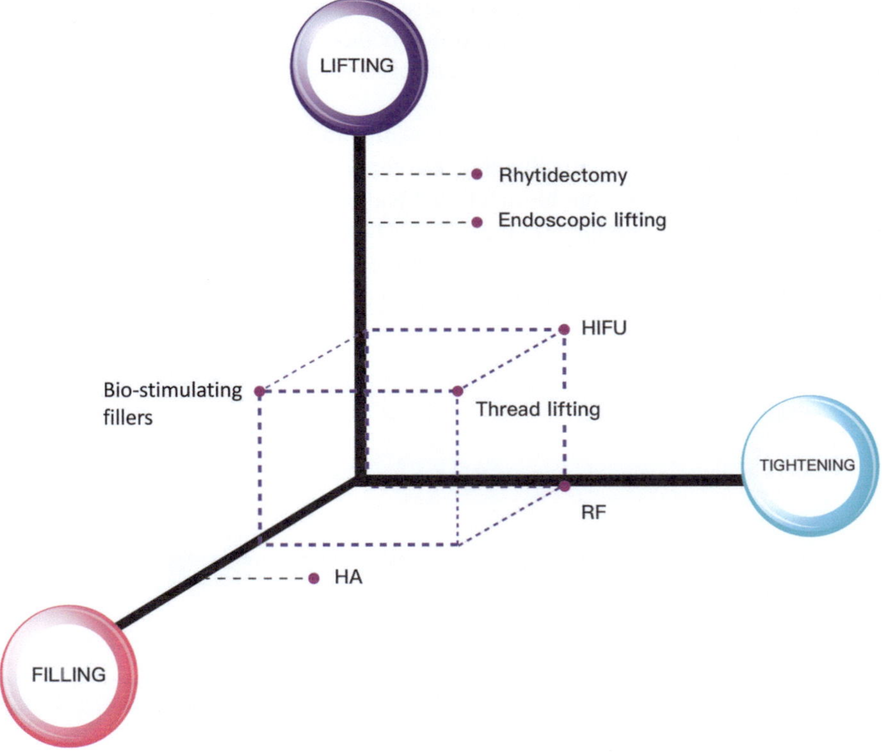

Fig. 12.1 Illustration demonstrating the role of various nonsurgical antiaging treatments

- Uni-directional lifting vs. Bi-directional lifting
- Antegrade lifting vs. Retrograde lifting
- Point lifting vs. Area lifting
- Tension balance
- Segmental lifting
- Volume shifting
- Vector extension
- Knotted vs. Unknotted sutures
- Other anchoring methods
- Superficial or deep plane lifting

By comprehending and incorporating these concepts, practitioners can optimize the outcomes of thread lifting procedures, tailoring treatment approaches to meet the unique needs and goals of individual patients.

Uni-directional Lifting vs. Bi-directional Lifting

Uni-directional barbed threads feature barbs that are oriented in a single direction, enabling tissue repositioning. However, these threads lack inherent anchoring capabilities. Consequently, additional anchoring methods, such as securing the threads to the scalp periosteum or knotting them together, are often necessary to ensure stable fixation.

In contrast, bi-directional threads possess the ability to both reposition tissues and provide anchorage, eliminating the need for additional knotting.

It is important to note that bi-directional barbed threads bring the skin and soft tissues together at the midpoints of the barbs on both sides (Fig. 12.2). Consequently, tissue accumulation and protrusion occur at the turning points of the barbs on the thread. This property can be effectively employed for tissue realignment and volumization effects.

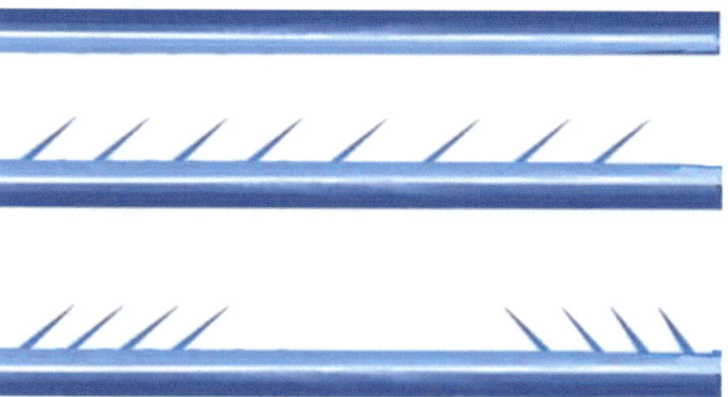

Fig. 12.2 Example of smooth, uni-directional, and bi-directional barbs

Antegrade vs. Retrograde Insertion (Fig. 12.3)

Antegrade Insertion

The technique of embedding the thread "top to bottom" offers distinct advantages as it allows the insertion points of the thread to be concealed within the hairline or scalp. However, this technique is highly sensitive to precision, and achieving a more superficial placement of the threads can pose challenges.

Retrograde Insertion

Conversely, embedding the thread from "bottom to top," known as retrograde insertion, provides the advantage of producing a more substantial lifting effect. However, it should be noted that this technique results in visible thread insertion points on the skin. Additionally, there is an increased risk of side effects such as depression and pigmentation at the entry sites.

The selection of either antegrade or retrograde insertion technique depends on several factors, including patient preferences, the desired outcome, and individualized treatment considerations.

Tension Balance (Fig. 12.4)

Understanding the dynamics of tension within the skin and different tissues is crucial to avoid post-insertion irregularities in thread lifting procedures.

Fig. 12.3 Antegrade vs. retrograde. (Image credit: CanStockPhoto)

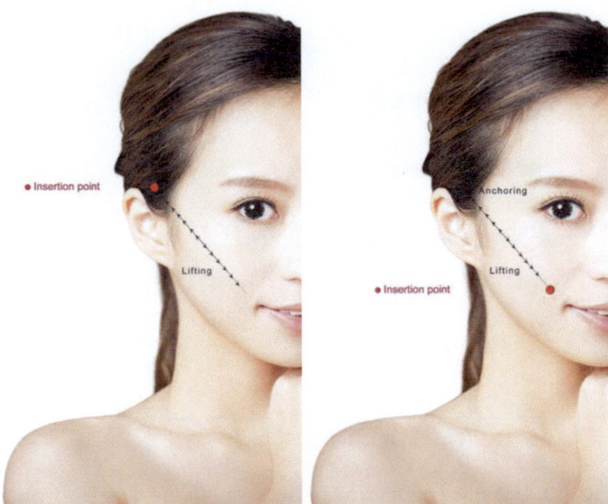

Creating a balanced tension starts with the principles of physics. Simply put, it involves achieving equilibrium in thread tension within the same area. The most straightforward approach is to ensure that each thread enters the skin from the same point with the same length.

Similarly, wrinkles are primarily caused by muscle contraction, resulting in their perpendicular orientation to the direction of the muscle fibers. This principle holds true for thread lifting as well. To minimize the impact of muscle contraction, it is essential to orient the threads as perpendicular as possible to the direction of the wrinkles.

In the case of sector lifting, where multiple threads are employed, it is crucial to ensure that the length of each thread entering the skin is consistent while applying the same force to each thread. Failure to maintain uniformity in thread length can lead to an imbalance of tension, resulting in skin depression or irregularities (Fig. 12.3).

To ensure optimal outcomes, it is imperative to carefully assess and adjust the tension applied during thread lifting procedures. By achieving a harmonious balance of tension, the risk of surface irregularities, such as convex and concave areas on the skin, can be minimized. This underscores the importance of meticulous technique and precise tension adjustment throughout the procedure to maintain a smooth and even appearance of the treated area.

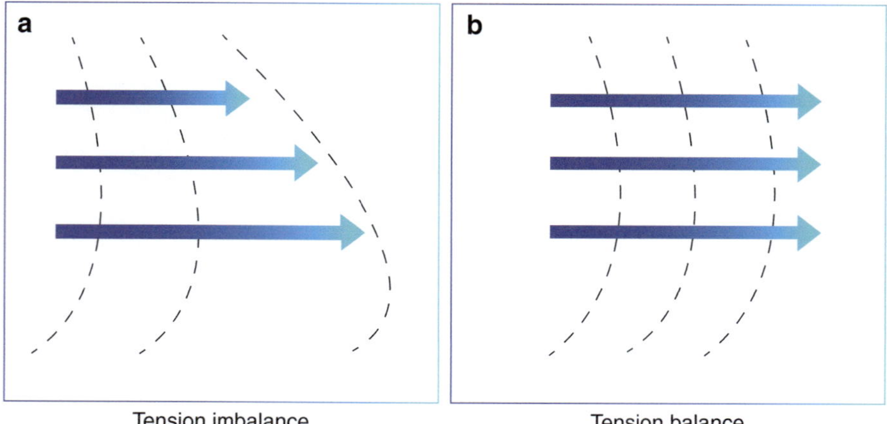

Fig. 12.4 Achieving tension balance within the skin is a critical consideration in thread lifting procedures. Failing to attain proper tension balance can result in convex and concave surface irregularities on the skin following the treatment

Point Lifting vs. Sector Lifting (Figs. 12.5 and 12.6)

Point Lifting: Small Target Area

All threads inserted are focused on one point and one target, for example, only one small facial area and target area.

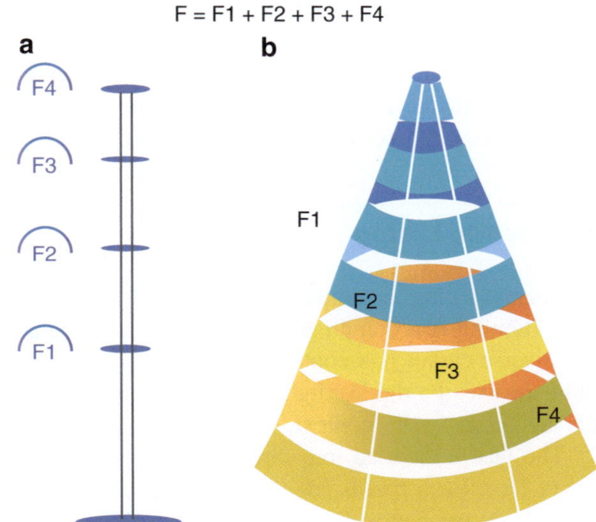

Fig. 12.5 (**a**) Point lifting, (**b**) sector lifting

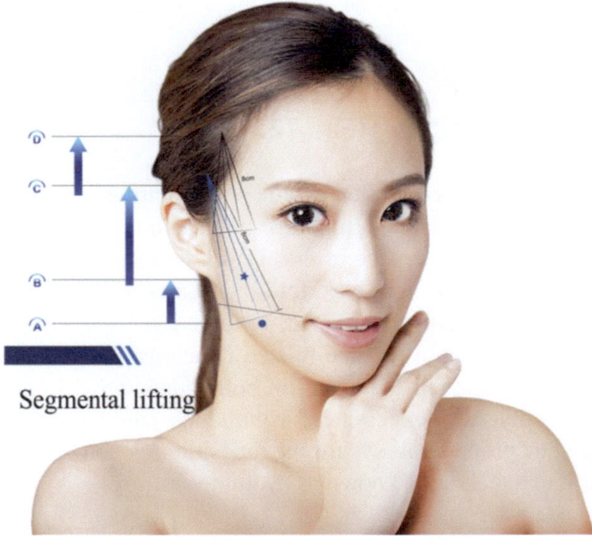

Fig. 12.6 Segmental lifting. (Image credit: CanStockPhoto)

Sector Lifting

The method described focuses on the treatment of large areas in thread lifting procedures. By strategically aligning the threads in a sector pattern, tissue repositioning can be achieved. This pattern allows for a balanced and controlled distribution of tension within the skin, thereby preventing skin depression or dimpling.

It is important to note that in this method, not all of the mechanical forces exerted by the threads are directed uniformly in the same direction. This intentional variation in force distribution helps to manage tension and optimize results. However, it should be acknowledged that this approach may result in a reduction in the overall strength of the threads. Therefore, careful consideration should be given to thread selection and placement techniques to ensure the desired outcomes while maintaining the necessary mechanical integrity of the threads.

Segmental Lifting

Segmental lifting technique can be likened to a game of tug-of-war, where tissue repositioning is accomplished in a step-by-step manner, section by section. Given the diverse curves and contours of the face, ranging from the scalp to the jaw and chin, the use of a rigid straight cannula may inadvertently penetrate unintended layers and areas. In this context, segmental lifting provides an effective solution.

The face is divided into three distinct parts: the upper face, middle face, and lower face. Each part is addressed individually, and the lifting process progresses from the lower part to the upper part (Fig. 12.6). This segmented approach allows for precise targeting of specific areas while ensuring optimal outcomes. By addressing each segment separately, the overall lifting effect can be achieved in a controlled and comprehensive manner, taking into consideration the unique characteristics and needs of each facial region.

Volume Shifting (Fig. 12.7)

The aging process often entails redistribution and loss of volume in specific facial regions, such as the temporal, suborbital, and buccal fat areas. These changes can impact the appearance of the cheeks, temples, and nasolabial folds, contributing to the formation of wrinkles, folds, and lines on the aging face [5].

As previously mentioned, bi-directional barbed threads play a crucial role in addressing these volume-related concerns. By gathering the target tissues at the turning points of the barbs on both sides, these threads effectively bring together areas that have experienced volume loss and have become hollow over time. This unique property allows for the repositioning and realignment of ptotic areas, resulting in a technique known as "volume shifting."

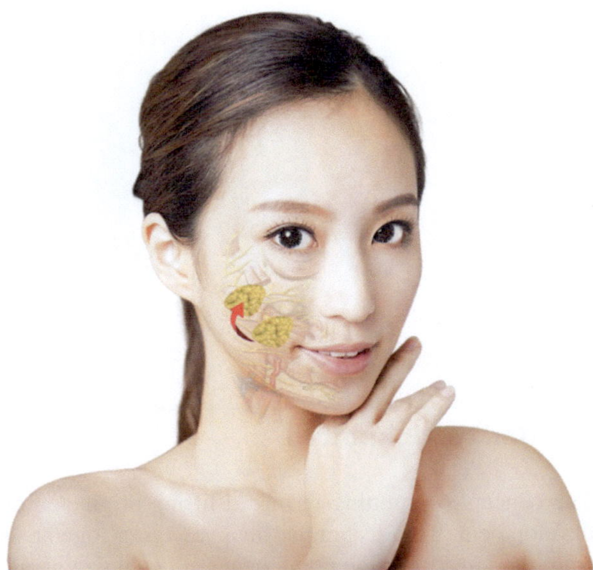

Fig. 12.7 Volume shifting. (Image credit: CanStockPhoto)

Utilizing this method enables clinicians to achieve both volumization and recontouring of the facial features (Fig. 12.6). By strategically placing bi-directional barbed threads, the targeted areas can be revitalized and restored, leading to a more harmonious and youthful appearance.

Vector Extension

During thread insertion in thread lifting procedures, it is crucial to select the appropriate layer within the facial anatomy. The complexity of facial anatomy necessitates careful consideration to avoid adverse effects, including facial nerve injury and disruptions to natural facial expressions following treatment.

The concept of vector extension is employed to address distant target areas without directly inserting threads into those specific regions. This approach allows for the treatment of point C by performing procedures at points A and B, thereby leveraging the force generated to extend and reposition the tissue at point C (Fig. 12.8). By strategically planning and implementing vector extension techniques, clinicians can achieve desired outcomes in distant target areas, expanding the scope and efficacy of thread lifting procedures.

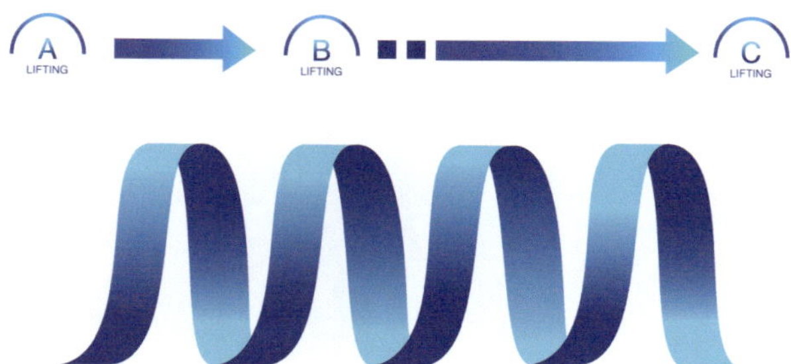

Fig. 12.8 Vector extension

Knotted vs. Unknotted

The concept of knotting in thread lifting originated during the early stages of its development. This technique involves tying together two threads that are placed from the same insertion point, generating a restraint and anchoring effect. Knotting serves to reduce the risk of thread migration and immediate relapse of the treatment, thereby enhancing the longevity of results.

Based on the authors' experience, when threads are knotted together, the outcomes tend to exhibit prolonged durability. This knotting process is typically performed when the insertion points can be discreetly hidden within the hairline.

It is important to note that this method is highly technique sensitive. The knots should be delicately executed, avoiding excessive size and looseness. Failure to achieve proper knotting can result in palpability, pain, or infection. Utmost care must be taken to prevent hair entanglement within the knot, necessitating meticulous attention and precision during the procedure.

Other Anchoring Methods

Among the various anchoring methods in thread lifting, one approach involves utilizing a curved needle to bury the exposed thread back into the scalp while simultaneously securing it to the deep fascia or periosteum.

This concept allows for the utilization of multiple methods, such as triangular fixation and combining fascia fixation with knotting, among others. By employing these techniques, clinicians can achieve effective anchoring and stabilization of the threads, contributing to the longevity and desired outcomes of the thread lifting procedure.

Superficial Lifting vs. Deep Plane Lifting

A recently published technique involves the use of threads for repositioning the buccal fat pad [6]. This procedure requires a high level of technical proficiency and is best performed by experienced surgeons. The threads are carefully passed through the deep buccal fat pad, positioned under the zygomatic arch and above the temporalis muscle.

Executing this technique demands precise anatomical knowledge, extensive experience, and expertise. Furthermore, patient cooperation and comprehension of the procedure are vital. It is important to note that potential side effects following this technique may include deep hematoma, lymphatic swelling, and temporary restriction of mouth movement.

The sub-zygomatic approach (Fig. 12.9) offers distinct advantages, including a more natural outcome, minimal widening of the cheekbones, and reduced susceptibility to the effects of muscle contraction, resulting in longer-lasting results. The limited widening of the zygomatic width holds particular appeal for individuals of East Asian descent [7–12].

Moreover, a combination of superficial and deep plane lifting techniques can be employed synergistically to achieve optimal outcomes in thread lifting procedures.

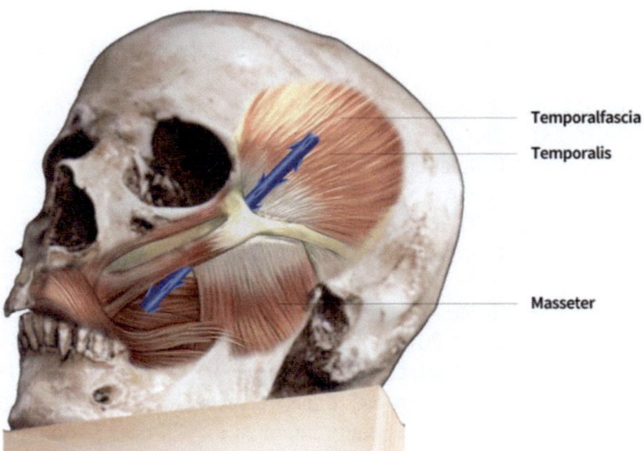

Fig. 12.9 The sub-zygomatic lifting technique presents a novel approach to address sagging skin in the peri-oral region or nasolabial fold while preserving the integrity of the superficial skin structure. This method specifically targets the sub-zygomatic area, allowing for precise lifting and repositioning of the sagging skin without impacting the superficial layers. By focusing on the sub-zygomatic region, this technique offers a targeted solution to address localized concerns, providing natural-looking results while minimizing disruption to the surrounding skin structure

Conclusion

In conclusion, thread lifting has gained significant popularity, particularly in Asia. However, it is essential to acknowledge the existing lack of consensus and systematic training for this procedure. East Asian medical practitioners who offer thread lifting services often employ their own customized facial contouring and rejuvenation methods.

To achieve desirable outcomes in contouring and rejuvenation, several key factors must be considered. These include thorough patient selection, a comprehensive understanding of facial anatomy, adherence to meticulous aseptic techniques, and the utilization of appropriate threads and techniques tailored to individual patient needs.

Addressing these considerations in a well-informed and precise manner can contribute to the successful execution of thread lifting procedures, resulting in satisfactory contouring and rejuvenation outcomes. Further research, standardization of techniques, and interdisciplinary collaboration are necessary to enhance the understanding and utilization of thread lifting in aesthetic medicine.

References

1. Sulamanidze M, Sulamanidze G. Facial lifting with aptos methods. J Cutan Aesthet Surg. 2008;1:7–11.
2. Sulamanidze M, Sulamanidze G. APTOS suture lifting methods: 10 years of experience. Clin Plast Surg. 2009;36:281–306.
3. Sulamanidze M, Paikidze T, Sulamanidze G, Neigel JM. Facial lifting with "APTOS" threads: featherlift. Otolaryngol Clin N Am. 2005;38(5):1109–17.
4. Sulamanidze M, Paikidze T, Sulamanidze G. Lifting of soft tissues: old philosophy, new approach—a method of internal stitching (Aptos needle). Aktuelle Dermatologie. 2004;30(10):82.
5. Fitzgerald R, Graivier MH, Kane M, Lorenc ZP, Vleggaar D, Werschler WP, Kenkel JM. Update on facial ageing. Aesthet Surg J. 2010;30(Suppl):11S–24S.
6. Tsai Y-T, Zhang Y, Wu Y, Yang H-H, Chen L, Huang PP-H, et al. The surgical anatomy and the deep plane thread lift of the buccal fat pad. Plast Reconstr Surg Glob Open. 2020;8(6).
7. Samizadeh S, Wu W. Ideals of facial beauty amongst the Chinese population: results from a large national survey. Aesthet Plast Surg. 2018;1–11.
8. Samizadeh S. The ideals of facial beauty among Chinese aesthetic practitioners: results from a large national survey. Aesthet Plast Surg. 2018;1–13.
9. Samizadeh S. Chinese facial physiognomy and modern day aesthetic practice. J Cosmet Dermatol. 2019.
10. Samizadeh S. Beauty standards in Asia. In: Non-surgical rejuvenation of Asian faces. Springer; 2022. p. 21–32.
11. Samizadeh S. Facial ageing in east Asians. In: Non-surgical rejuvenation of Asian faces. Springer; 2022. p. 97–106.
12. Samizadeh S. Facial physiognomy. In: Non-surgical rejuvenation of Asian faces. Springer; 2022. p. 33–9.

Thread Lifting: Essential Principles and Practices

13

George Sulamanidze, Kajaia Albina,
Konstantin Sulamanidze, Marlen Sulamanidze,
and Souphiyeh Samizadeh

Abstract

The rising appeal of thread lifting in non-surgical rejuvenation is notable among aesthetic practitioners. Despite widespread discussion, a gap remains in comprehensive scientific evidence on its safety, effectiveness, longevity, and potential risks. This chapter discusses the critical aspects essential for achieving lasting success with thread lifting. It emphasizes the importance of meticulous patient selection, detailed preoperative planning, choosing the right sutures, and mastering the insertion technique. These elements are pivotal for ensuring the procedure's efficacy, safety, and durability, addressing both practitioners' and patients' expectations for minimally invasive aesthetic enhancements.

G. Sulamanidze (✉)
Clinic of Plastic and Aesthetic Surgery and Cosmetology, Total Charm Clinic,
Tbilisi, Georgia
e-mail: aptos@aptos.ge

K. Albina
Department of Clinic of Plastic Surgery and Dermatology, Total Charm Clinic,
Tbilisi, Georgia

K. Sulamanidze · M. Sulamanidze
Total Charm Clinic, Tbilisi, Georgia
e-mail: const@aptos.ru; gracia@aptos.ru

S. Samizadeh
King's College London, London, UK

University College London, London, UK

Great British Academy of Aesthetic Medicine, London, UK
e-mail: info@baamed.co.uk

© Springer Nature Switzerland AG 2024
S. Samizadeh (ed.), *Thread Lifting Techniques for Facial Rejuvenation and Recontouring*, https://doi.org/10.1007/978-3-031-47954-0_13

Keywords

Thread lifting · Thread lift · Facial rejuvenation · Face thread lift · Facelift · Non-surgical facelift · Insertion technique · Thread landmarks · Thread selection

Thread lifting has garnered substantial attention for its potential in facial rejuvenation and lifting. However, the discourse often outpaces the available scientific evidence regarding its safety, effectiveness, and longevity. Thread lifting's rise in aesthetic medicine comes with challenges, necessitating precise approaches for success. Key aspects include:

1. Varied Thread Quality: The market's diverse thread origins necessitate stringent selection based on chemistry, manufacturing, and sterility.
2. Systematic Training Deficit: A gap in comprehensive training on insertion techniques underscores the reliance on manufacturer-provided education.
3. Consensus Lack: The absence of agreement on the most effective techniques for varied indications complicates practice.

Addressing these through individualized patient assessment, procedural rigor, technique customization, a deep knowledge of facial anatomy and understanding anatomical changes with aging is crucial for optimal outcomes. Key considerations include:

1. Individualized Patient Assessment: Avoid generalizations; tailor approaches to each patient. Generalized landmarks and guidelines cannot be applied to all and will not result in a good outcome if individual patient factors are not considered.
2. Procedural Rigor for Safety and Efficacy:
   (a) Patient selection
   (b) Correct indication
   (c) Procedure conditions
       (i)   Clinical environment
       (ii) Aseptic technique
       (iii) The implantation procedure
   (d) Choosing effective products
   (e) Thread implantation technique
3. Technique Customization: Select techniques based on the patient's unique condition and establish individual treatment protocols.
4. Anatomical and Physiological Considerations:When considering the optimal thread and insertion technique for facial rejuvenation, beyond gravitational effects, it's crucial to account for:
   (a) Soft Tissue Compartments: Analogous to balloons, soft tissue compartments they provide volume in youth but atrophy over time, leading to volume loss (Figs. 13.1 and 13.2).

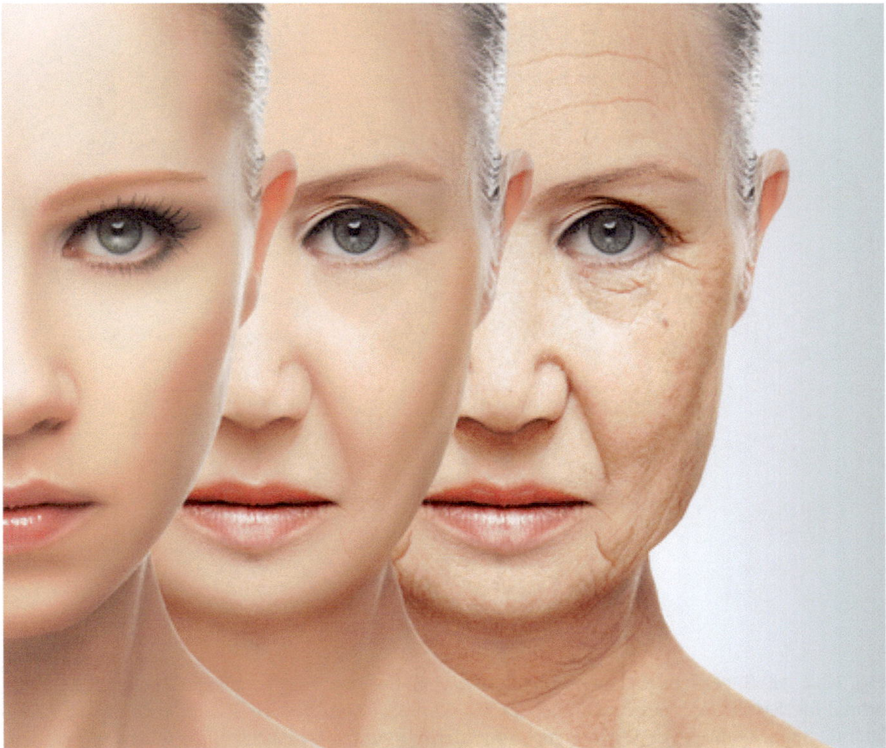

Fig. 13.1 Different aspects of facial ageing should be understood, including skeletal, muscular, ligament, fat pad, and skin changes. (Image credit: Shutterstock)

  (b) Ligaments: These structural components connect soft tissue to bone, losing
      elasticity and support with age.
  (c) SMAS Laxity and Skeletal Remodeling: Changes in the Superficial
      Musculoaponeurotic System and bone structure significantly contribute to
      facial aging. [1].

Therefore, a reproducible and optimal outcome can be achieved by paying attention
to the above factors and fundamentals of thread lifting.

Building on the anatomical and physiological considerations for thread lifting,
practitioners must also focus on these universal aspects for all patients, regardless of
the specific indications or thread types used: (Fig. 13.3):

1. Thread Implantation Trajectory: Determine the optimal path for thread insertion
   to achieve the desired lifting effect.
2. Correct Anatomical Layer for Implantation: Identify the correct anatomical layer for
   placing threads. This is crucial for effectiveness and minimizing complications.
3. Thread Fixation Points: Establish secure anchoring points for threads to ensure
   longevity and stability of the lifting effect.

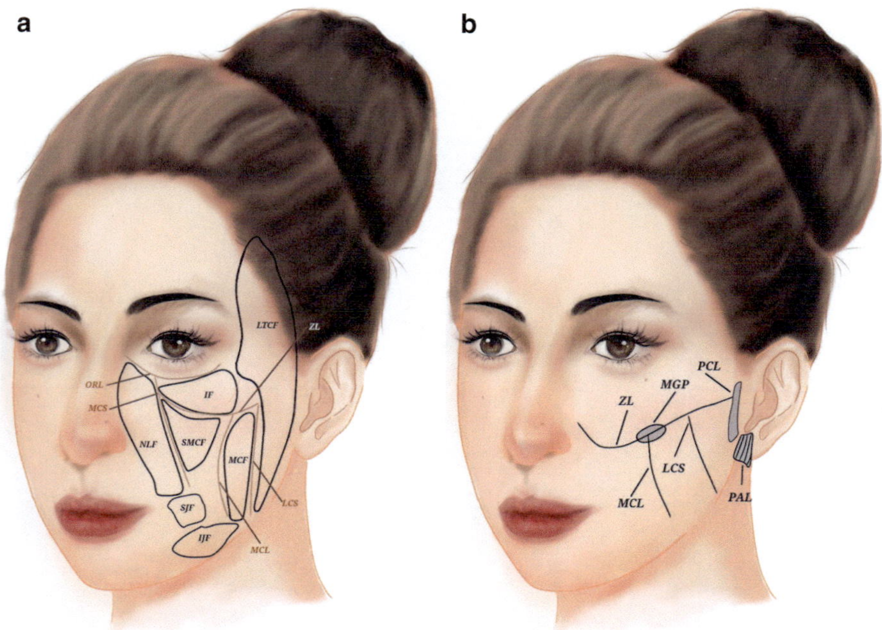

Fig. 13.2 (**a**) Superficial fat compartments. (**b**) Main ligaments used as anchoring points. *IF* infra-orbital fat, *SMCF* superficial medial cheek fat, *NLF* nasolabial fat, *MCF* middle cheek fat, *LTCF* lateral temporal-cheek fat, *SJF, IJF* superior, inferior jowl fat, *ORL* orbicularis retaining ligament, *ZL* zygomatic ligament, *MCS* medial cheek septum, *MCL* masseteric cutaneous ligament, *LCS* lateral cheek septum, *ZL* zygomatic ligament, *MGP* Mc Gregor patch, *PCL* parotid cutaneous ligament, *PAL* platysma auricular ligament

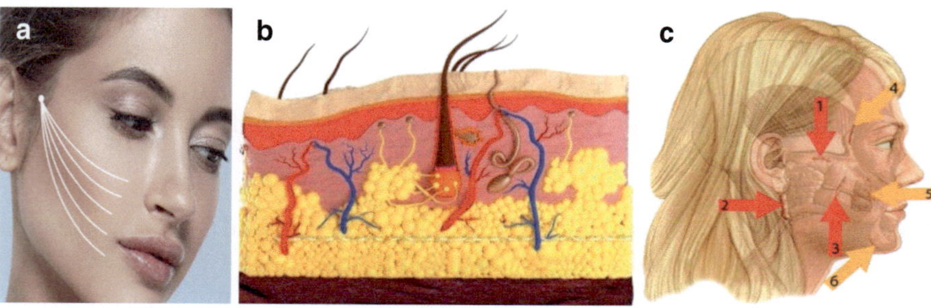

Fig. 13.3 Key Pillars of Thread Lifting: Demonstrating the essentials across all procedures and thread types (**a**) Thread vector, (**b**) layer of placement, (**c**) fixation point. (Image credit APTOS)

The Trajectory of Thread Implantation

To ensure a successful thread-lifting procedure, understanding its fundamentals is essential:

1. Aim: Re-position and align facial tissues against aging vectors.

Aging Vectors (Fig. 13.4):

- In the upper third, almost vertically
- In the middle third, obliquely and vertically
- In the lower third, horizontal.

2. I Influence of Facial Muscles: The facial muscles set the boundaries for effective soft tissue repositioning.

Fig. 13.4 Vectors of facial ageing. Upper face: vertical, periorbital: inferior and inferolateral vector. Midface and lower face: anteromedially

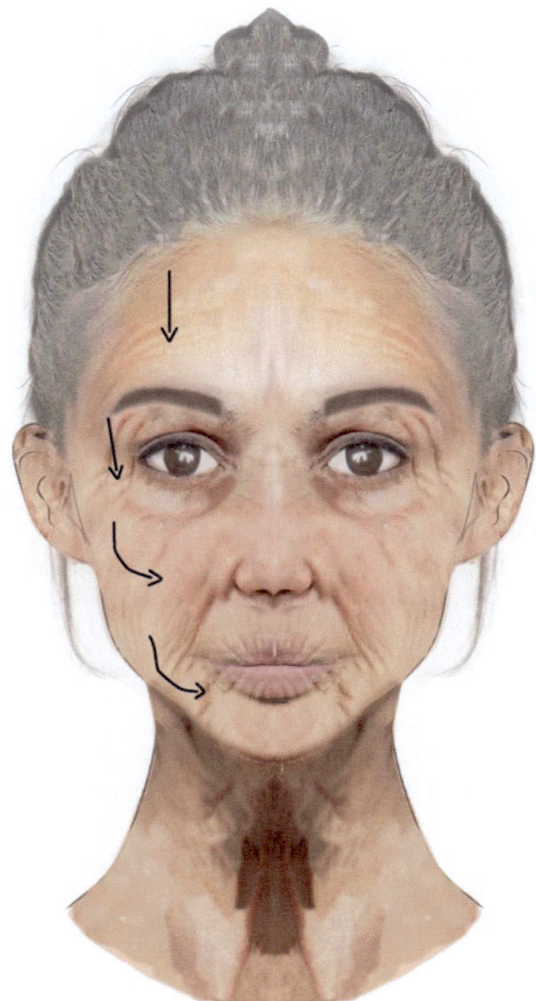

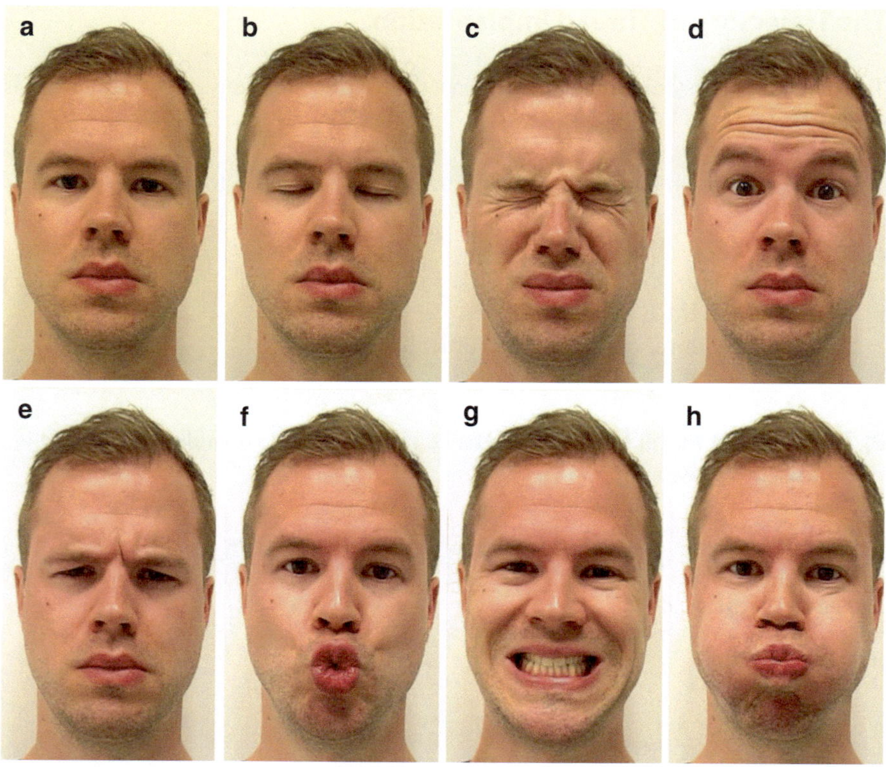

Fig. 13.5 Face at rest and during animation. (**a**) Resting position; (**b**) closing the eyes gently; (**c**) closing the eyes firmly; (**d**) raising the eyebrows; (**e**) frowning; (**f**) pursing the lips; (**g**) showing the teeth and (**h**) puffing of the cheeks. (Reproduced with permission from Loonen, T.G.J., Horlings, C.G.C., Vincenten, S.C.C., et al. Characterizing the face in facioscapulohumeral muscular dystrophy. *J Neurol* 268, 1342–1350 (2021) [2])

Consideration of muscle movement vectors is essential. Avoid vertical threads in the midface to reduce tension on threads. Opt for a curved trajectory for a more effective and lasting outcome (Fig. 13.5)

In thread lifting, it's crucial to acknowledge that threads can't lift muscles directly. Implantation should avoid areas of active facial expression to prevent muscle movements from compromising thread stability. Thus, choosing the right trajectory for thread implantation is vital for maximizing the effectiveness and durability of the lift.

The trajectory for thread implantation is critical to the procedure's longevity and efficacy. Understanding and strategic planning of thread insertion paths, aligned with facial contours and muscle movements, are imperative. This careful consideration ensures the lift remains effective over time, enhancing both the aesthetic result and the duration of the benefits. Selecting the optimal path not only maximizes the lift's longevity but also minimizes potential complications, making it a fundamental aspect of successful thread lifting. (Several examples are showcased in Fig. 13.6).

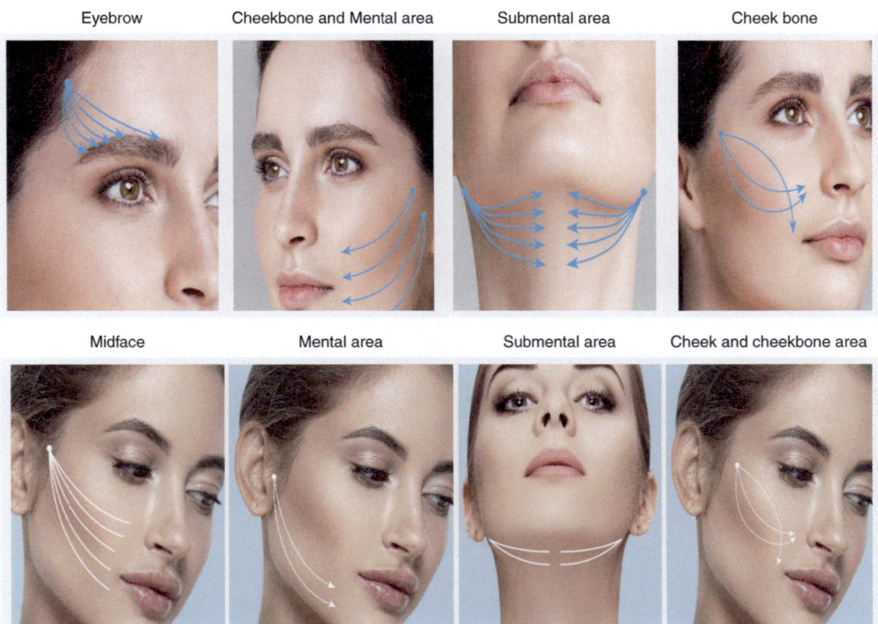

Fig. 13.6 The trajectory of thread insertion

Optimal Anatomical Layers for Thread Implantation in Aesthetic Procedures

Correct placement of threads is critical for achieving the desired aesthetic outcomes in thread lifting procedures. Key considerations include:

- For Bio-Stimulation and Skin Rejuvenation
- For Lifting Effect: Placement in the subcutaneous adipose tissue layer is optimal for lifting and repositioning facial tissues.

The APTOS threads and techniques work at the level of subcutaneous adipose tissue (Fig. 13.7), not in the dermis and muscles [3]. This strategic placement is critical for minimizing risks and achieving the intended aesthetic results. [4].

A youthful and healthy facial appearance relies on adequate and well-distributed adipose tissue, facilitating smooth transitions across facial zones. Displacement, atrophy and hypertrophy in these fat compartments can lead to aesthetic contour irregularities and contribute to facial ptosis, more pronounced in medial than lateral areas due to the structural support of facial ligaments.

APTOS threads can be placed superficially sub-dermally but not in the dermis. They can also be inserted relatively deep, near muscles but NOT in the muscles. This strategic layering achieves distinct outcomes: subcutaneous

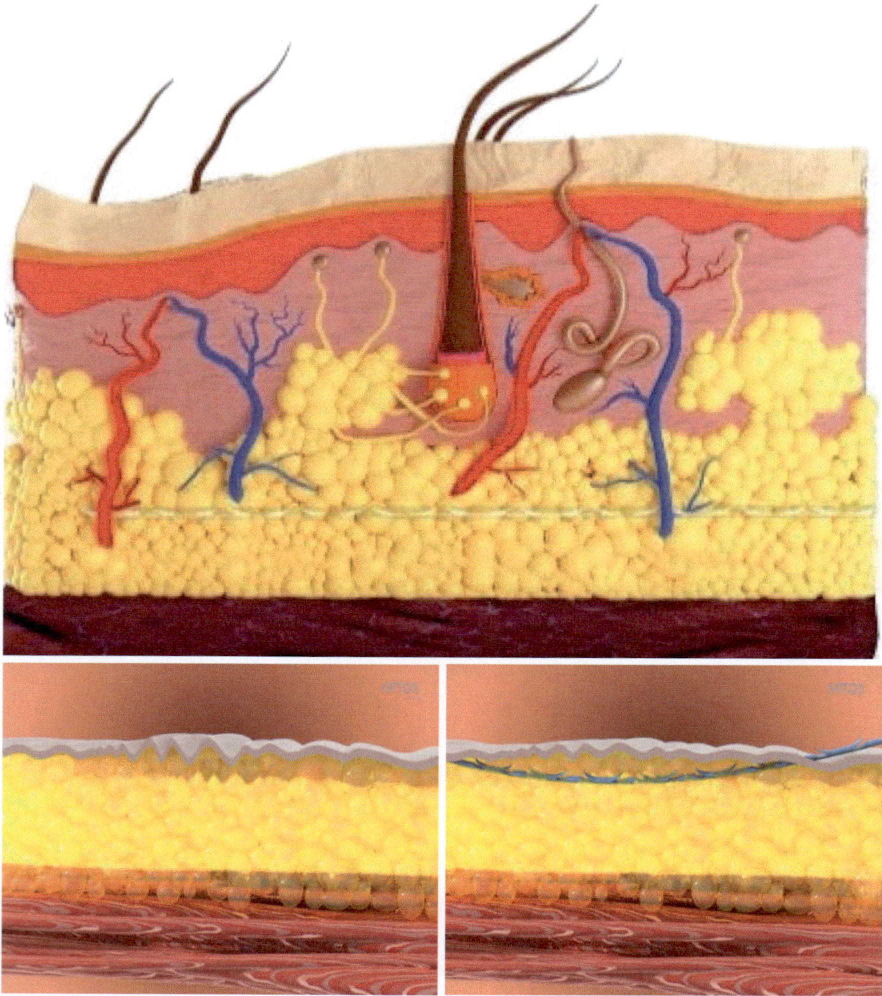

Fig. 13.7 Images illustrating Thread implantation in the subcutaneous layer

placement enhances lifting, while deeper placement allows for soft tissue volumization. Such precise positioning, especially for mid-face volume enhancement, optimizes facial fat compartment repositioning and volumization. The technique's success hinges on correct area, layer, and vector selection, underlining the procedure's adaptability to achieve desired aesthetic effects through meticulous application (Fig. 13.8) [5, 6].

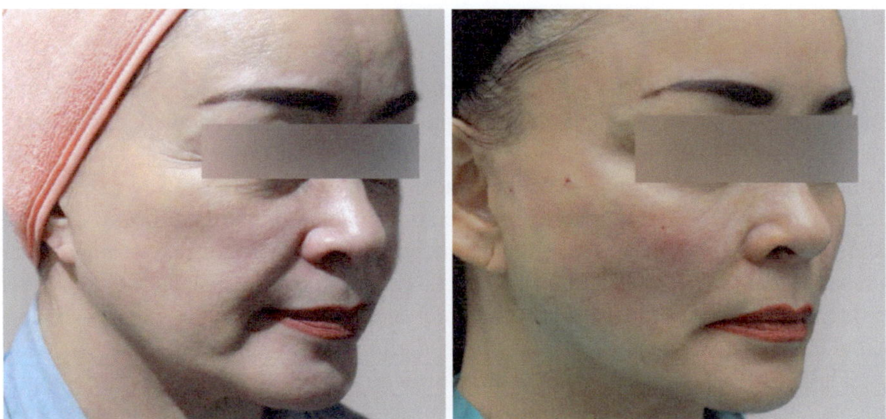

Age: 40; Area Treated: Jawline, Cheekbone area, Mid Face Nasolabial fold

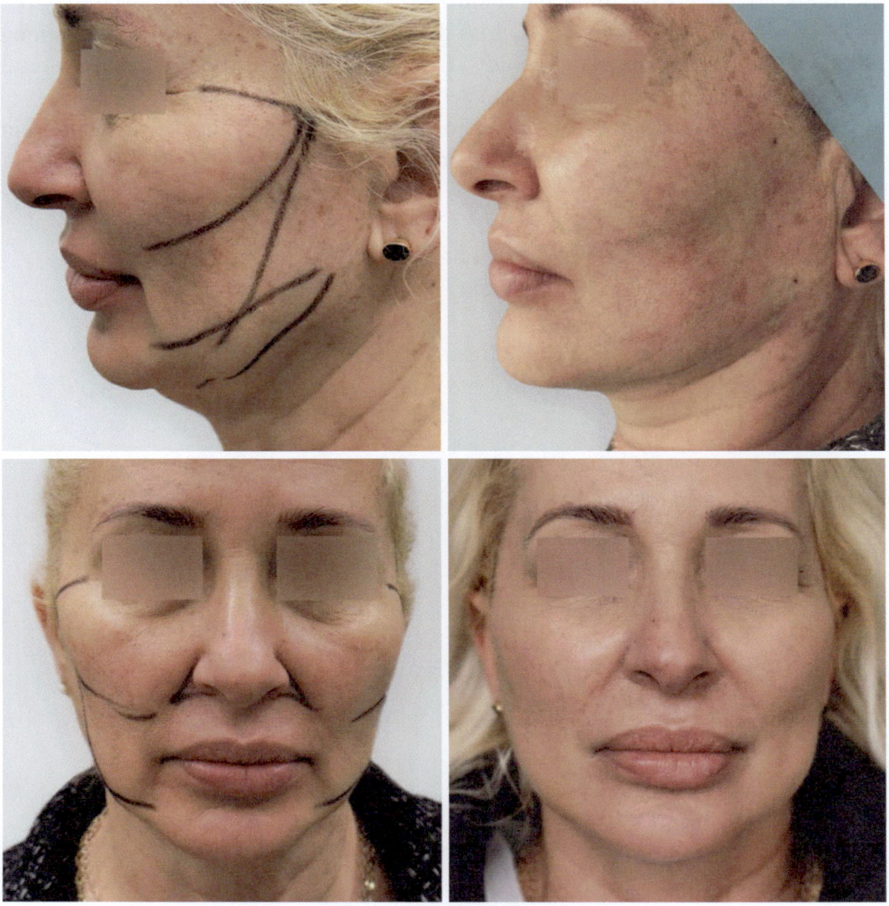

Age: 57; Area Treated: Midface and lower face

Fig. 13.8 Examples of repositioning of the soft tissues in the midface and periorbital area using APTOS threads

Fixation Points for Threads

For effective thread lifting, identifying stable fixation points is crucial due to the facial fatty tissue's loose nature. Techniques typically target subcutaneous adipose tissue, which is segmented into compartments by connective tissue septa. These compartments, which can lose volume and coherence with age, are key to restoring facial structure through thread lifting. Fixation points often align with facial septa and ligaments, which serve as reliable anchors due to their consistent anatomical presence and role in connecting skin and fascia to the deeper facial structures. This strategic placement of threads at anatomical anchor points, like the malar and mandibular ligaments, ensures the longevity and effectiveness of the lift.

Thread lifting aims to reestablish the structural harmony of facial fat compartments, anchoring at points that align with facial septa and ligaments. These ligaments serve as reliable anatomical structures for fixation due to their consistent locations, effectively retaining and stabilizing the skin and SMAS against the deeper facial structures. Key ligaments such as the malar, mandibular, and orbital, among others, are utilized as anchorage points, facilitating the repositioning and structural integrity of facial tissues for a rejuvenated appearance.

The ligaments serve as essential anchor points in thread lifting, securing the skin and SMAS layer to the facial structure beneath. They include (Fig. 13.9):

- Malar ligament
- Platysma-auricular (false ligament not fixated to the periosteum)
- Masseteric cutaneous (false ligament)
- Orbital ligament
- Buccal maxillary retaining (false ligament)
- Mandibular ligament

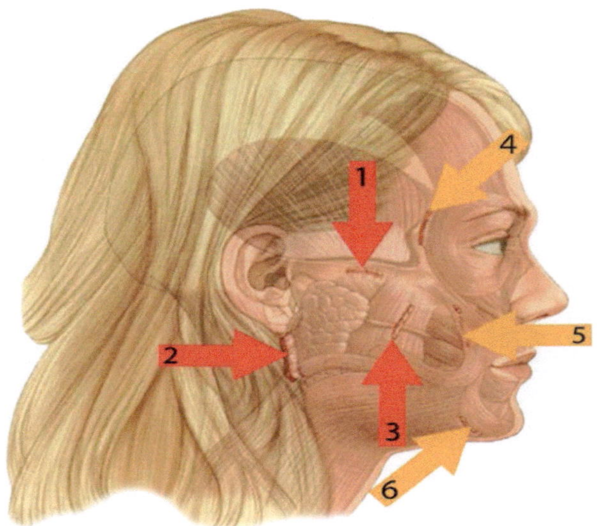

Fig. 13.9 Facial ligaments. Malar ligament (1); platysma-auricular (false ligament not fixated to the periosteum) (2); masseteric cutaneous (false ligament) (3) orbital ligament (4); buccal maxillary retaining (false ligament) (5); mandibular ligament (6). (Image credit: APTOS)

Figure 13.8 shows the main fixing points or defining points for most thread-lifting methods.

The significance of ligaments in thread lifting underlines the necessity for aesthetically favorable outcomes, with an emphasis on selecting threads supported by scientific evidence. The global trend towards non-surgical, minimally invasive rejuvenation techniques, exemplified by APTOS threads, demands meticulous application, including proper patient evaluation and thread selection. Achieving safety and efficacy in thread lifting depends on strict adherence to established techniques, accurate indication identification, and patient selection. The choice of implantation trajectory, anatomical layer, and fixation points plays a crucial role in ensuring the durability and success of the lifting effect.

Conclusion

In conclusion, the global shift towards non-surgical, minimally invasive techniques for lifting ptotic facial and neck tissues highlights a preference for procedures like thread lifting, with APTOS threads standing out for their ability to reposition and realign soft tissues effectively. This chapter underscores the importance of selecting threads backed by research for their safety and efficacy. Successful thread lifting requires strict adherence to proper implantation techniques, patient selection, and the use of appropriate products. The implantation trajectory, anatomical layer, and fixation points are critical factors that influence the long-term success and efficiency of thread lifting.

References

1. Okuda I, Yoshioka N, Shirakabe Y, Akita K. Basic analysis of facial ageing: the relationship between the superficial musculoaponeurotic system and age. Exp Dermatol. 2019;28(S1):38–42.
2. Loonen TGJ, Horlings CGC, Vincenten SCC, Beurskens CHG, Knuijt S, Padberg GWAM, et al. Characterizing the face in facioscapulohumeral muscular dystrophy. J Neurol. 2021;268(4):1342–50.
3. Sulamanidze M, Sulamanidze G. APTOS suture lifting methods: 10 years of experience. Clin Plast Surg. 2009;36(2):281–306.
4. Sulamanidze M, Sulamanidze G, Vozdvizhensky I, Sulamanidze C. Avoiding complications with Aptos sutures. Aesthet Surg J. 2011;31(8):863–73.
5. Sulamanidze M, Paikidze T, Sulamanidze G, Neigel JM. Facial lifting with "APTOS" threads: featherlift. Otolaryngol Clin N Am. 2005;38(5):1109–17.
6. Sulamanidze M, Fournier P, Paikidze T, Sulamanidze G. Removal of facial soft tissue ptosis with special threads. Dermatol Surg. 2002;28(5):367–71.

Thread Lifting: Criteria for Optimal Candidate Selection

Patient Selection

Souphiyeh Samizadeh, George Sulamanidze, Kajaia Albina, Konstantin Sulamanidze, and Marlen Sulamanidze

Abstract

Multiple factors govern a successful and optimal outcome for thread-lifting procedures. These include patient-related factors, product-related factors, and operator factors, including the clinical environment and techniques used. Correct patient selection is a critical factor in determining an optimal outcome when using threads for facial rejuvenation and recontouring. Regarding patient selection, many factors such as general health, mental health, social history, and expectations are overlooked by the practitioners. Only when these are assessed and established, the practitioner can look at the indications for the actual procedure and examine if the patient is suitable for the thread-lifting procedure.

S. Samizadeh

University College London, London, UK

King's College London, London, UK

Great British Academy of Aesthetic Medicine, London, UK
e-mail: info@baamed.co.uk

G. Sulamanidze (✉)
Clinic of Plastic and Aesthetic Surgery and Cosmetology Total Charm, Tbilisi, Georgia
e-mail: aptos@aptos.ge

K. Albina
Department of Clinic of Plastic Surgery and Dermatology "Total Charm", Tbilisi, Georgia

K. Sulamanidze · M. Sulamanidze
Total Charm Clinic, APTOS, Tbilisi, Georgia
e-mail: const@aptos.ru; gracia@aptos.ru

© Springer Nature Switzerland AG 2024
S. Samizadeh (ed.), *Thread Lifting Techniques for Facial Rejuvenation and Recontouring*, https://doi.org/10.1007/978-3-031-47954-0_14

"

Keywords
Thread lifting · Thread lift · Facial rejuvenation · Face thread lift · Patient selection · Expectations · Facelift · Non-surgical facelift

The efficacy of thread lifting in addressing the signs of aging and facial contouring hinges upon a thorough comprehension of individual characteristics, anatomy, and the diverse aging processes affecting different tissue layers. Consequently, meticulous planning and consideration of patient-specific factors are imperative to achieve optimal treatment outcomes.

General Health

Patients deemed suitable for thread treatment procedures typically exhibit good general health, a positive psychological outlook, and realistic treatment expectations. It is not advisable to carry out the procedure in patients with an active skin infection in the treatment area, open wounds or lesions, acne, or cold sores.

There are absolute contraindications, and caution is advised in some cases. In many scenarios, the clinician's clinical judgment should be practised. Examples include:

- Acute inflammatory processes or dermatological conditions affecting the treatment area
- Acute/active respiratory viral infection
- Chronic diseases in their acute phase
- Hypertension
- Infectious diseases including HIV and viral hepatitis
- Autoimmune disorders and other systemic diseases
- Coagulation disorders such as hemophilia
- Predisposition to keloid formation
- Multiple allergies or a history of anaphylaxis
- Oncological conditions
- Concurrent anticoagulant or antiplatelet therapy
- Mental health disorders
- Pregnancy, breastfeeding
- Prior placement of non-biodegradable implants or injections in the treatment area
- Immunocompromised/Immunodeficiency conditions

Patients should be advised **against** discontinuing prescribed medications unless instructed by a healthcare professional. However, it is advisable to suspend the use of over-the-counter supplements known to increase the risk of bruising, including:

- Ginseng
- Garlic

- Vitamin E
- Vitamin D
- Vitamin B6
- Co-enzyme Q10
- Fish oil/Omega-3 fatty acids
- Ginkgo Biloba
- Sweet Clover
- Sweet Woodruff
- St. John's Wort

Thorough documentation of allergies is paramount, with any known sensitivities to thread materials, coatings, or anesthetics warranting careful consideration. Atopic individuals may manifest heightened reactions post-procedure, necessitating extended healing periods. Special attention should be paid to asthmatic patients, those prone to stress-induced asthma, and individuals with panic disorders. During menstruation, heightened sensitivity, hormonal fluctuations affecting skin sensitivity and vascular response, as well as discomfort, and mood changes, could impact patient tolerance, increasing the risk of adverse reactions or complications during and after threadlifting procedures.

Mental Health

Screening for mental health, encompassing psychiatric history and current mental state, should constitute an integral component of the initial consultation for threadlifting procedures. This comprehensive evaluation benefits both the patient and the practitioner, fostering an in-depth discussion to ascertain the motivations for seeking cosmetic interventions [1]. Additionally, exploring all potential outcomes and alternative solutions is imperative to identify and safeguard vulnerable patients, thereby facilitating informed consent.

Expectations

Unrealistic expectations regarding treatment outcomes strongly correlate with poor responses and adverse psychosocial outcomes [2]. Establishing realistic expectations is paramount for successful threadlifting procedures. Patients often oversimplify the procedure in their minds, expecting it to be painless, straightforward, and devoid of visible signs or downtime. Misleading marketing by product companies, practices, and practitioners, compounded by social media influences, contribute to these misconceptions. Engaging in comprehensive discussions about treatment options, potential outcomes, pre- and post-procedural expectations, as well as rare side effects and complications, while utilizing before and after images, aids in cultivating more realistic patient expectations. It's noteworthy that expectations may vary based on cultural and ethnic backgrounds [3].

Correct Indication

Thread lifts are most suitable for patients exhibiting mild to moderate rather than severe ptosis and skin laxity. To tailor the appropriate thread technique for each patient, physicians should prioritize individual patient characteristics and primary areas of concern. Therefore, practitioners should diligently consider patient preferences to establish realistic outcome expectations (in Fig. 14.1).

Optimal candidates for thread lifts typically exhibit mild to moderate signs of aging, primarily between the ages of 35 and 55, encompassing both women and men. However, individuals with excessively sagging skin, particularly at advanced ages, may experience limited improvement. Similarly, individuals who are obese or have thick, dimpled skin texture may experience minor improvements. In such cases, combining thread lifts with liposuction may be beneficial (Table 14.1).

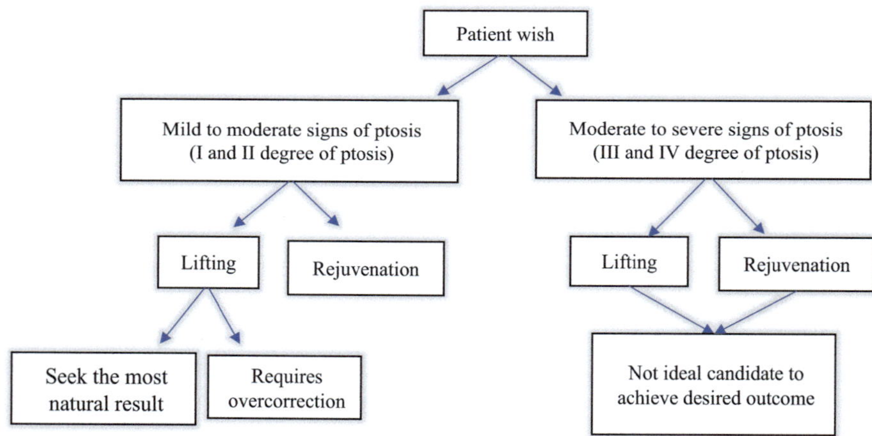

Fig. 14.1 Patient Wishes and Expectations, Integral Considerations for the Physician

Table 14.1 Criteria of suitable candidates for thread treatment procedure

Suitable candidates for procedure:	
Face-Mild to moderate ptosis (I and II degree of ptosis)	Yes
Sufficient skin thickness to prevent thread palpability	Yes
Absence of significant facial adiposity	Yes
Loss of volume	Yes
Fine lines and wrinkles	Yes
Loss of skin elasticity and tone	Yes
Ptotic eyebrows	Yes
Mild mi-face ptosis	Yes
Relapse from a previous procedure such as a facelift or neck lift	Yes
Thin skin	No
Excessive skin laxity	No
Obesity or very heavy, rugged skin	No
Permanent implants and fillers (e.g. PMMA and silicone) in and around area of treatment	No

Conclusion

In conclusion, the increasing interest in thread lifting underscores its significance as a minimally invasive modality for facial lifting, recontouring, and rejuvenation. The cornerstone of achieving optimal outcomes lies in meticulous patient selection, involving a comprehensive assessment of signs of aging, patients' overall health status, and mental well-being. Equally indispensable is the provision of comprehensive patient education, encompassing procedural intricacies, anticipated outcomes, potential side effects, downtime, and post-treatment care. Furthermore, the adherence to correct technique through continuous education and training among physicians is imperative. Central to success is the cultivation of realistic patient expectations and a profound understanding of the aging process. By prioritizing these elements in patient selection, treatment planning, and procedural execution, surgeons can consistently deliver the desired outcomes in thread lifting procedures, ensuring both efficacy and patient satisfaction.

References

1. Brunton G, Paraskeva N, Caird J, Bird KS, Kavanagh J, Kwan I, et al. Psychosocial predictors, assessment, and outcomes of cosmetic procedures: a systematic rapid evidence assessment. Aesthet Plast Surg. 2014;38(5):1030–40.
2. Rumsey N, Harcourt D. The psychology of appearance. McGraw-Hill Education; 2005.
3. Schofield M, Hussain R, Loxton D, Miller Z. Psychosocial and health behavioural covariates of cosmetic surgery: Women's health Australia study. J Health Psychol. 2002;7(4):445–57.

Thread Lifting: Treatment Procedure

15

George Sulamanidze, Kajaia Albina,
Konstantin Sulamanidze, Marlen Sulamanidze,
and Souphiyeh Samizadeh

Abstract

Thread lifting represents a significant advancement in facial and body rejuvenation and contouring, straddling the boundary between non-surgical and surgical aesthetic interventions. This chapter delineates the spectrum of thread lifting techniques, emphasizing the importance of a clinical setting for these procedures due to their minimally invasive to invasive nature. Critical to achieving desirable outcomes are thorough patient selection, precise thread choice, and adept technique application. Highlighted are the prerequisites for successful thread lifting: a deep understanding of facial anatomy and aging, meticulous planning of insertion patterns based on individual anatomical considerations and morphology, and adherence to strict aseptic protocols. Through addressing the complexities

G. Sulamanidze (✉)
Clinic of Plastic and Aesthetic Surgery and Cosmetology Total Charm, Tbilisi, Georgia
e-mail: aptos@aptos.ge

K. Albina
Department of Clinic of Plastic Surgery and Dermatology "Total Charm", Tbilisi, Georgia
e-mail: albina@aptos.ru

K. Sulamanidze · M. Sulamanidze
Total Charm Clinic, APTOS, Tbilisi, Georgia
e-mail: const@aptos.ru; gracia@aptos.ru

S. Samizadeh
King's College London, London, UK

University College London, London, UK

Great British Academy of Aesthetic Medicine, London, UK
e-mail: info@baamed.co.uk

© Springer Nature Switzerland AG 2024
S. Samizadeh (ed.), *Thread Lifting Techniques for Facial Rejuvenation and Recontouring*, https://doi.org/10.1007/978-3-031-47954-0_15

involved in thread lifting, including patient expectations, treatment planning, and post-procedure care, this chapter offers healthcare professionals a detailed road-map for executing thread lift procedure with optimal standards.

Keywords

Thread lifting · Thread lift · Facial rejuvenation · Face thread lift · Facelift · Non-surgical facelift · Insertion technique · Thread landmarks · Thread selection

Emphasizing the critical importance of thorough patient evaluation, it becomes clear that success hinges not merely on identifying the correct indications—such as mild to moderate skin laxity, ptosis, superficial rhytids, and volume loss—but on a comprehensive understanding of the patient's medical, social, and cosmetic history, alongside mental health considerations, aesthetic desires, and post-procedural expectations. This foundational approach ensures a tailored treatment, where the selection of suitable threads and strategic planning of insertion patterns are intimately aligned with the natural aging vectors, facial musculature, and the unique anatomical and morphological characteristics of each patient.cknowledging the patient's ideals of beauty, cultural nuances, and ensuring they fully comprehend the procedure's scope, alternative options, associated risks, and benefits are pivotal steps in the consultation process. This comprehensive dialogue aims to align the treatment plan with the patient's expectations, fostering a mutual understanding that lays the groundwork for a successful outcome. It is essential for the practitioner to meticulously explain the importance of adhering to aftercare instructions to optimize healing and enhance the longevity of the results. This chapter systematically outlines the thread lifting procedure, emphasizing the technical execution. It abstracts from specific thread types, indications, or anatomical considerations, focusing instead on the procedural framework essential for all thread lifting interventions. This chapter equips practitioners with a foundational understanding applicable across the diverse spectrum of thread lifting applications, ensuring consistency in prevention of complications and achieving optimal results. Addressing the appropriate indications for thread lifting is paramount, as suboptimal results are often attributed to poor selection of indications, threads, or technical execution. Ensuring a meticulous evaluation process can significantly enhance the likelihood of achieving desired aesthetic outcomes and patient satisfaction.

Indications include [1, 2]:

- Mild-moderate skin laxity
- Mild-moderate ptosis
- Superficial rhytids
- Mild-moderate volume loss
- Adequate subcutaneous fat, quantified as more than 1.5 cm upon gentle pinching, to ensure sufficient tissue support for the threads and durability of the lifting effect.

Following the establishment of clear indications for thread lifting, the subsequent step is the meticulous selection of the appropriate threads and the careful determination of treatment landmarks, crucial for guiding the thread insertion pattern. This phase requires an in-depth understanding of facial aging, encompassing the general principles of thread lifting techniques alongside the specific aims and objectives of the treatment. Critical considerations during this process include:

- The vectors of aging, which vary across different facial areas, highlighting the need for a customized approach to address the unique patterns of ptosis and volume loss.
- The aging process affecting various facial layers, necessitating a strategy that considers the complexity of facial structures and their interactions.
- The significance of facial musculature, where an understanding of muscle function is essential for achieving natural-looking results without compromising facial expressions.
- The dual objectives of thread lifting: bio-stimulation for enhancing skin quality and texture, and lifting/recontouring for adjusting the physical contours of the face.
- A critical understanding of the patient's individual facial anatomy and ethnic characteristics and considerations is essential for the successful customization of the thread lifting procedure.
- Ideals of beauty: The patient's personal ideals of beauty should be thoroughly discussed during the consultation process. This dialogue ensures that the treatment plan aligns with the patient's aesthetic goals and expectations.

Building upon the foundational understanding of a patient's individual facial anatomy and ethnic considerations, it's imperative to engage in thorough discussions regarding standards and ideals of beauty during the consultation phase. This dialogue ensures that the thread lifting procedure aligns with the patient's aesthetic desires. For instance, in the context of East Asian facelifts, where individuals often present with a naturally wider midface and lower face, it's crucial to strategically plan the procedure to avoid further widening these areas, as this does not align with the aesthetic preferences typically held by this demographic. [3–6].

Overall stages of the thread treatment procedure can be seen in Fig. 15.1.

The thread lift procedure is a minimally invasive surgical intervention that necessitates rigorous adherence to aseptic technique to prevent infection and ensure patient safety. Maintaining optimal hand hygiene practices is crucial for all healthcare professionals involved in the procedure. Detailed protocols and guidelines, including a comprehensive summary, are presented in Table 15.1.

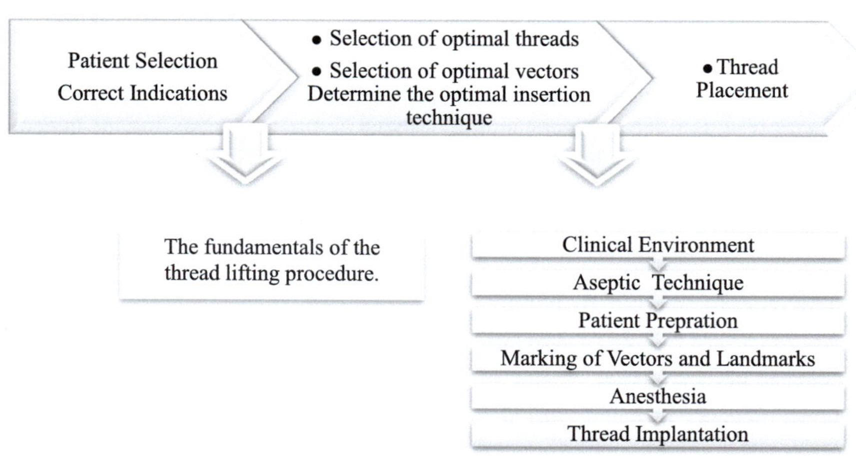

Fig. 15.1 Overall stages of thread treatment procedure

Table 15.1 Summary of guidelines for thread lifting procedure

Facility Prepration	• Thread lifting treatment should be carrived out in a clinical or a surgical room. • Sterile medical tools and consumables are to be prepared beforehand.
Patient Prepration	• On the day of the procedure, comprehensive medical and cosmetic history should be taken again from the patient. • Patient should be informed and educated regarding the procedure, its risks and benefits, potential complications, and the rehabilitation period. • Informed consent to be taken-verbal and written. • Patients are advised to attend without any makeup. All makeup should be removed before the procedure. • The patient's face should be cleansed thoroughly using an antiseptic solution, starting from the center and moving towards the periphery. • A sterile drape should be applied over the patient's face, with an aperture cut to expose the treatment area.
Healthcare Professional Preparation	• It is recommended to wear a surgical gown • Meticulous hand hygiene should be practiced following surgical hand hygiene guidelines. • Sterile gloves should be worn. Utilize a non-touch aseptic technique.

Most surgical site infections often stem from commensal and pathogenic microorganisms originating from the patient's microbiota, which may include antibiotic-resistant strains. Key steps in prevention include:

- Conducting the procedure in a clinical environment conducive to sterility.
- Ensuring the utilization of sterile consumables, instruments, and gloves throughout the procedure.
- Preparing the patient according to surgical standards, including the use of a sterile drape to isolate the treatment area.

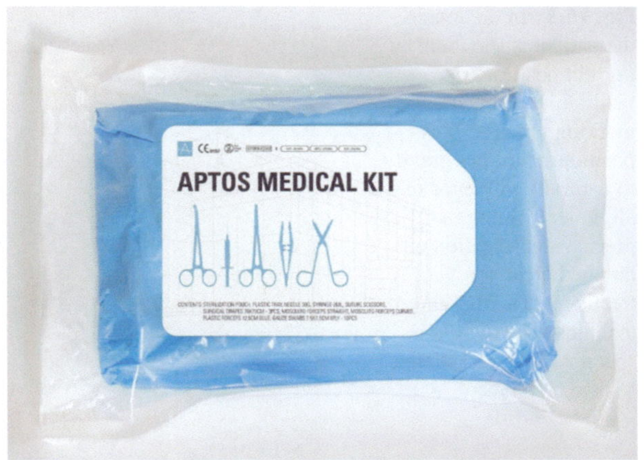

Fig. 15.2 Sterile instruments for the procedure. The APTOS medical kit contains all the required instruments. (Image credit APTOS)

Instruments and Consumables for the Procedure

- The Procedure Room: Ensure the availability of a dedicated medical procedure room equipped for the task.
- Medical Kits and Surgical Procedure Trays: Ensure the availability and organization of medical kits and surgical procedure trays containing all necessary instruments and consumables for the procedure.
- Sterile instruments: forceps, scissors, a clip for skin procedures (if necessary, you can add two mosquito-type clips and two hats to the kit), or use the APTOS Medical Kit (Fig. 15.2).
- 5- or 10-mL syringe—2 pcs., 30G needle, 18G needle (if not included with threads); APTOS threads are enclosed with all required attributes: 18G × 40 mm lancet point needle (to make an entry point), round tip cannula (for infiltration anaesthetic and thread insertion).
- Skin disinfection solution (Octenisept, Betadine, Chlorhexidine).
- Adrenaline-containing anaesthetic 1:100,000 to 1:200,000 (ultracaine, ubistesin, septanest, etc.).
- Sterile gloves, gown, cap, and mask.
- Surgical drape and cap for the patient.

Landmarks and Insertion Path Determination

Thread lifting necessitates thorough pre-planning. Following development of an individualized treatment plan, precise pathways for thread implantation are demarcated using medical marking pens (Fig. 15.3). The marking is performed with the patient in an upright position to ensure accurate assessment of gravitational effects. Following identification of the target tissue for lifting, referred to as the 'zone of action,' precise marking of entry points and implantation trajectories for each thread

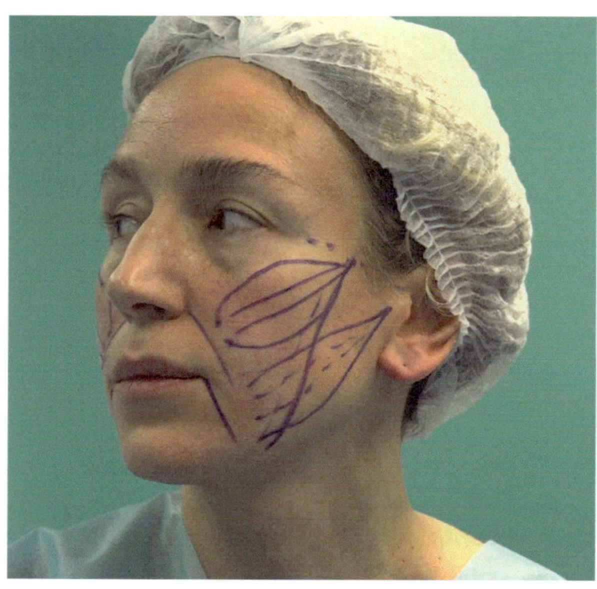

Fig. 15.3 In the image, the patient is shown in an upright position, facilitating an accurate marking process. This positioning allows gravity to naturally influence tissue alignment, aiding in precise identification of targeted areas for treatment. The marking technique showcased is specific to the Excellence Visage method.

is undertaken. The primary objective of this marking procedure is to ensure symmetrical alignment between the right and left sides.

Skin Preparation

- Stage 1: To remove organic debris, dirt, makeup, skin secretions (sweat and sebum), and superficial microorganisms.
  - Remove makeup completely (recommend patients to attend with no makeup)
  - Carefully wash and clean the skin
- Stage 2: To reduce resident skin flora substantially and achieve residual antiseptic activity. It is not possible to completely sterilize the skin.
- Main antiseptic agents used for pre-operative skin preparation (aqueous or alcohol-based form):
  - Chlorhexidine gluconate (CHG)
  - Iodophors (povidone iodine; PI)

Both agents exhibit efficacy against a broad spectrum of skin microorganisms and provide persistent activity, preventing regrowth for several hours post-application. Adequate application of the chosen antiseptic solution is essential, extending from the area of operation to adjacent sites. Gauze swabs are utilized for even distribution of antiseptic agents. Caution should be exercised with the use of CHG, as it can be inactivated by soaps and shampoos, irritate the eyes, and cause corneal burns or ototoxicity if it enters the eyes or ears. Application should proceed outward from the treatment area, followed by the placement of a surgical drape (Figs. 15.4 and 15.5).

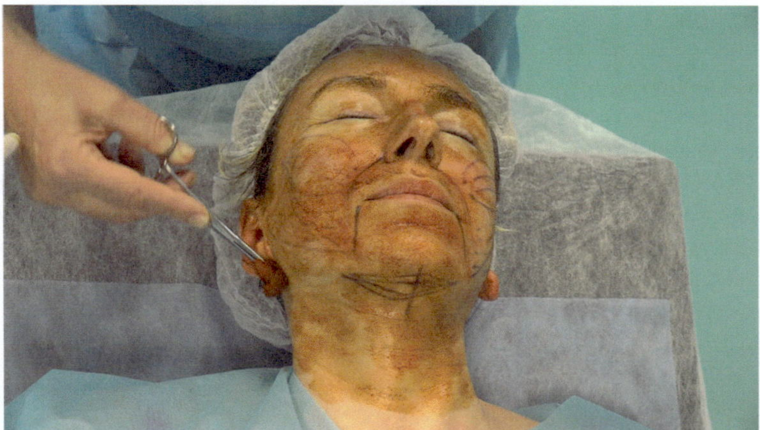

Fig. 15.4 Skin preparation using iodophor solution, applied with a gauze swab and sterile forceps, exemplifying the meticulous process of pre-operative skin preparation.

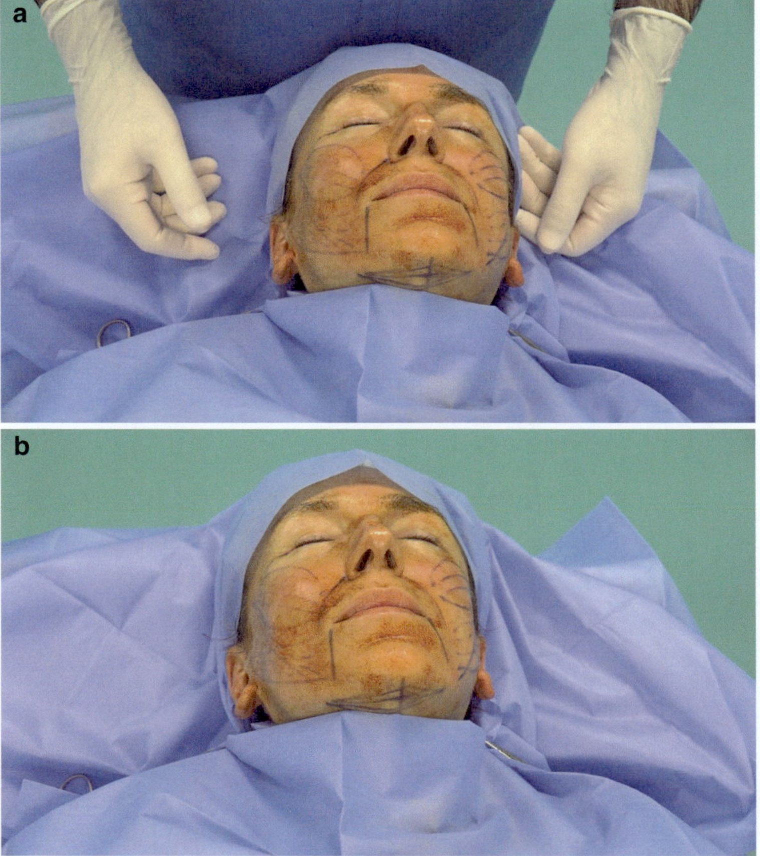

Fig. 15.5 Isolation of area of treatment

Anaesthesia

Post disinfection and placement of the surgical drape, local anesthesia is administered. Initially, entry points are infiltrated with 1% lidocaine combined with epinephrine (adrenaline) at a ratio of 1:100,000 to 1:200,000, facilitating analgesia (Fig. 15.6). Epinephrine serves the dual purpose of inducing vasoconstriction, unless contraindicated, and prolonging the anesthetic's duration of action. Following a brief interval (1–2 minutes), an 18G × 40 mm needle can be used to establish entry points. A cannula can then be used for infiltration and to anesthetize the delineated areas according to previously marked pathways, administering the anesthetic retrogradely (0.1–0.5 mL per path) (Figs. 15.6 and 15.7).

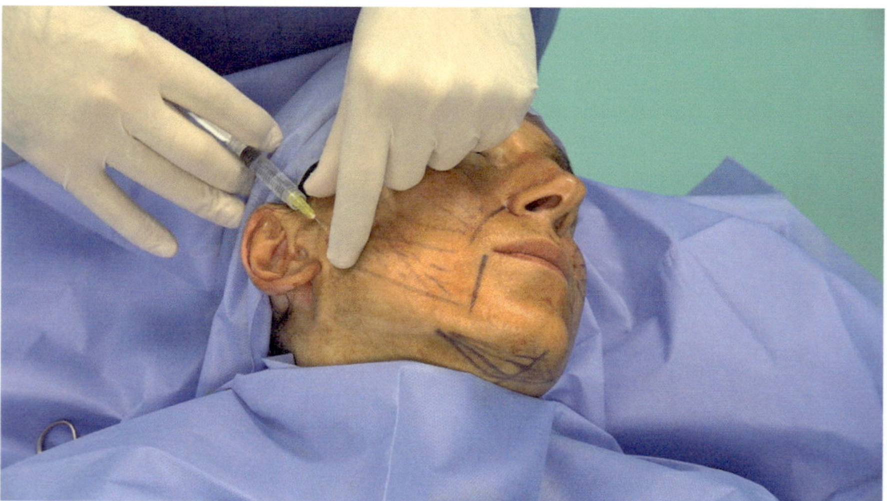

Fig. 15.6 Initial administration of local anaesthesia for the entry point using a 30G needle

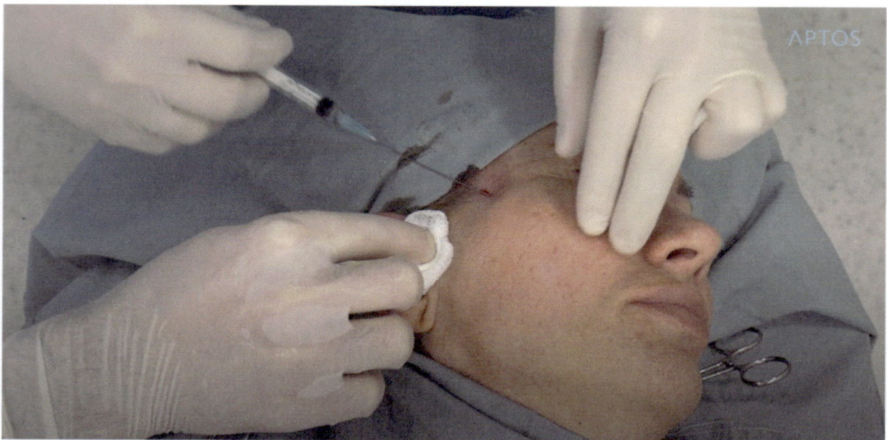

Fig. 15.7 Anaesthesia of the area to be treated using a cannula

Insertion Techniques

The method of suture insertion significantly influences the outcome of thread treatment.

Insert the needle or cannula at a 90-degree angle to the skin, gently gathering it into a fold (Fig. 15.8). Advance the cannula/needle in the subcutaneous tissue under the skin parallel to its surface. Progress the cannula/needle under the skin parallel to its surface. Always assess the depth of the needle or cannula movement during

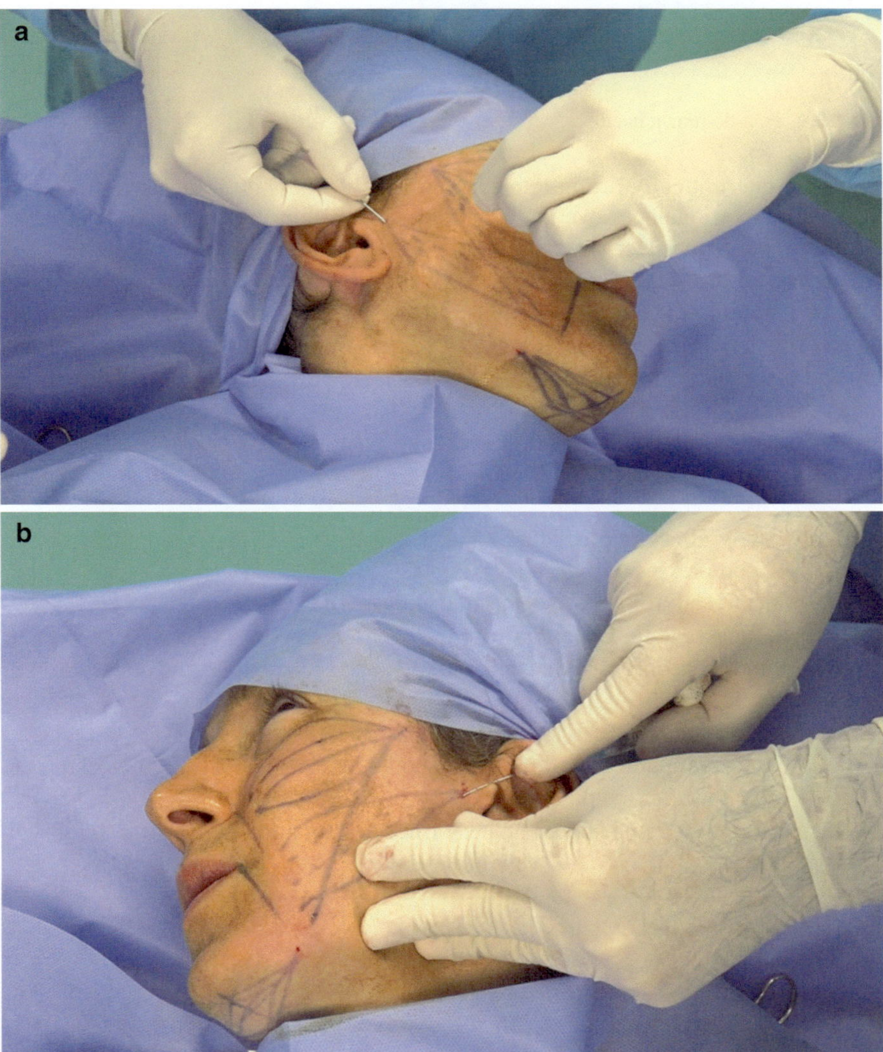

Fig. 15.8 Insertion and advancing of thread with a cannula/needle into the subcutaneous layer

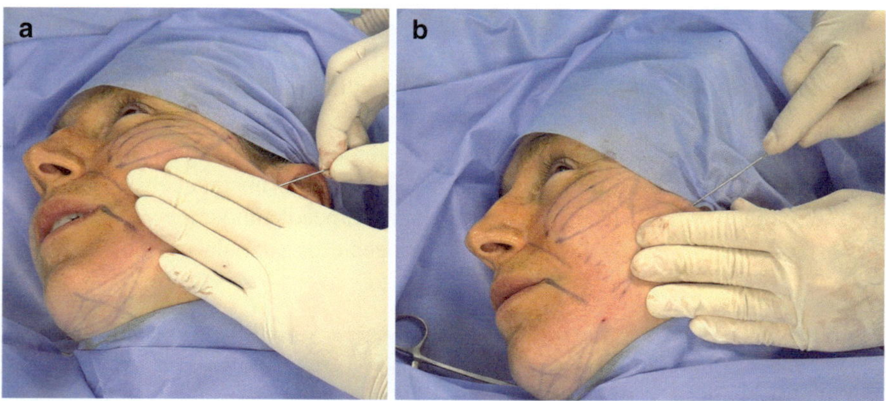

Fig. 15.9 Non-dominant hand

insertion, intermittently lifting it to evaluate the thickness of tissue above it (elevation test). Additionally, move the cannula/needle within the implantation plane to ensure proper layer placement (oscillating test). Correct placement within the subcutaneous tissue is confirmed when the guide moves smoothly along the path. Incorrect options include intradermal insertion or advancing the guide to deeper layers, which may encounter resistance. The non-dominant hand can assist in guiding and positioning the threads (Fig. 15.9).

Rehabilitation

- Immediately after the procedure and for 2–3 days after that, the patient should use cold compresses (e.g. Icepack).
- The patient is advised not to apply makeup for 48 h.
- No facial massage for 2 months.
- No thermal procedures (steam bath, bathtub, and sauna) and avoid direct sunlight for 1 month.
- No sports or intensive activity for 2 weeks.
- Follow-up examinations of the patient should be carried out 1, 2, 4 weeks, 3, 6, and 12 months after the procedure;
- Control photographing should be performed at 3, 6, and 12 months.

Combination with Other Treatments

- Botulinum toxin—2 weeks before the procedure
- Light and laser devices—1 month before or after the procedure
- On the day of the procedure, chemical peels, micro-needling, or other dermatological procedures
- Fillers—2–3 weeks after the procedure

- Biorevitalization—2 weeks before the procedure
- PRP—1 week before, on the day and 1 week after the procedure
- Further thread-lifting procedure—after 12–18 months

Conclusion

Thread lifting is a term encompassing a broad range of procedures, from the placement of a few thin surgical sutures beneath the skin to the use of numerous long threads with diverse surface characteristics for repositioning soft tissues. As such, thread lifting techniques can vary significantly in their invasiveness, spanning from minimally invasive approaches to those that are more complex and require precise surgical intervention. The efficacy of thread lifting as a versatile and effective method for facial rejuvenation and recontouring places it uniquely between non-invasive therapies and traditional surgical facelifts. However, the success of these procedures is critically dependent on meticulous patient evaluation, the selection of appropriate threads, and the precision of the technique applied.This chapter has highlighted the paramount importance of conducting thread lifting within a clinical setting to ensure the highest standards of safety and asepsis are maintained, reflecting the procedure's complexity and its position on the spectrum of invasive interventions. Adherence to the detailed guidelines and principles discussed is essential for complication prevention and optimal outcomes.This comprehensive approach to thread lifting not only ensures the safety and well-being of patients but also enriches the practitioner's toolkit with a procedure that harmonizes science, art, and technique in the pursuit of beauty and youthfulness.

References

1. Halepas S, Chen XJ, Ferneini EM. Thread-lift sutures: anatomy, technique, and review of current literature. J Oral Maxillofac Surg. 2020;78(5):813–20.
2. Kim B, Kim B, Oh S, Jung W. The art and science of thread lifting. Springer; 2019.
3. Samizadeh S. The ideals of facial beauty among Chinese aesthetic practitioners: results from a large national survey. Aesthet Plast Surg. 2018;43:102–14.
4. Samizadeh S, Wu W. Ideals of facial beauty amongst the Chinese population: results from a large national survey. Aesthet Plast Surg. 2018;42:102–14.
5. Liew S, Wu WT, Chan HH, Ho WW, Kim H-J, Goodman GJ, et al. Consensus on changing trends, attitudes, and concepts of Asian beauty. Aesthet Plast Surg. 2016;40(2):193–201.
6. Liew S. Discussion: Microbotox of the lower face and neck: evolution of a personal technique and its clinical effects. Plast Reconstr Surg. 2015;136(5 Suppl):101s–3s.

Part IV

Threadlifting Techniques and Combination Treatments

Thread Lift for East Asian Facial Rejuvenation

16

Chia-Hsien Hsieh, Hsien-Li Peter Peng, and Souphiyeh Samizadeh

C.-H. Hsieh
Diamond Cosmetic Clinic, Taipei, Taiwan, R.O.C.

Diamond-biotechnology Co., Ltd., Taipei, Taiwan, R.O.C.

H.-L. P. Peng (✉)
P-Skin Professional Clinic & Hair Restoration Center, Kaohsiung, Taiwan, R.O.C.

Department of Dermatology, Tri-Service General Hospital, National Defense Medical Center, Taipei, Taiwan

Laser and Photonics Medicine Society of Taiwan (LMSTW), Taipei, Taiwan

Taiwanese Dermatological Association (TDA), Taipei, Taiwan

Taiwanese Society for Dermatological & Aesthetic Surgery (TSDAS), Taipei, Taiwan

Taiwan Society of Hair Restoration Surgery (TSHRS), Taipei, Taiwan

Chinese Across the Strait Association of Plastic and Aesthetic (CASAPA), Beijing, China

ISDS, Darmstadt, Germany

DASIL, Milwaukee, WI, USA

International Medicine Affairs Committee, Kaohsiung City Medical Association, Kaohsiung, Taiwan, R.O.C.

S. Samizadeh
King's College London, London, UK

University College London, London, UK

Revivify London Clinic, London, UK

Great British Academy of Aesthetic Medicine, London, UK
e-mail: info@baamed.co.uk

© Springer Nature Switzerland AG 2024
S. Samizadeh (ed.), *Thread Lifting Techniques for Facial Rejuvenation and Recontouring*, https://doi.org/10.1007/978-3-031-47954-0_16

Abstract

Thread lifting has gained significant popularity in Asia as a minimally invasive option for facial rejuvenation and recontouring, reflecting the region's unique beauty ideals that often vary from Western preferences. This chapter discusses the application of Polydioxanone (PDO) threads for enhancing and rejuvenating various facial areas, including the upper face, midface, and lower face. It provides a comprehensive overview of use of PDO threads in achieving a lifted, more youthful appearance by addressing concerns such as sagging eyebrows, nasolabial folds, and the appearance of a double chin. Additionally, the chapter emphasizes the importance of understanding the anatomical and morphological nuances of the Asian face and East Asian ideals of beauty to tailor treatments that align with regional aesthetic preferences. It also covers critical aspects of complications prevention and management, offering insights into ensuring patient safety and optimizing outcomes. Through a detailed exploration of PDO thread-lifting, this chapter aims to equipt healthcare professionals with the knowledge to apply these techniques effectively in their practice, considering the diverse beauty standards and facial features prevalent in Asia.

Keywords

Thread lift · Thread lifting · Thread-lift method · Thread-lift technique · Thread-lift procedure · Threading · Facial rejuvenation · Asian facial rejuvenation · East Asian facelift · East Asian face thread lift

The quest for minimally invasive techniques that promise youthful rejuvenation with minimal downtime has led to the widespread adoption of threadlifting. This procedure, particularly embraced in Asia, not only reflects the unique beauty standards of the region but also aligns with the global trend towards less invasive cosmetic interventions. The market offers a wide array of threadlifting products, yet not all meet the rigorous standards of sterility or have the endorsement of regulatory bodies such as the FDA in various countries. It is crucial for practitioners to exercise diligence in sourcing their materials, prioritizing threads that are not only sterile but also backed by reputable manufacturers. These providers are distinguished not only by their commitment to quality and safety but also by their support for medical professionals through both initial and advanced training programs. Such educational opportunities are invaluable, ensuring that practitioners are well-versed in the latest techniques and supported throughout their practice.

A profound understanding of facial anatomy underpins the success of threadlifting techniques. Practitioners are urged to enhance their anatomical knowledge through specialized training, ideally supplemented with cadaver dissection, beyond their initial medical or dental education. This deepened anatomical insight is critical in avoiding complications such as nerve damage, facial asymmetry, or unnatural expressions, ensuring that the placement of threads in target layers accurately for optimal aesthetic outcomes [1].

Ensuring all procedures are carried out in a clinical setting with strict adherence to aseptic practices is paramount. For anesthesia, a 2% lidocaine solution is recommended, tailored to the specific area of the face being treated. For instance, in procedures targeting the upper face, anesthesia can be achieved through sensory blocks of the supratrochlear and supraorbital nerves, utilizing 1% or 2% lidocaine with epinephrine for effective numbing at the insertion points. This approach to anesthesia is integral to a pain-free, comfortable experience for the patient, facilitating precise and effective thread placement. This chapter discusses the intricacies of using Polydioxanone (PDO) threads for enhancing and rejuvenating different areas of the face. It aims to provide practitioners with a comprehensive understanding of how to effectively apply these threads to meet the diverse aesthetic desires of their patients. Through detailed guidance on technique, anatomical considerations, and safety protocols, this chapter serves as a valuable resource for achieving superior results in facial rejuvenation with PDO threads, reinforcing the practitioner's commitment to excellence in patient care.

Forehead and Eyebrows

The application of threads in the upper face primarily targets forehead and eyebrow elevation, and skin rejuvenation through biostimulation. For addressing volume loss in the forehead, dermal fillers are more appropriate, while neuromodulators, can be used to address rhytids by relaxing the underlying muscles. This combination approach allows for a nuanced treatment plan that addresses both structural and aesthetic concerns, providing a tailored solution to meet individual patient needs. The upper facial area presents unique challenges for thread lifting, including:

1. The skin's thinness, which demands precise handling.
2. The strong, active frontalis muscle.
3. Adherent tissues with minimal fat pads and limited spacing between layers, requiring careful navigation.
4. A complex vasculature that increases the risk of bruising and vascular injury.
5. The proximity to the supraorbital and supratrochlear nerves, necessitating caution to avoid nerve damage.

Although lifting the forehead with threads presents challenges due to anatomical complexities, it remains a viable option for achieving subtle rejuvenation. Threads not only offer a means for collagen stimulation and elevation of the eyebrows but are also effective in enhancing the glabella complex for a more youthful appearance.

For elevation, practitioners have two primary strategies. The initial approach involves inserting the thread cannula from the hairline, advancing it deeply along the periosteum towards the eyebrows. At this juncture, the decision to pierce the

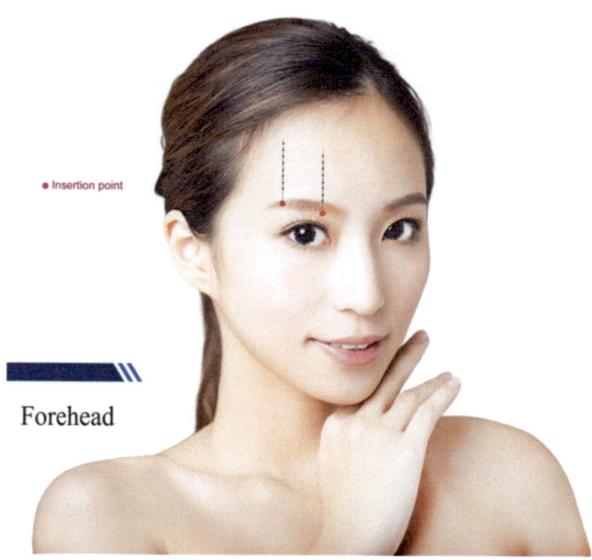

Fig. 16.1 Insertion points.
(Image credit:
CanStockPhoto)

skin and exit the thread or not can be made. The former approach can enhance the lifting effect, though it may lead to temporary dimpling. For this technique, the use of robust, thicker threads like barbed 1-0 threads is preferable, given their placement in a deeper tissue layer (Figs. 16.1 and 16.2).

Alternatively, the cannula may be inserted starting from the eyebrows and directed back towards the hairline, allowing the thread to lie within the subcutaneous layer. This method accommodates finer threads, such as 3-0 threads, but necessitates the use of a greater number of threads. Due to their size, these threads present a reduced risk of becoming visible, palpable and extrsion. However, given the frontalis muscle's strength and frequent movement, there is a heightened chance of thread displacement and diminished efficacy. Consequently, augmenting thread lifts in this region with energy-based devices (EBD) like High-Intensity Focused Ultrasound (HIFU) or Radiofrequency (RF), or using botulinum toxins to reduce muscle activity, can enhance outcomes.

Both smooth and non-smooth Polydioxanone (PDO) threads offer a viable solution for filling in static wrinkles. This approach is particularly appealing for the upper face, where the risk associated with dermal filler treatments is higher. For treating static wrinkles, 1-0 multi-directional wedge-shaped PDO sutures/threads, inserted via an 18G cannula, can be effective. Employing two to six barbed PDO threads in a 'stacked pattern' per site within the subcutaneous layer optimizes results. Depending on the depth of the wrinkles, two to four-folded barbed PDO threads are suitable for superficial lines, while three to six threads may be required for more pronounced wrinkles, arranged in an overlapping fashion for every 3–4 cm segment of the targeted area and static rhytid [2] (Fig. 16.3).

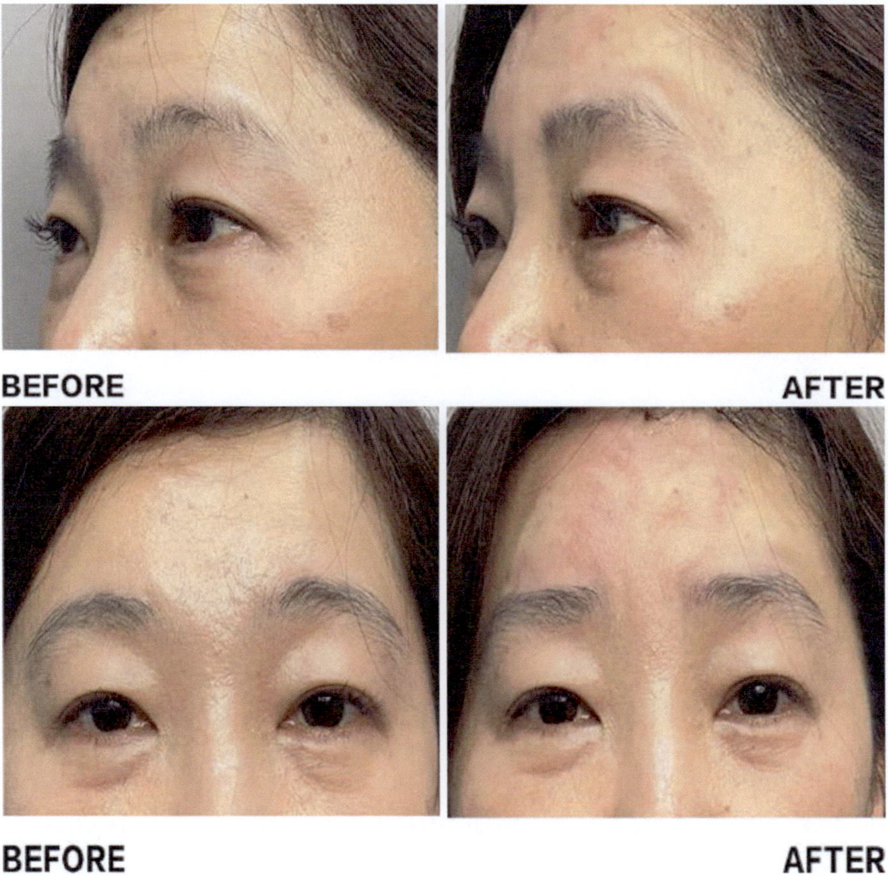

BEFORE   **AFTER**

BEFORE   **AFTER**

Fig. 16.2 Before and after photos illustrating eyebrow elevation in a 50-year-old lady who underwent thread lifting with eight 3-0 bi-directional PDO cog threads on each side of her forehead. A mild torsion of the forehead was observed post-treatment but spontaneously resolved within 3 to 7 days

Fig. 16.3 (**a**) Multi-directional wedge-shaped PDO sutures. (**b**) Short (3–4 cm), barbed PDO threads in a folded configuration can be placed in the subcutaneous layer. Gentle pressure can be applied to the overlying skin with the non-dominant hand while simultaneously rotating and withdrawing the cannula with the working hand [2]

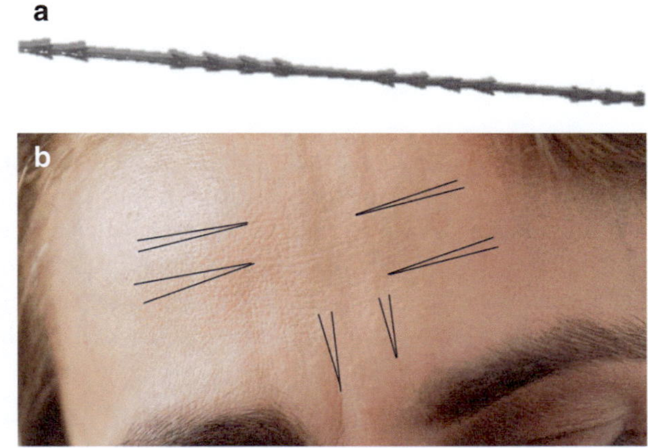

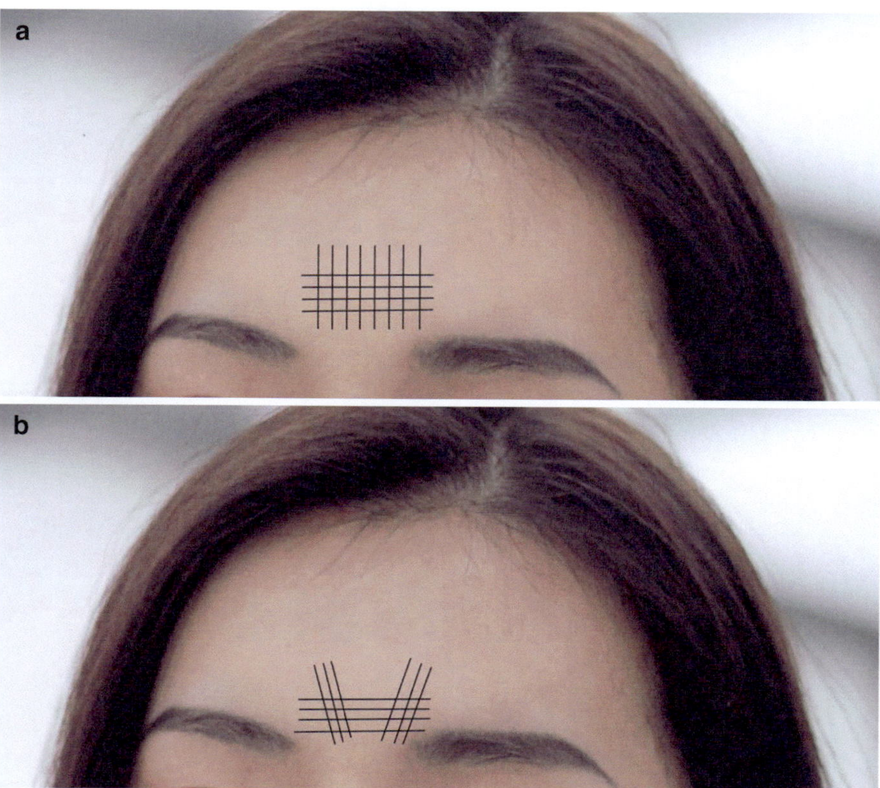

Fig. 16.4 (**a**) Crosshatch technique for biostimulation and skin improvement. (**b**) Technique for biostimulation and skin improvement in the glabella region

Other commonly used patterns for bio-stimulation and rhytids can be seen below (Fig. 16.4a, b). These are just examples; the number of threads, the pattern used, and their exact location depends on patient factors and the type of threads used. The recommended space between threads is 1 cm.

Clinical cases of wrinkle reduction treatment are shown in Figs. 16.5 and 16.6.

Eyebrows

The eyebrows serve as a critical feature of the face, framing the eyes and significantly influencing facial expression and overall appearance. Their shape, position, and fullness are not just markers of beauty but also convey emotions and contribute to the perception of age. Well-defined, appropriately positioned eyebrows can lift the appearance of the face, creating a more alert and rejuvenated look (Fig. 16.7). With age, the eyebrow position, shape and hair density changes, leading to a tired or sad appearance.

Fig. 16.5 Preoperative and postoperative clinical photographs of a patient who received thread augmentation with short, folded, wedge-shaped PDO sutures for the static wrinkles on the forehead and glabella: (**a**) initial; (**b**) 2-month follow-up. White circle indicated treatment areas before and after procedure. Reproduced with permission from Kang SH, Moon SH, Rho BI, Youn SJ, Kim HS. Wedge—shaped polydioxanone threads in a folded configuration ('Solid fillers'): A treatment option for deep static wrinkles on the upper face. *Journal of Cosmetic Dermatology.* 2019;18(1):65–70 [2]

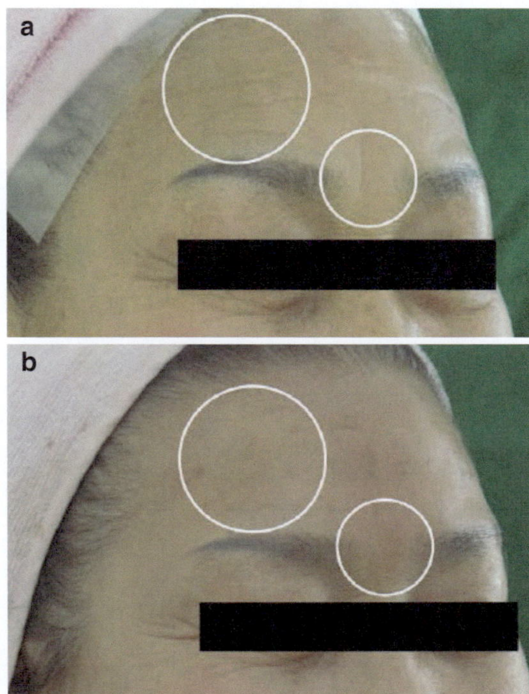

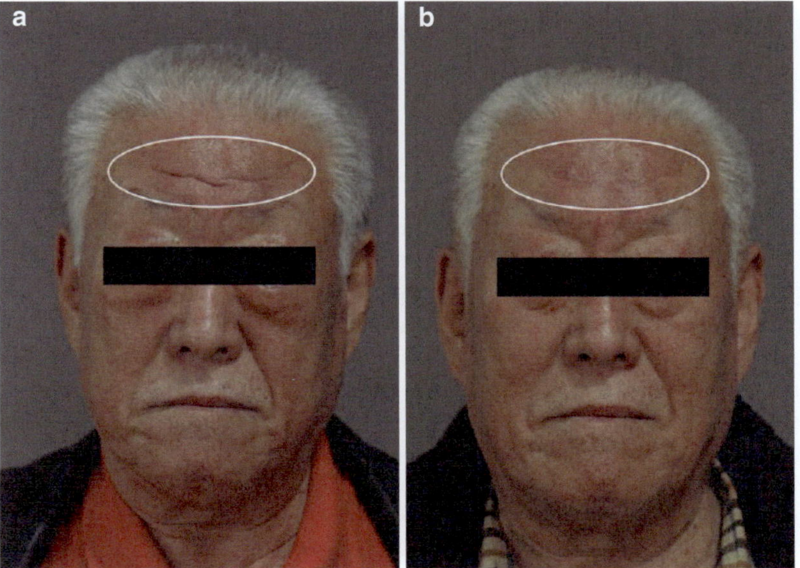

Fig. 16.6 Preoperative and postoperative clinical photographs of a patient who received thread augmentation with short, folded, wedge-shaped PDO sutures for the static wrinkles on the forehead and glabella: (**a**) initial; (**b**) 2-month follow-up. White circle indicated treatment areas before and after procedure. Reproduced with permission from Kang SH, Moon SH, Rho BI, Youn SJ, Kim HS. Wedge—shaped polydioxanone threads in a folded configuration ('Solid fillers'): A treatment option for deep static wrinkles on the upper face. *Journal of Cosmetic Dermatology.* 2019;18(1):65–70 [2]

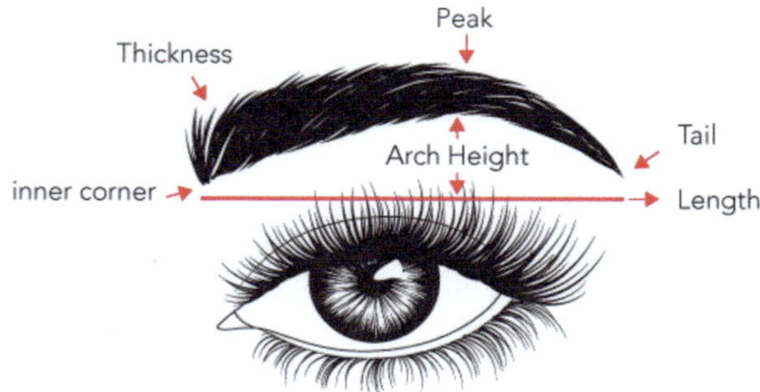

Fig. 16.7 Ideal position and shape of eyebrows

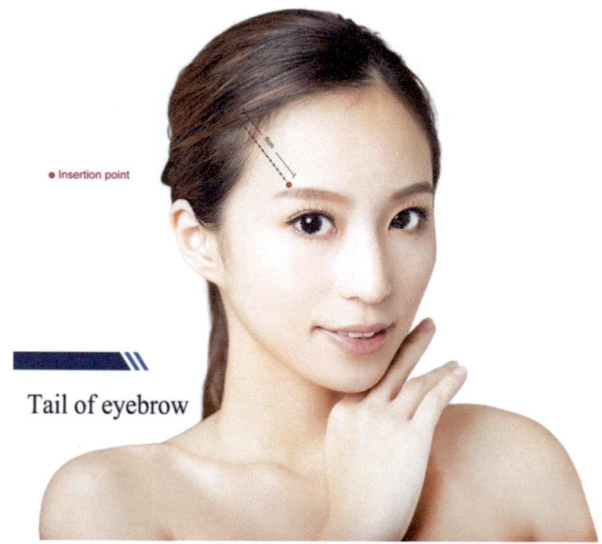

Fig. 16.8 Different thread-lifting method targeting the eyebrow tails for subtle elevation and contouring. (Image credit: CanStockPhoto)

Eyebrows can be lifted using thread-lifting methods (Fig. 16.8). In Western and Middle Eastern beauty ideals, a pronounced eyebrow arch or a lifted tail is frequently desired for its aesthetic appeal. However, these specific modifications are generally not preferred among East Asian women. Over-emphasizing the arch or lifting the tail in this demographic can unintentionally convey expressions of perplexity, irritation and anger, diverging from the subtle, natural enhancements, and the "soft look" more commonly valued in East Asian beauty standards.To circumvent this, the thread lift procedure can be strategically tailored with subtle adjustments in eyebrow position, ensuring results that harmonize with the individual's aesthetic preferences and cultural standards. Threads can be placed either from the hairline down towards the eyebrows or vice versa.

The position of the lateral canthus can be very slightly and temporarily elevated (Figs. 16.9 and 16.10). Due to the eyelids' exceptionally thin skin, it is strongly advised to use a 3-0 thread for treatment in this delicate area. As demonstrated in

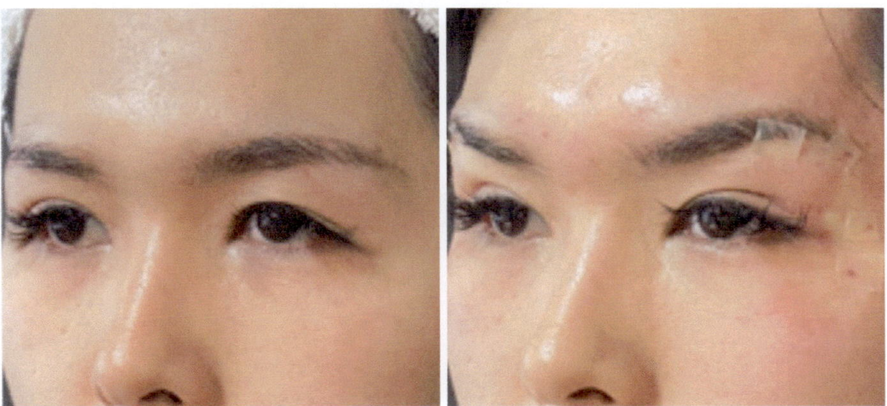

Fig. 16.9 Before and after (immediately) pictures of a 30-year-old lady had thread lifting of the eyebrow's tail using four 1-0 bi-directional cogged threads on each side, retrograde

Fig. 16.9, the technique involves inserting the thread and subtly yet directly lifting the lateral part of the eyelid, offering a potent and effective approach for achieving an immediate lift. This area has a rich capillary network, making it susceptible to bruising during interventions. To enhance treatment outcomes, it is recommended to combine the procedure with carefully calibrated injection of botulinum toxins.

Figure 16.11 represents a comprehensive technique for eyebrow lifting using PDO threads through a double-layer sequential insertion, as outlined in the study 'Immediate treatment of botulinum toxin type A-induced brow ptosis' by Kyoung et al. Morphometric measurements crucial for evaluating brow position and incorporating anatomical landmarks for accurate intervention are provided. This technique is meticulously outlined by the ordered placement of threads from 1 to 12, utilizing both 9-cm and 6-cm multi-directional cogged threads. The approach integrates a deep layer technique, placing threads into the subperiosteal layer and the galeal fat pad, alongside a superficial layer method, entering through the same point into the subcutaneous fat. Following the procedure, protocols include securing the forehead with 3M tape for three days and applying cold compression for two days.

This innovative use of PDO cog thread insertion for the immediate treatment of brow ptosis induced by botulinum toxin type A, offers a promising approach for addressing eyebrow ptosis [3].

Additionally, various other techniques have been explored and documented by different authors, catering to a wide range of aesthetic preferences and anatomical considerations. Among these, the A-PDO technique stands out for its particular appeal to the Caucasian demographic, showcasing the diversity and customization potential of thread lifting procedures in meeting the specific aesthetic goals of different populations [4].

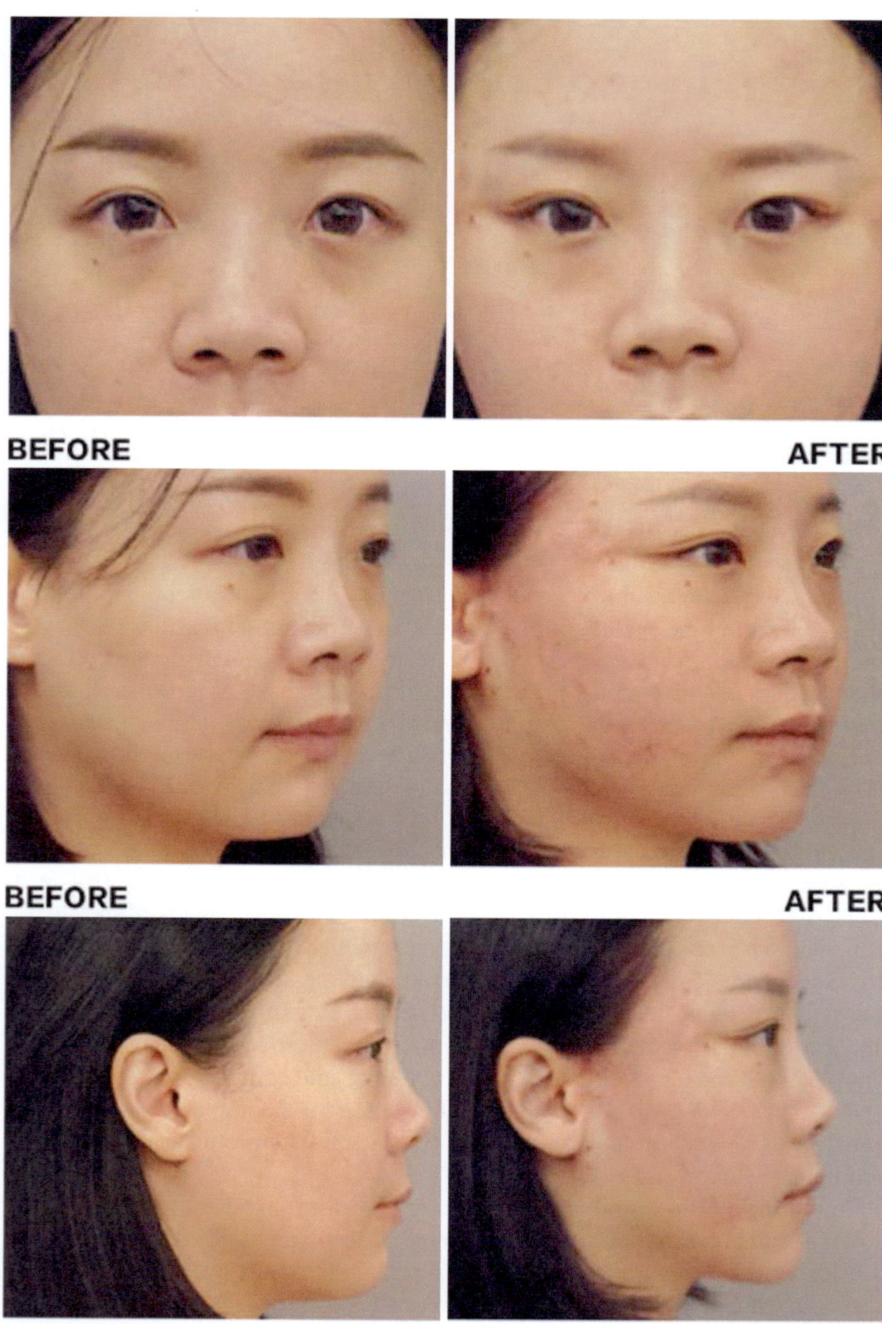

Fig. 16.10 Before and after (immediately) photos of a 35-year-old lady following a thread lift procedure aimed at elevating the lateral aspects of the eyebrows. Four 1-0 bi-directional cogged threads were used on each side, retrograde insertion. Additionally, treatment of the mid-face is evident. Any skin puckering and slight overcorrection observed typically resolves within 1-3 days following the procedure

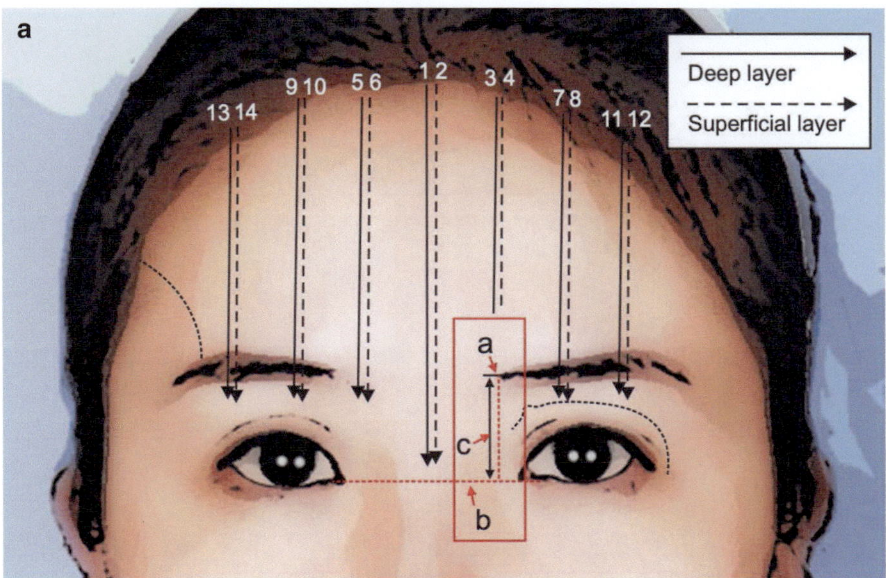

Fig. 16.11 (**a**) Double-layer sequential insertion of multi-directional cogged PDO thread. The numbers (i.e. 1–12) represent the insertion of the thread in order. Numbers 1 and 2 are 9-cm-long threads, and the others are 6-cm-long threads. Morphometric measurement of the brow position (red square): a superomedial angle of the eyebrow; b connecting line between both medial canthi; c, the distance between a and b. In this technique, the author places threads into the subperiosteal layer in the upper half of the forehead and into the galeal fat pad and brow fat (i.e. the deep layer approach) in the lower half of the forehead. Threads were also inserted into the subcutaneous superficial fat layer through the same entry site (i.e. the superficial layer approach). 3 M tape was used to fix the forehead for 3 days post-procedure, and cold compression was applied for 2 days [3]. Reproduced with permission from Kyoung-Jin Ka, Kang, K.J. and Chai, C.Y., 2017. Immediate treatment of botulinum toxin type A-induced brow ptosis with polydioxanone cog thread insertion. *Journal of Cosmetic Medicine*, 1(1), 46–51. (**b**) Morphological changes of the ptotic brows and their surrounding soft tissues by brow lifting using cogged PDO threads. Four women (1, 2, 3, and 4) underwent botulinum toxin injection to improve the forehead, glabella, or/and crow's feet. Side effects happened 2–3 days after the procedure. Three-to-seven days after the botulinum toxin injection, all three patients received brow lifting using PDO threads. The patients were followed up for 2 weeks (1′, 2′, 3′, and 4′) to a maximum of 3 months (1″, 2″, 3″, and 4″) after the brow lifting procedure. a–a″, forehead volume deficiency; b–b″, swelling and sagging of glabella, nasion, and upper eyelid; and c–c″, transverse wrinkle. Reproduced with permission from Kyoung-Jin Ka, Kang, K.J. and Chai, C.Y., 2017. Immediate treatment of botulinum toxin type A-induced brow ptosis with polydioxanone cog thread insertion. *Journal of Cosmetic Medicine*, 1(1), 46–51 [3]

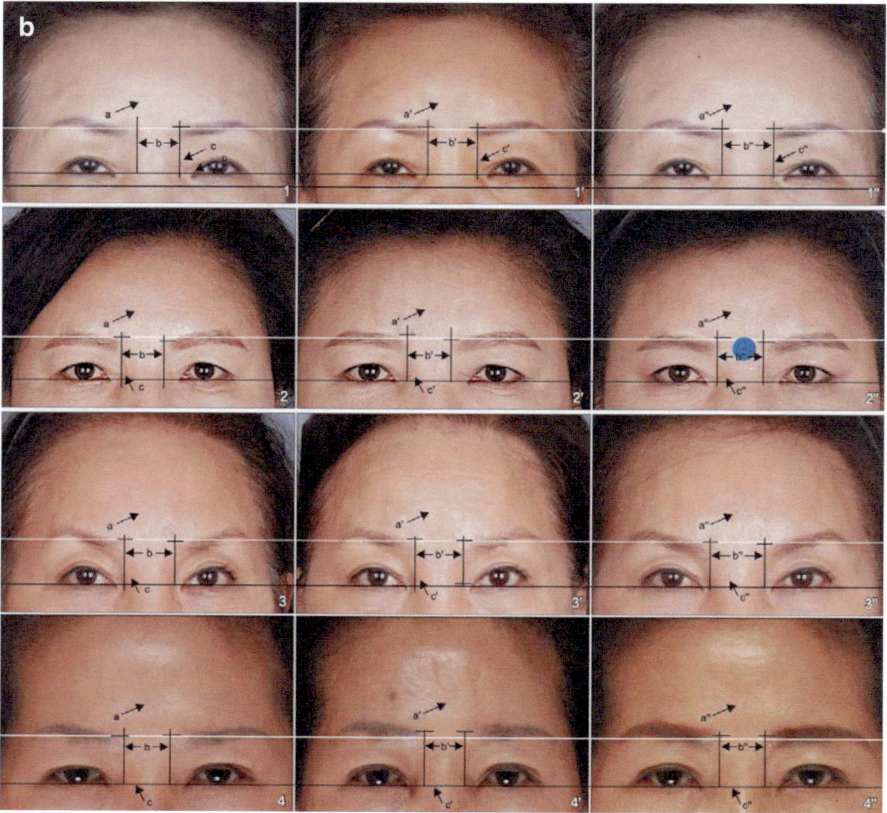

Fig. 16.11 (continued)

Nasolabial Fold

Nasolabial folds often emerge as a primary concern among individuals seeking cosmetic enhancements and anti-aging treatments. With mid-face aging, several key morphological changes take place: the descent of attenuated lower eyelid skin below the inferior orbital rim, a downward shift of the malar fat pad leading to diminished malar prominence, a more pronounced tear trough deformity, and deepening of nasolabial folds. These changes collectively contribute to the more visible signs of aging [5].

The underlying causes of pronounced nasolabial folds are multifaceted, encompassing factors such as bone resorption, muscle contraction, fat accumulation, and skin sagging. These elements contribute to the complexity of effectively treating deep nasolabial folds [6, 7].

Thread lifting offers a solution to mitigate ptosis, while fillers can address volume loss [8]. Botulinum toxin injections are effective in relaxing overactive muscles, and techniques like high-intensity focused ultrasound (HIFU) can reduce fat deposits. Given the distinct targets of these treatments, a combined therapeutic approach is often advocated, especially for addressing the unique aesthetic concerns prevalent in the Asian demographic.

Thread lifting yields a trifecta of benefits: immediate lifting through mechanical action, cellular rejuvenation via collagen stimulation, and enhanced skin texture through neovascularization [9].

For treating ptotic tissue, the technique involves inserting threadain a cannula from the scalp in the temporal region to the nasolaboal folds.This strategic placement allows for the repositioning and lifting of midface tissues, including the nasolabial folds, also affecting the lower face, leveraging the principle of vector extension to exert lifting effects on the lower midface (Figs. 16.12, 16.13, 16.14).

An alternative approach to lifting the nasolabial fold involves the sub-zygomatic method, where the cannula is guided from the temporal scalp, passing through the deep buccal fat pad, and extending to the nasolabial area. This technique preserves natural facial expressions by avoiding alterations in muscle dynamics. Due to its technical complexity, it requires a high level of precision and understanding of facial anatomy, making it suitable exclusively for practitioners with extensive experience in facial surgery.

Fig. 16.12 Nasolabial fold thread placement. (Image credit: CanStockPhoto)

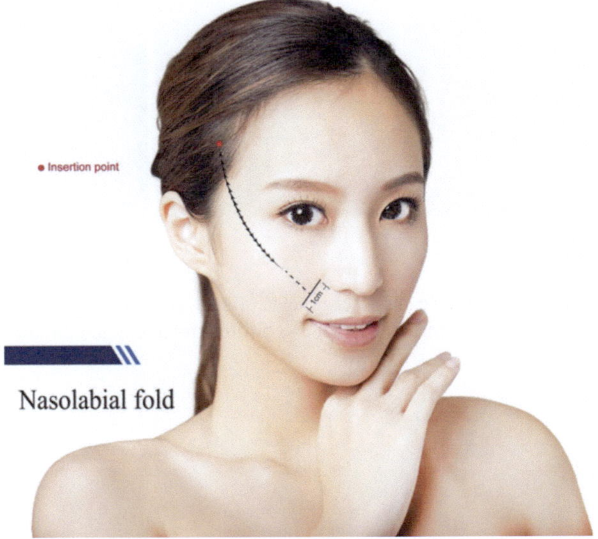

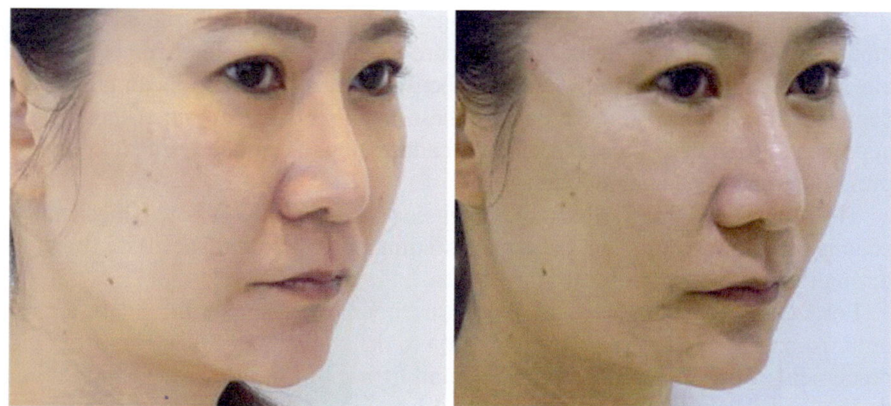

Fig. 16.13 Before and after images of a 40-year-old lady who underwent thread lifting for naso-labial fold correction with four 1-0 bi-directional cogged threads on each side

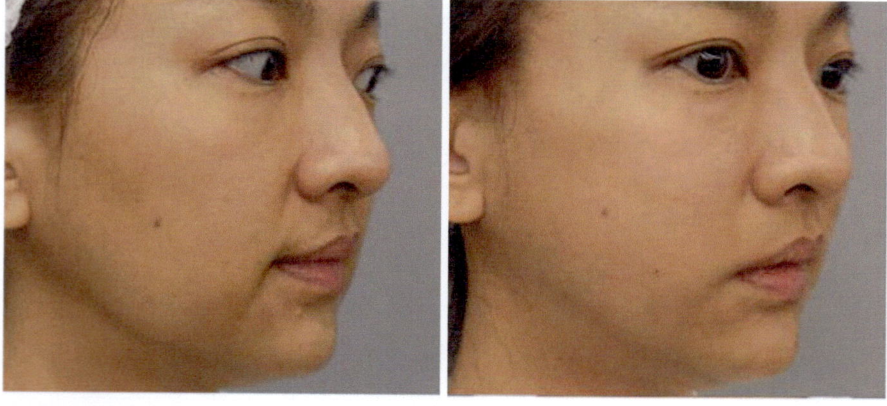

Fig. 16.14 Before and after images of a 38-year-old lady who underwent thread lifting for naso-labial fold correction with four 1-0 bi-directional cogged threads on each side

Fig. 16.15 Medical cheek thread placement

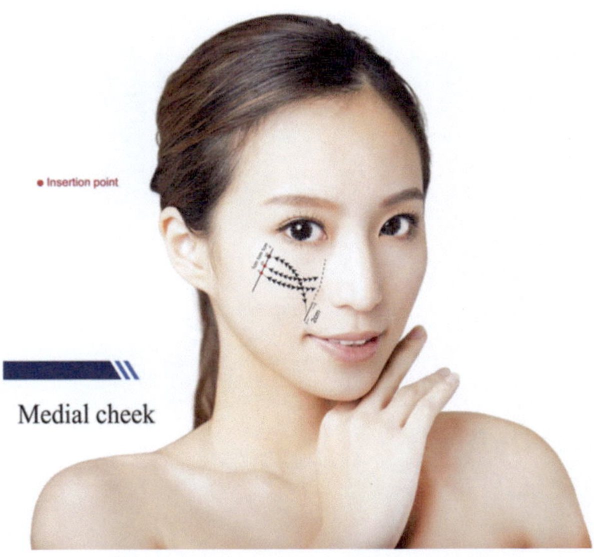

Medial Cheek

 Genetic predispositions and the natural aging process can lead to volume loss in the medial cheek area, contributing to an appearance that may seem aged and fatigued. However, specific parameters can guide the assessment and determination of whether elevation or volumization is necessary for restoring midface harmony [10].

For treatment, the approach targets the deep fat layer to facilitate bidirectional tissue repositioning and restore the area's natural curvature. As depicted in Fig. 16.15, threads are strategically placed following a curvilinear pattern. Adjusting the tension of these threads allows for the soft tissues to be effectively compressed, achieving both volumization and suspension of the medial cheek area [11]. Additionally, two horizontal threads are utilized to secure and stabilize the achieved improvements—clinical examples of medial cheek thread lifting as shown in Figs. 16.16 and 16.17.

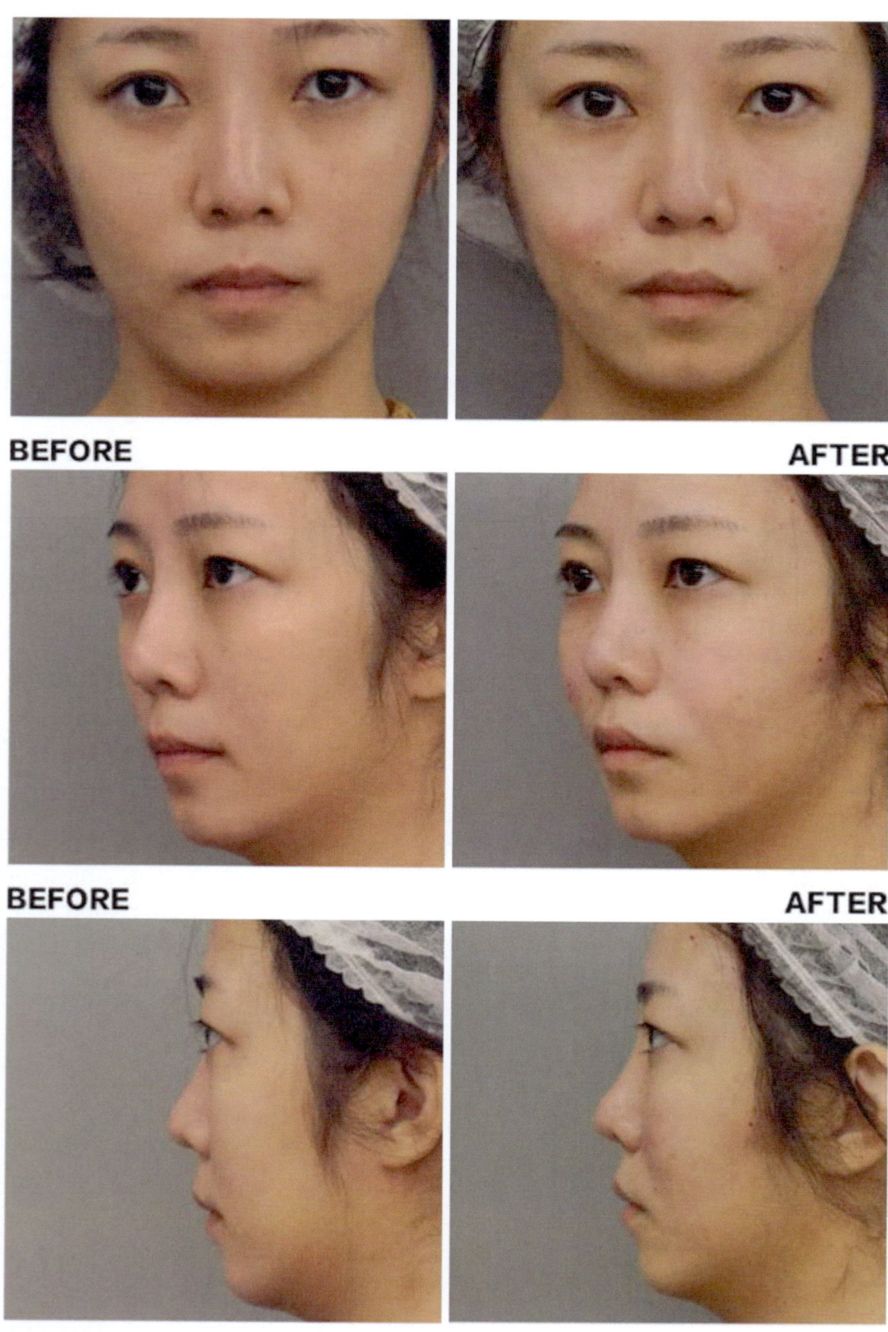

Fig. 16.16 Before and after images showcase a 32-year-old lady who underwent medial cheek thread lifting, utilizing three 1-0 bi-directional cogged threads on each side

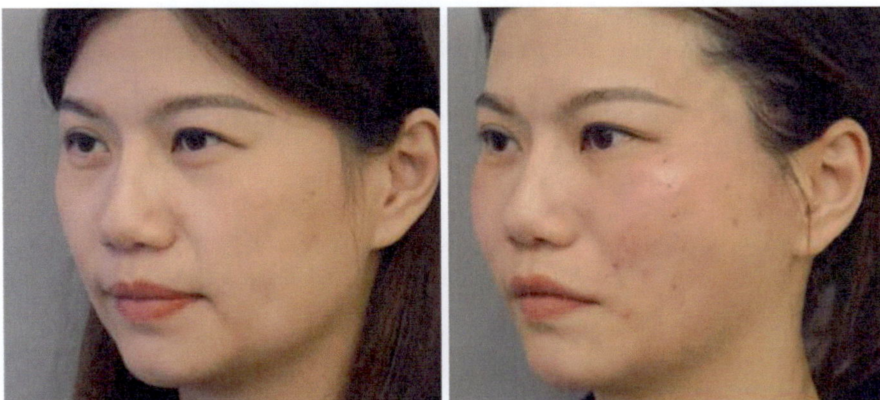

Fig. 16.17 Before and after images depict a 34-year-old lady who received medial cheek thread lifting with three 1-0 bi-directional cogged threads on each side. Initial dimpling occurred immediately post-treatment, resolved naturally within one week

Fig. 16.18 Thread lifting technique targeting jowling and jawline contouring. (Image credit: CanStockPhoto)

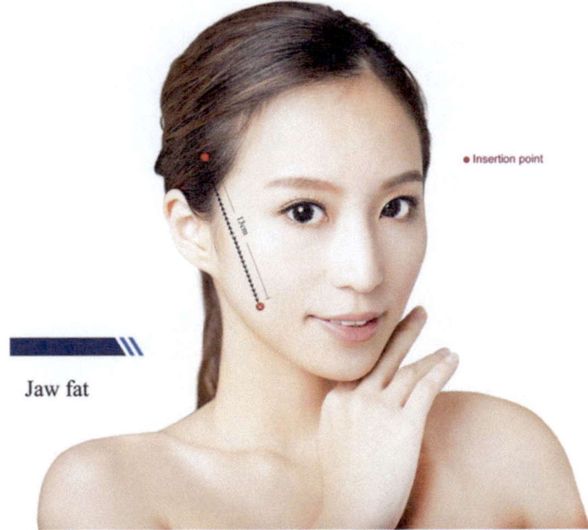

Jawline

Jowling results from a complex interplay of age-related changes, including fat redistribution, bone structure alterations, and the sagging of soft tissues against the facial ligaments.

To address jowling, the initial step involves identifying the most prominent point of jawline fat and the deepest concave point on the cheek. These two points are then connected and extended upwards towards the hairline to determine the optimal insertion point for the thread lifting procedure (Fig. 16.18).

Bi-directional barbed threads are inserted from the hairline through the identified points to gather the skin at the concave point, effectively redistributing volume from the areas of ptosis to areas lacking volume. This method proves particularly advantageous for individuals exhibiting minimal ptosis, offering a subtle yet effective lift and volume enhancement.

For cases of moderate to severe ptosis, a more comprehensive approach is necessary, involving multiple threads and varied paths of insertion. This strategy ensures a more pronounced correction by addressing the extensive soft tissue laxity and volume loss, tailoring the lift to accommodate the degree of sagging present (Fig. 16.19).

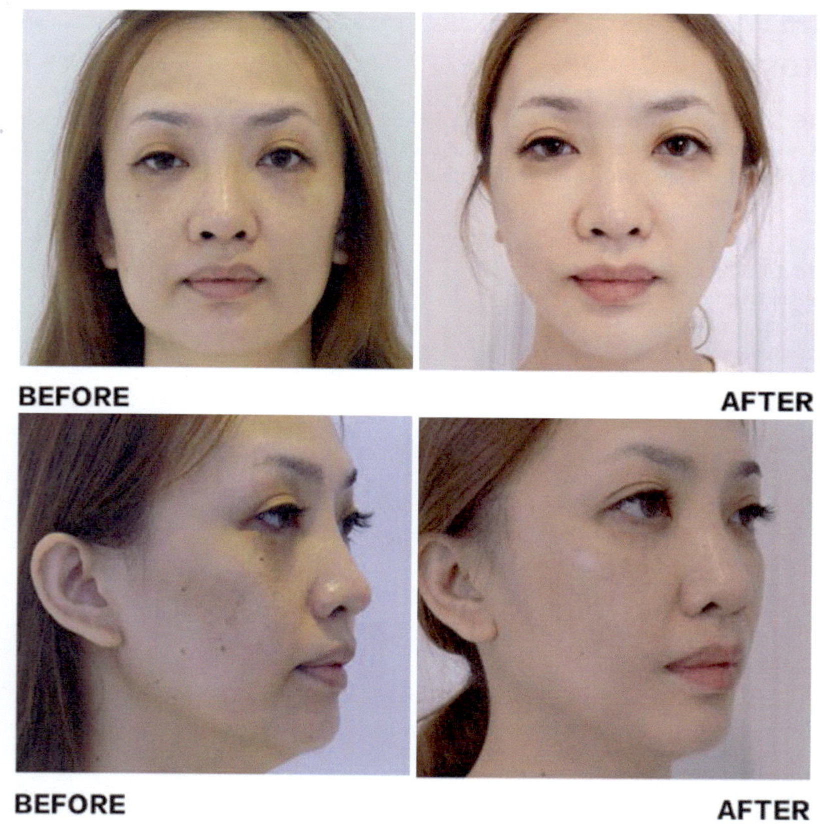

Fig. 16.19 Before and after images of a 42-year-old lady who underwent thread lifting for jowling, employing one 1-0 bi-directional cogged thread on each side. The after picture showcases results 2 months post-treatment

Jawline and Facial Recontouring

Thread lifting serves as an effective technique for redefining the jawline in individuals experiencing minimal to moderate ptosis, as illustrated in Fig. 16.20. This method is particularly successful in sculpting a V-shaped facial contour in East Asian patients and enhancing facial contours in young patients with little to no ptosis.

Following the definition of the superficial musculoaponeurotic system (SMAS) by Mitz and Peyronie, facial rejuvenation techniques have advanced significantly. The evolution from skin-only rhytidectomy to comprehensive soft tissue repositioning and SMAS lifting techniques has marked a significant progression in aesthetic surgery [12, 13].

Employing four to eight threads, practitioners can perform lifts from the temporal scalp down to the jawline in a sectoral approach to maintain an even tension across the mid-face area. Each thread exerts uniform force, intertwined and secured beneath the entry point to ensure stability. The placement depth is calibrated above the superficial temporal fascia in the temple and extends to the SMAS in the cheek area. Clinical cases of the jawline and facial re-contouring are shown in Figs. 16.21, 16.22, 16.23, 16.24.

Fig. 16.20 Thread lifting for jawline redefinition. (Image credit: CanStockPhoto)

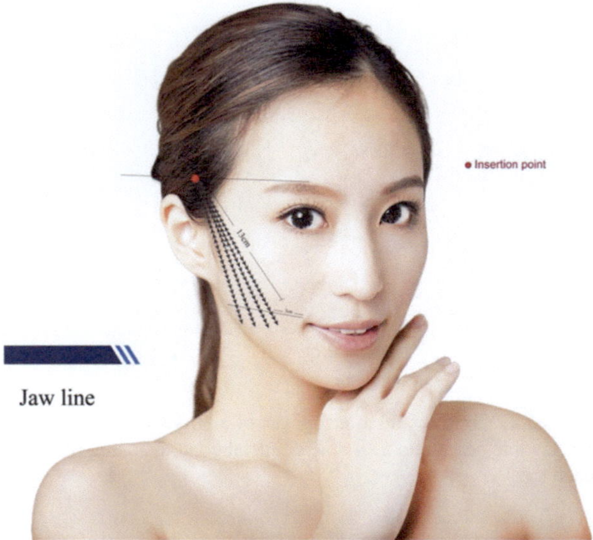

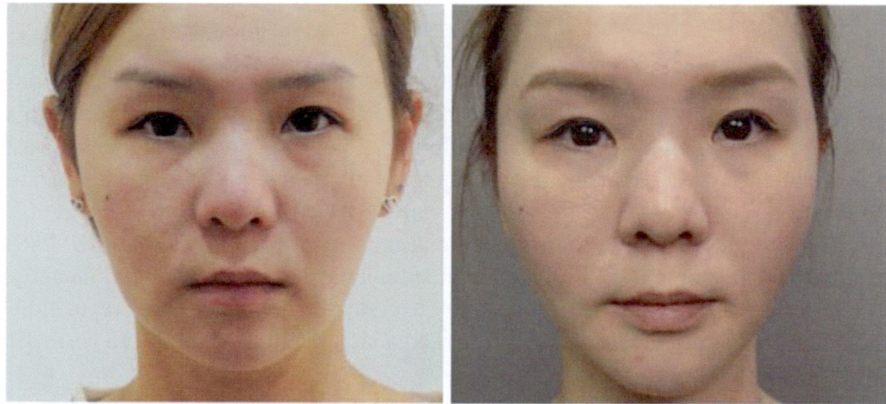

Fig. 16.21 Before and after images of a 34-year-old lady who underwent thread lifting to refine her jawline and attain a 'V-shaped facial contour' using four 1-0 bi-directional cogged threads on each side

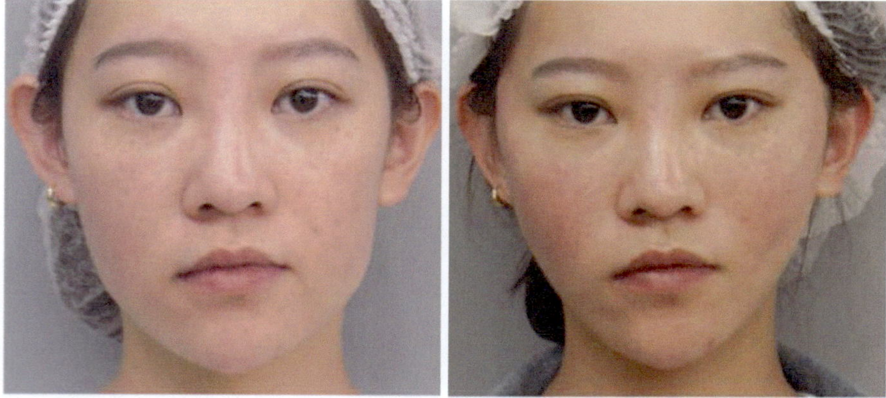

Fig. 16.22 Before and after images of a 36-year-old lady who underwent thread lifting to refine her jawline and attain a 'V-shaped facial contour' using four 1-0 bi-directional cogged threads on each side

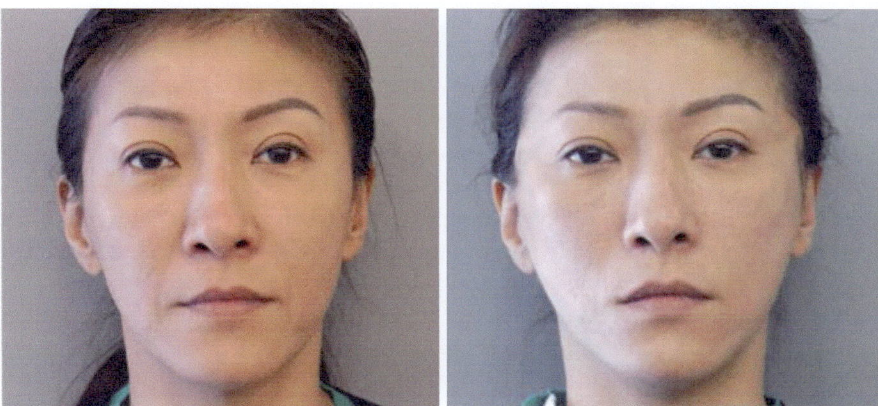

Fig. 16.23 Before and after images of a 48-year-old lady who underwent thread lifting to refine her jawline and attain a 'V-shaped facial contour' using four 1-0 bi-directional cogged threads on each side

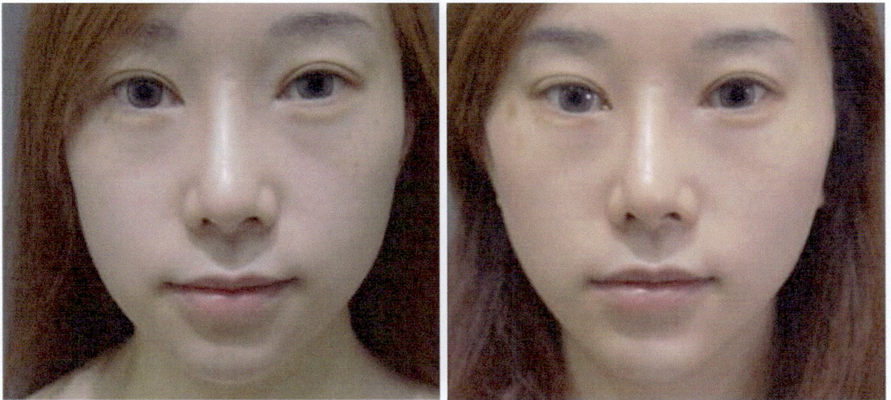

Fig. 16.24 Before and after images of a 34-year-old lady who underwent thread lifting to refine her jawline and attain a 'V-shaped facial contour' using four 1-0 bi-directional cogged threads on each side

Marionette Folds

The deepening of marionette folds arises from a complex interplay of factors, including skeletal restructuring, fat redistribution with atrophy and deposition near the marginal mandibular ligament adhesions, and the activity of the depressor anguli oris muscle. Consequently, addressing these concerns requires a nuanced, multimodal approach that extends beyond simplistic interventions.

Thread lifting can effectively improve this area. Threads can be inserted from the hairline to the marionette folds (Fig. 16.25).

It is crucial to ensure that threads near the corners of the mouth are not inserted too deeply to avoid the risk of them encroaching into the oral cavity. Clinical cases are shown in Figs. 16.26 and 16.27.

Fig. 16.25 Thread lifting for reducing the appearance of the marionette folds. (Image credit: CanStockPhoto)

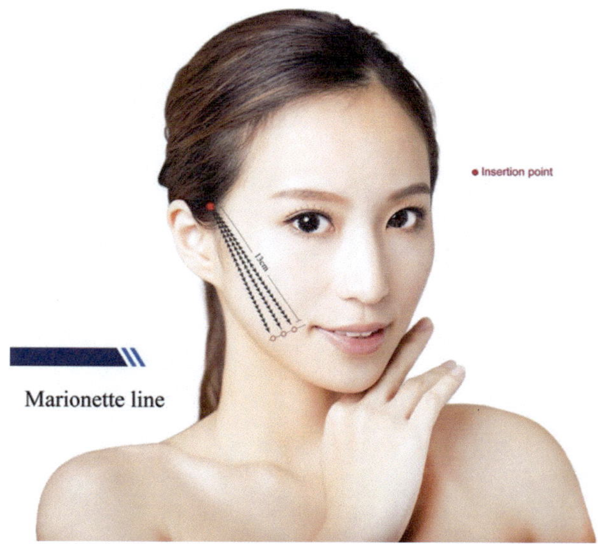

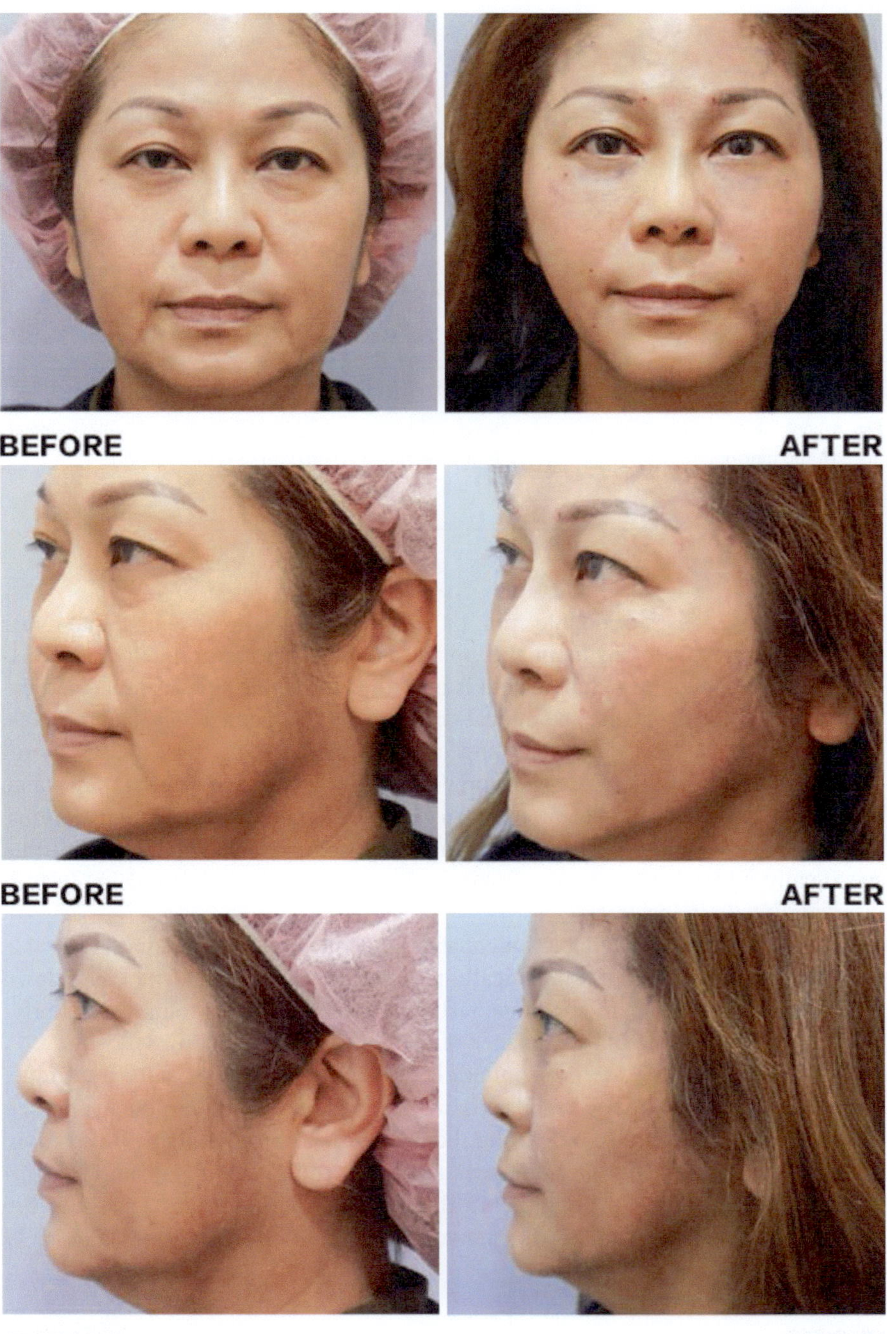

Fig. 16.26 Before and after images of a 55-year-old lady had thread lifting to reduce appearance of the marionette folds using three 1-0 bi-directional cogged threads on each side

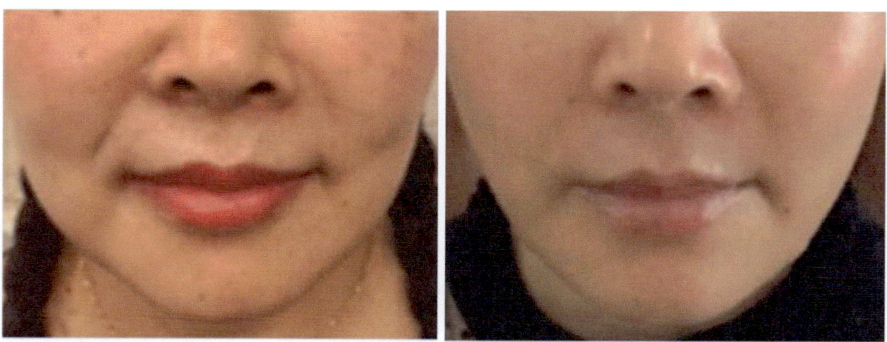

Fig. 16.27 Before and after images of a 56-year-old lady who had thread lifting to reduce appearance of the marionette folds using three 1-0 bi-directional cogged threads on each side

Double Chin

There are three causes of double chin: fat accumulation, skin loosening, and hyoid bone displacement. Among them, the thread can only solve the problem of skin laxity. The development of a double chin is attributed to factors such as fat accumulation, skin and muscle laxity, anatomical structure, weight fluctuations, and genetics, each affecting the submental area's appearance.Understanding these causes is crucial for determining the most appropriate treatment approach, which may range from lifestyle modifications and non-invasive procedures to surgical interventions, depending on the underlying factors contributing to the double chin. Thread lifting specifically addresses the issue of skin laxity and can result in mild lipolysis if inserted directly in the area.

Two approaches are available for enhancing the jawline and reducing the double chin: Firstly, threads can be strategically placed from the hairline, extending down to the mandibular angle, to simultaneously tighten the skin and compress underlying fat, thereby refining the appearance of the double chin (Fig. 16.28).

Secondly, threads can be applied locally using a crosshatch technique, designed to facilitate lipolysis and further tighten the skin. This targeted approach significantly contributes to redefining the cervicomental angle, achieving a more sculpted and aesthetically pleasing neck and chin profile. Clinical examples demonstrating the efficacy of double chin thread lifting through these methods are showcased, illustrating the transformative potential of these techniques (Fig 16.29 and 16.30).

Fig. 16.28 Bi-direction cog PDO thread lifting for double chin. (Image credit: CanStockPhoto)

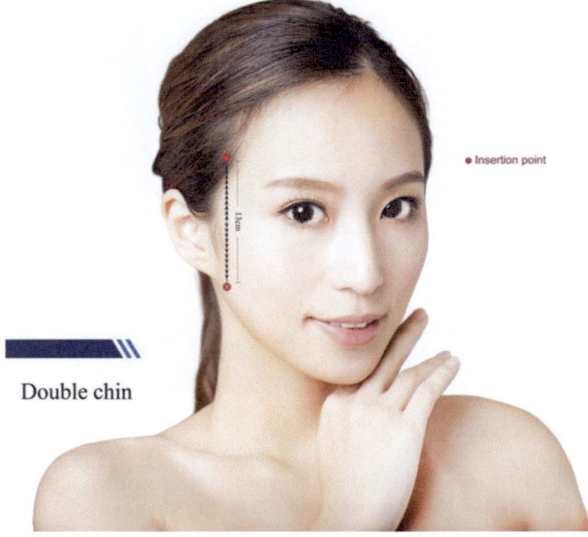

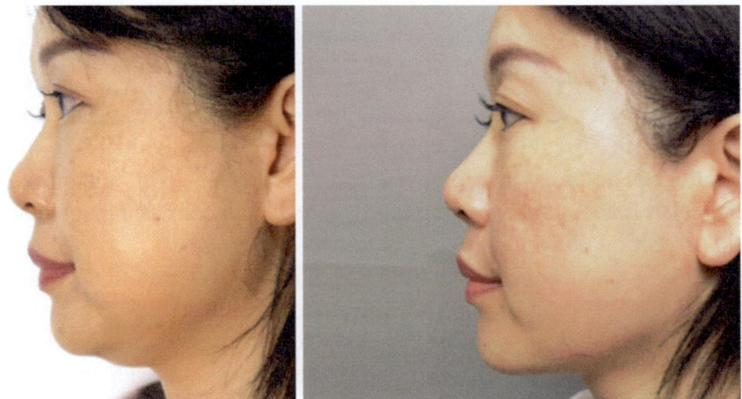

Fig. 16.29 Before and after images of a 55-year-old lady who had thread lifting to reduce appearance of the double chin using two 1-0 bi-directional cogged threads on each side

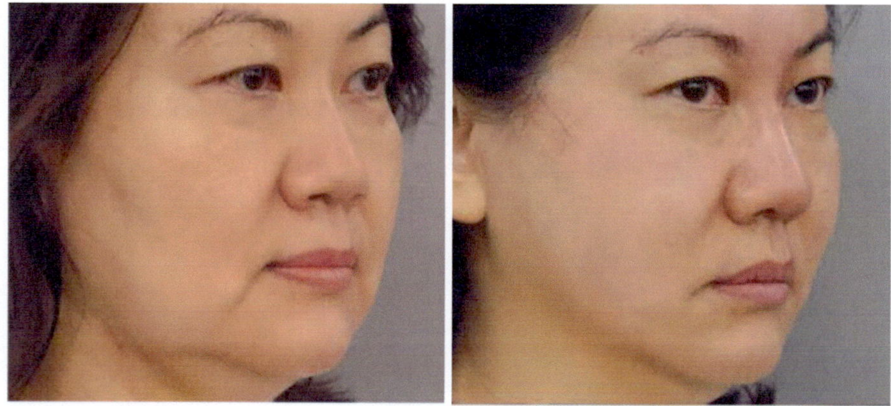

Fig. 16.30 Before and after images of a 42-year-old lady had thread lifting to reduce appearance of the double chin using two 1-0 bi-directional cogged threads on each side

Nose

The nose can be divided into four parts: nasion, nasal bridge, and columella.

Threads can be utilised to elevate the nasal tip, increase nasal bridge height, and correct minor irregularities, catering especially to individuals seeking subtle modifications. The thread can be used as a "solid filler". This method holds particular appeal in East Asian demographics, where desires for nasal height enhancement and tip projection prevail.

A significant benefit of employing threads over traditional fillers is the minimized risk of vascular thrombosis, ischemia, and the severe complications such as blindness that have been reported with filler injections globally. Additionally, threads maintain their size, preventing the unwanted broadening of the nasal structure over time—a notable drawback associated with filler expansion. Consequently, thread lifting for nasal enhancement offers a comparatively safer alternative. For nose reshaping, the use of barbed threads is advocated, as demonstrated in images below (Fig. 16.31).

Clinical cases of thread lifting for nose reshaping are shown in Figs. 16.32, 16.33, 16.34, 16.35, 16.36.

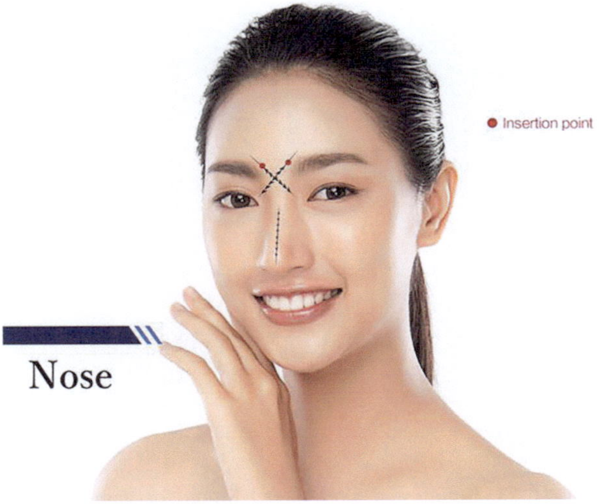

Fig. 16.31 Thread lift for nose reshaping

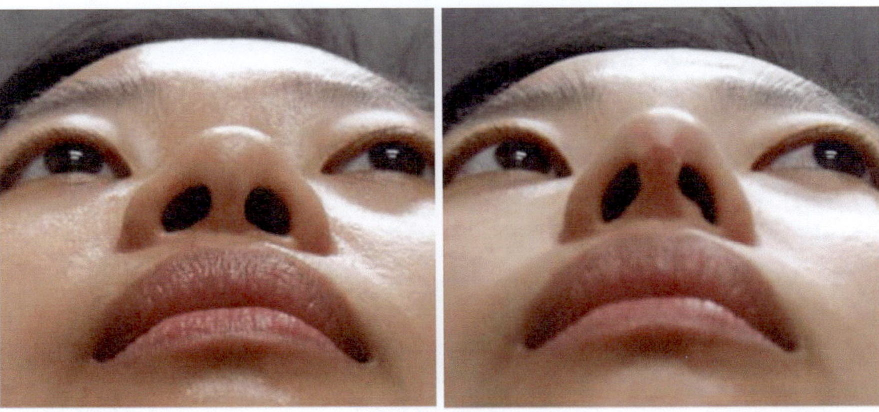

Fig. 16.32 Before and after images showcase a 28-year-old lady who underwent thread lifting for nasal columella enhancement, utilizing two 1-0 bi-directional cogged threads

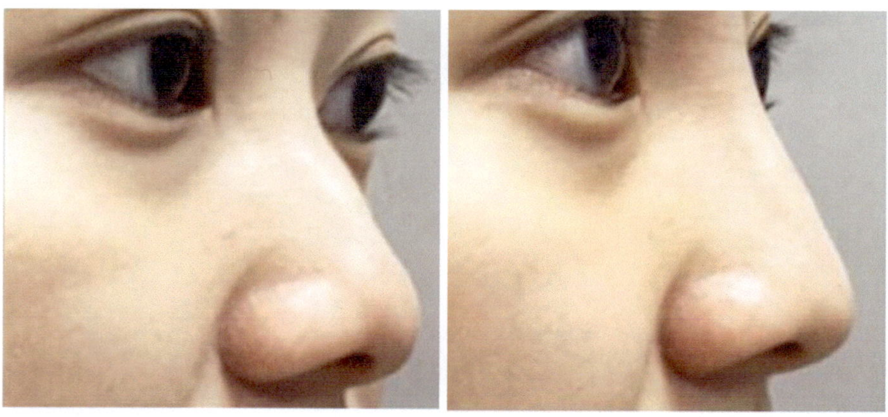

Fig. 16.33 Before and after thread lifting for nasal bridge enhancement with four 1-0 bi-directional cogged threads on a 30-year-old lady

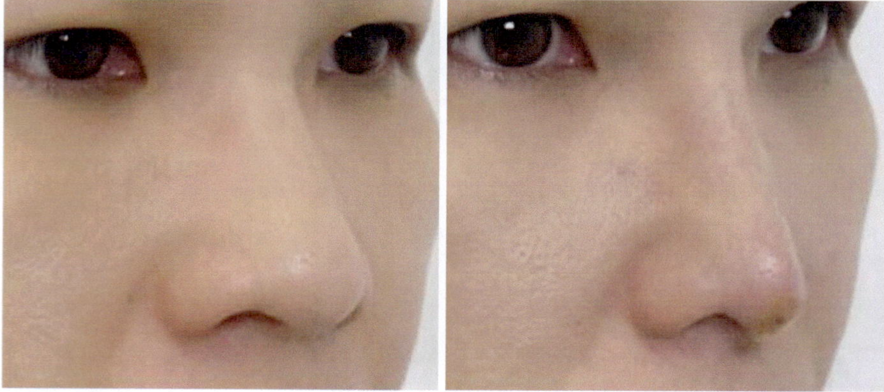

Fig. 16.34 Before and after images of a 35-year-old lady had thread lifting for enhancement of thenasal bridge and nasion using six 1-0 bi-directional cogged threads

Combination Therapy

Combination therapies in aesthetic medicine have significantly evolved, now embracing a multi-modal approach that synergizes different treatment modalities for enhanced outcomes. This approach goes beyond the mere use of various thread types in lifting and contouring procedures to include fillers, collagen-stimulators, and energy-based devices. The rationale behind combining treatments lies in their ability to address multiple facets of facial aging and skin degradation

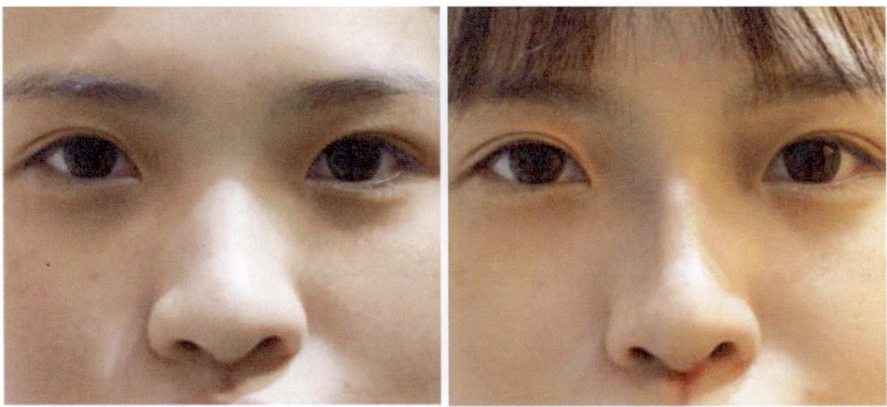

Fig. 16.35 Before and after images of a 24-year-old lady who had thread lifting to improve the nasal bridge and nasion using six 1-0 bi-directional cogged threads

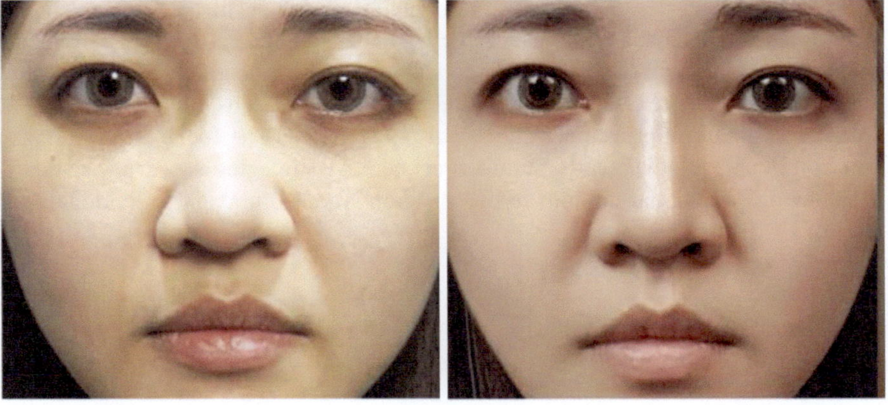

Fig. 16.36 Before and after images of a 23-year-old lady had thread lifting to improve the nasal bridge and nasion using six 1-0 bi-directional cogged threads

simultaneously, providing a more comprehensive rejuvenation. Incorporating regenerative medicine into a multi-modal treatment plan underscores the shift towards treatments that not only aim to correct aesthetic concerns but also restore and maintain the health and vitality of the skin at a cellular level. This holistic approach ensures that the outcomes are not just superficially appealing but are underpinned by healthier, more resilient skin tissue. By adopting a comprehensive strategy that combines lifting, volumizing, stimulating, and regenerating, practitioners can deliver tailored treatments that address the individual needs of their patients more effectively. Such an approach underscores the importance of a thorough understanding of the various modalities at a practitioner's disposal, and the synergies between them, to achieve the best possible results in facial aesthetics.

Conclusion

In summarizing this chapter on the versatile application of Polydioxanone (PDO) threads for facial rejuvenation and recontouring, particularly tailored for East Asian aesthetics, it is evident that the strategic use of varying PDO thread types is critical for achieving the best aesthetic outcomes. No single thread type has emerged as universally superior; rather, the effectiveness lies in a tailored approach that considers the unique anatomical and aging-related characteristics of each patient. Moreover, this chapter underscores the significance of embracing a multimodal treatment strategy. Incorporating a combination of PDO threads, along with other complementary modalities such as fillers, energy-based devices, and advancements in regenerative medicine, significantly enhances the efficacy of anti-aging and lifting treatments. This integrated approach not only offers a broader spectrum of anti-aging benefits but also aligns with the evolving paradigm in aesthetic medicine towards treatments that are not just corrective but also regenerative. By fostering an environment of continuous innovation and adopting a holistic treatment philosophy, practitioners can more effectively meet individual patient needs, driving forward the fields of aesthetic improvement and facial rejuvenation. The focus on customization, combined with the incorporation of regenerative strategies, sets a new standard in achieving natural, harmonious results that honor the cultural and individual identities of East Asian patients.

References

1. Halepas S, Chen XJ, Ferneini EM. Thread-lift sutures: anatomy, technique, and review of current literature. J Oral Maxillofac Surg. 2020;78(5):813–20. https://doi.org/10.1016/j.joms.2019.11.011.
2. Kang SH, Moon SH, Rho BI, Youn SJ, Kim HS. Wedge-shaped polydioxanone threads in a folded configuration ("solid fillers"): a treatment option for deep static wrinkles on the upper face. J Cosmet Dermatol. 2019;18(1):65–70.
3. Kang K-J, Chai C-Y. Immediate treatment of botulinum toxin type A-induced brow ptosis with polydioxanone cog thread insertion. J Cosmetic Med. 2017;1:46–51.
4. Arora G, Arora S. Neck rejuvenation with thread lift. J Cutan Aesthet Surg. 2019;12(3):196–200.
5. Doumit G, Gharb BB, Rampazzo A, et al. Surgical anatomy relevant to the transpalpebral subperiosteal elevation of the midface. Aesthet Surg J. 2015;35(4):353–8.
6. Ezure T, Amano S. Involvement of upper cheek sagging in nasolabial fold formation. Skin Res Technol. 2012;18(3):259–64.
7. Cotofana S, Fratila A, Schenck T, et al. The anatomy of the aging face: a review. Facial Plast Surg. 2016;32(03):253–60.
8. Kapoor KM, et al. Treating Aging Changes of Facial Anatomical Layers with Hyaluronic Acid Fillers. Clin Cosmet Investig Dermatol. 2021;14:1105–18.

9. Lots TCC. Effect of pdo facelift threads on facial skin tissues: An ultrasonographic analysis. J Cosmet Dermatol. 2023;22(9):2534–41. https://doi.org/10.1111/jocd.15761. Epub 2023 May 2

10. YH, Ali. Two years' outcome of thread lifting with absorbable barbed PDO threads: Innovative score for objective and subjective assessment. J Cosmet Laser Ther. 2018;20(1):41–9.

11. Alberto D. Gabriele R. Thread lifting of the midface: A pilot study for quantitative evaluation. Dermatologic Therapy; 2021. p. e14958.

12. Mitz V. The superficial musculoaponeurotic system: a clinical evaluation after 15 years of experience. Facial Plast Surg. 1992;8(1):11–7. https://doi.org/10.1055/s-2008-1064627.

13. Mitz V, Peyronie M. The superficial musculo-aponeurotic system (SMAS) in the parotid and cheek area. Plast Reconstr Surg. 1976;58(1):80–8. https://doi.org/10.1097/00006534-197607000-00013.

Poly-L-lactic Acid Cone Threads–Silhouette Soft Threads—Patient Selection and Treatment Procedure

Souphiyeh Samizadeh and Kyungkook Hong

Abstract

This chapter discusses the application of Silhouette Soft threads, a forefront innovation in aesthetic medicine, for facial rejuvenation and recontouring. Composed of biocompatible, biodegradable materials—poly-L-lactic acid (PLLA) and poly-L-glycolide (PLGA)—these resorbable sutures offer a novel approach to achieving a youthful and contoured facial appearance. The chapter provides an overview of the threads' material properties, mechanisms of action, and the biological process of resorption, highlighting their safety and efficacy for clinical use. It further explores the technique's application in lifting and redefining facial contours, detailing procedural steps, patient selection criteria, and post-procedure care. The chapter underscores the versatility of Silhouette Soft threads in addressing various signs of aging, such as mild-moderate soft tissue ptosis and loss of volume, thereby offering patients a minimally invasive option for facial enhancement.

Keywords

Polylactic acid threads · PLLA · Threads · Thread lifting · Non-surgical facial rejuvenation · Facial threads · Face thread lift · Non-surgical facelift · Silhouette soft

S. Samizadeh (✉)
University College, London, UK

King's College, London, UK

Great British Academy of Aesthetic Medicine, London, UK

K. Hong
Clinque hus-hu, Cheongdam, Seoul, South Korea

Thanks to Sinclair for providing the Silhouette Soft Safety Profile document.Terminology

Poly-L-lactic Acid (PLLA)

poly-L-glycolide (PLGA)

Silhouette soft threads are biocompatible, biodegradable suspension sutures made of poly-L-lactic acid (PLLA) and poly-L-glycolide (PLGA). The characteristics of these sutures enable their dual action for rejuvenation:

1. Immediate repositioning of the soft tissues
   (a) Compression and elevation of the soft tissues
2. Gradual tissue regeneration
   (a) Remodelling the target tissues by stimulating fibroblasts and activating collagen production and volume restoration

Each suture comprises two sets of cones that are equally spaced and oriented in opposing directions, along with a central monofilament (Fig. 17.1). The cones are separated by knots and can freely move between the cones. Following implantation, the cones get engaged by the subcutaneous tissue. This enables the soft tissue advancement over the distal cones and elevation of the soft tissue by the proximal cones.

Characteristics:

- Monofilaments 100% poly-lactic acid (PLLA)
- Cones in poly-lactic acid (82%) and glycolic polymer (18%) (PLGA)
- Bidirectional cones (face in opposite directions)
- Central monofilament: cones evenly spaced on either side of the cone-free central zone of 2 cm. Freely moving cones don't compromise the device's strength
- Each cone is separated by tied knots and is free-floating between them until tissue engagement
- A 12-cm needle is attached to both ends

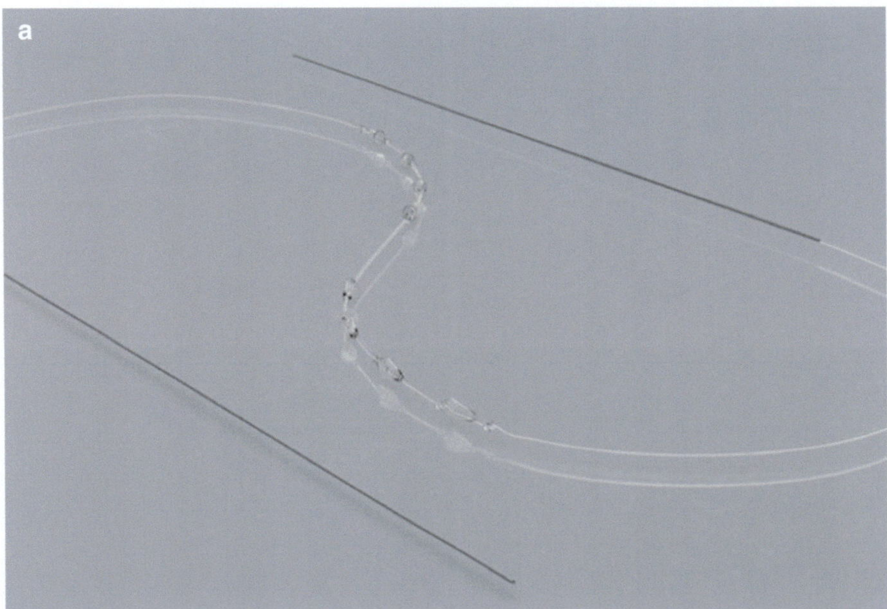

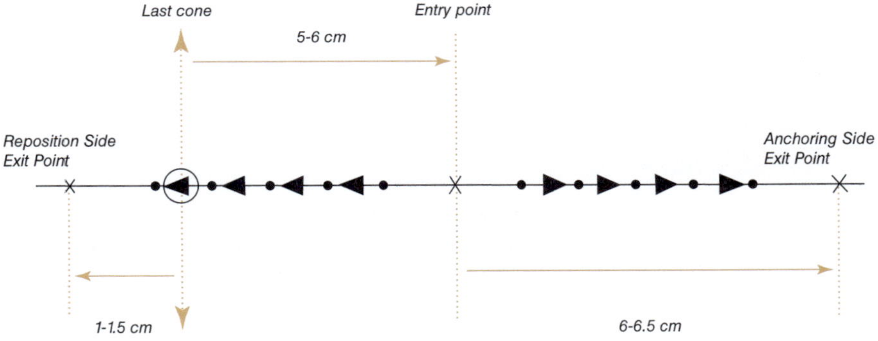

Fig. 17.1 (**a**) Silhouette soft thread, (**b**) 8 cone suture

Patient Selection and Treatment

Aim of the Treatment

The repositioning of the superficial fat compartments improves nasolabial folds, and marionette folds and reduces jowling, improving the jawline. Target fat pads for treatment with these threads include the nasolabial fat pad and superior and inferior jowl fat pads (Fig. 17.2). Volumization of the deep fat pads of the face should be carried out by filling agents.

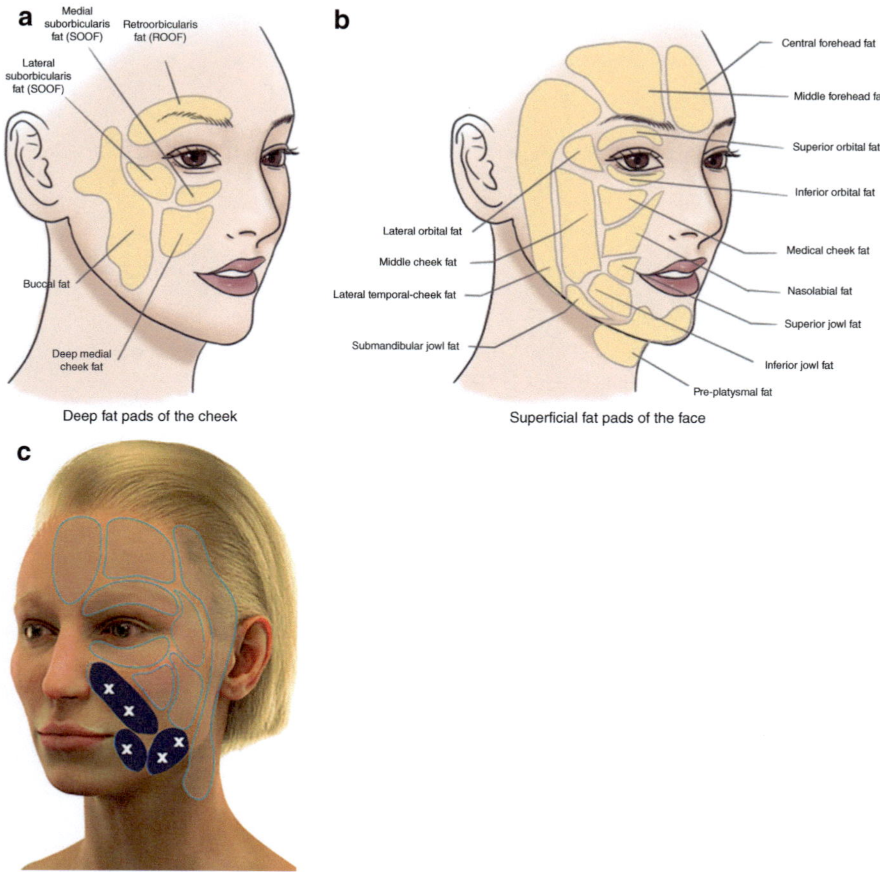

Fig. 17.2 (**a, b**) Superficial and deep fat pads of the face. C-Target fat pads for treatment with these threads include the nasolabial fat pad and superior and inferior jowl fat pads (marked in navy and white crosses) (Image C-With permission from Sinclair Pharma)

Indications:
- Loss of malar volume
- Minimal to moderate ptosis of:
  - Midface
  - Jawline
  - Eyebrow
- Neck laxity-minimal to moderate

Good skin quality is an essential prerequisite of this treatment.

Treatment order:
1. Loss of volume—volumization of deep fat pads and compartments
2. Relaxation of counteracting muscles (optional)
3. Repositioning of tissues
4. Superficial biostimulation

Not recommended for:
- Excessive ptosis and jowling
- Excessive skin
- Hypertrophic type of ageing
- Thin skin in combination with loss of volume/lack of fat tissue
- Known or suspected allergies
- Permanent fillers
- Acute and chronic skin diseases
- Autoimmune diseases
- Pregnancy
- Breastfeeding
- Active infection

When treatment planning for threads, the following should be considered:

- Vector
- Gravity
- Facial movement
- Thread characteristics

Selecting the correct number of threads for a specific facial area is crucial for maximizing the lifting effect and ensuring long-term results. Often, a lack of desired outcomes and reduced longevity can be traced back to technique-related issues, such as placement of insufficient number of threads. Patient-related factors, including lifestyle choices, also play a critical role in the longevity and success of thread-lifting procedures. The choice depends on the severity of soft tissue ptosis and the structural support needed. Utilizing multiple threads enhances the overall lift, distributes tension more evenly, minimizes the risk of thread breakage, thread migration and maintains long-term results.This approach not only secures the lifted tissues in place but also fosters a stronger collagen framework beneath the skin. For more pronounced corrections, especially in male patients who may require a more robust intervention, a tailored, possibly more intensive thread application is recommended (Figs. 17.3 and 17.4). Therefore, the degree of ptosis and the 'suspending' power of threads should be considered. It is imperative to maintain a minimum inter-thread spacing of 1cm. This approach not only secures the lifted tissues in place but also fosters a stronger collagen framework beneath the skin. For more pronounced corrections, especially in male patients who may require a more robust intervention, a tailored, possibly more intensive thread application is recommended.

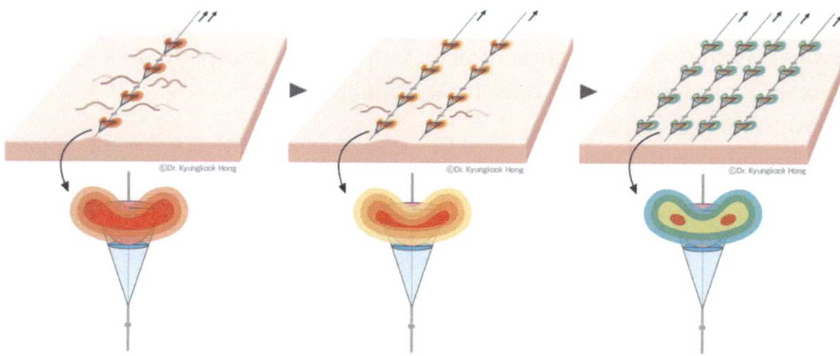

Fig. 17.3 The suspending 'power' of cones decreases laterally. Expecting a single suture to facilitate comprehensive midfacial elevation is clinically unfeasible. Optimal outcomes necessitate the deployment of an appropriate quantity of sutures, which serves to ensure adequate tissue repositioning, augment the overall mechanical lift capacity, diminish the potential for cone migration by alleviating stress on individual cones, and reinforce the collagenous scaffold essential for tissue stabilization post-repositioning. This strategy not only optimizes the mechanical efficacy of the lift but also promotes the structural integrity of the rejuvenated facial architecture, essential for sustained aesthetic enhancement. For optimal distribution and effectiveness in thread lifting procedures, each thread be positioned at a minimum distance of 1cm apart from adjacent threads

Fig. 17.4 Example of thread placement. Selecting the correct number of threads for a specific facial area is crucial for maximizing the lifting effect and ensuring long-term results. Often, a lack of desired outcomes and reduced longevity can be traced back to technique-related issues, such as the placement of an insufficient number of threads

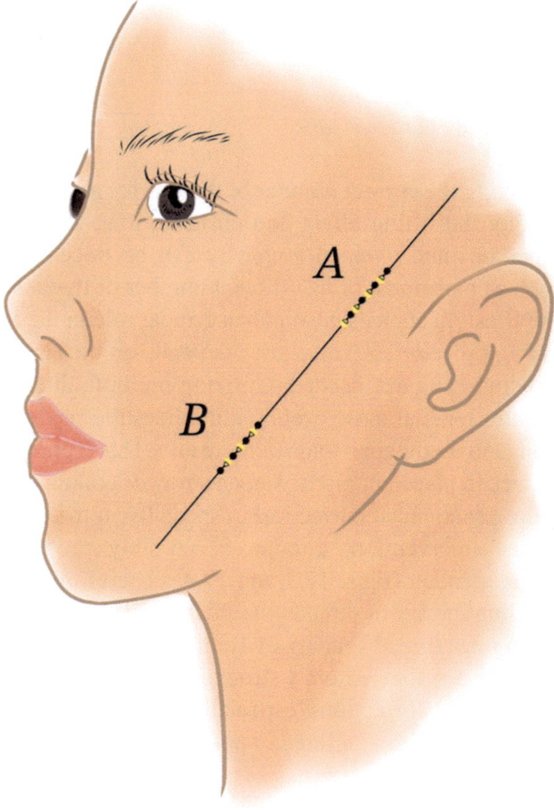

It is paramount to examine each patient individually and develop a personalized treatment plan. "Revised Planning and Insertion Patterns" are developed in collaboration with Dr. Francisco de Melo and Dr. A Carrijo and the recommended number of threads/sutures are as follows:

1. Midface
   (a) Mild: volume reposition with 3 sutures on each side of the face, 2 sutures of 8 cones, and 1 suture of 12 cones short
   (b) Moderate: volume reposition with 4 sutures on each side of the face, 3 sutures of 8 cones, and 1suture of 12 cones short
   (c) Severe: combination with volume replacement treatment in advance to volume reposition is recommended—4 sutures on each side of the face, 3 sutures of 8 cones, and 1suture of 12 cones short
2. Lower Face
   (a) Mild and moderate: volume reposition with 3 sutures on each side of the face, 3 sutures of 12 cones short. (In case of long face, 12 cones long could be considered.)
   (b) Severe: combination with volume replacement treatment in advance to volume reposition is recommended—4 sutures on each side of the face, 4 sutures of 12 cones short (in case of long face, some of 12 cones short could be replaced by 12 cones long)
3. Other Areas

   (a) Eyebrows: medial and lateral third could be treated with 8 cones or 12 cones short
   (b) Neck: 2 to 3 threads per side can be used in straight pattern per side or 2 to threads can be used in hammock pattern

Mild ptosis and localized tissues—e.g. loss of volume in the malar area resulting in deepening of the nasolabial folds and very mild labial commissure ptosis: 3 on each side of the face, a total of six sutures-8 cones

- Mild-moderate ptosis of the lower face and mild changes to the jawline: 6 on each side, a total of 12 sutures, one 12 cones to target the mild jowling and four eight cones to target the marionette fold area
- Moderate ptosis of facial soft tissues, to treat the full face-facial shape and contour changed due to ageing/loss of volume to target the jowling, nasolabial fold and treat the neck-10 sutures of 8 cones (for both sides) or 12 cones or four sutures of 12 cones and eight sutures of 8 cones targeting full face and the neck (for both sides)

Choosing the Correct Vector

Identifying the optimal vectors for thread lifting presents a significant challenge for practitioners. Careful evaluation is essential to determine the most effective direction and placement of threads to achieve the desired aesthetic outcome. This process involves assessing the target area's unique anatomical and aesthetic characteristics to ensure the threads enhance facial contours in a natural and harmonious manner. To ensure optimal outcomes in thread lifting, a detailed pre-procedural assessment is crucial. This involves evaluating the target area to understand the dynamics of facial animation, identifying the most effective points for thread tension, and determining the vectors that will produce a natural lift. Precise marking of entry and exit points, along with strategic placement of threads in relation to facial ligaments and fat pads, is essential for maximizing lift and minimizing risks. This comprehensive approach, tailored to each patient's anatomy, underpins the successful repositioning and rejuvenation of facial tissues. In summary:

1. Assess the Target Area: Begin by evaluating the target area's anatomy and understanding the dynamics of facial animation to identify how forces affect the skin and underlying structures (Fig. 17.5).
2. Identify the Optimal 'Pulling' Point: Locate the most efficient point for thread tension that will yield the desired lift, considering the unique characteristics of the target area.
3. Determine the "Pull" Direction: The thread should be as perpendicularly as possible to the target area to define the most effective treatment vector.
4. Mark Areas for Repositioning: Identify and mark superficial fat pads needing repositioning, such as the nasolabial fold and jowl areas, to guide the placement of the thread's distal end.

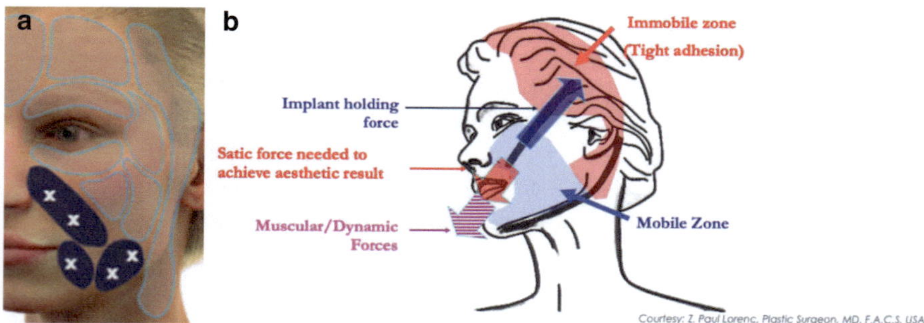

Fig. 17.5 (a) Identifying and marking the superficial fat pads crucial for repositioning, such as the nasolabial fold, superior jowl, and inferior jowl fat pads, is essential for a successful thread lifting procedure. These marks guide the placement of the thread's last cone, ensuring it anchors at the most strategic location for effective tissue repositioning. This precision is key to achieving the desired lift and contouring effects, as it ensures the thread engages with the target tissue at the optimal point for maximum aesthetic improvement. Image curtesy of Sinclair Pharma. (b) For optimal thread lifting outcomes, it is advised to position the anchoring point within denser, less mobile tissue located posterior to the masseteric ligament and superior to the zygomatic ligament. This strategic placement leverages the facial structure's natural stability, ensuring a secure and effective lift. This approach, developed and advocated by Dr. Z. Paul Lorenc, a renowned plastic surgeon, underscores the importance of understanding facial dynamics and the balance of forces for successful aesthetic enhancements. ChatGPT The image illustrates the forces at play in facial animation as conceptualized by Dr. Z. Paul Lorenc. This visualization, developed by Dr. Lorenc and reproduced here with his permission, serves as a crucial reference for understanding the strategic placement of anchoring points in thread lifting procedures, highlighting the significance of leveraging denser and less mobile tissue regions for effective aesthetic outcomes

5. Mark Entry and Exit Points: With the patient in an upright position, clearly mark where the thread will enter and exit the skin to ensure precision during the procedure.
6. Choose an Anchoring Point: Select an anchoring point in dense and relatively immobile tissue, ideally situated behind the masseteric ligament and above the zygomatic ligament for stability.

For example, for an eight cones suture and the treatment of the midface (Figs. 17.5 and 17.6):

(a) Define the position of the most distal cone—'The last cone'—over the fat compartment to be repositioned.
(b) Entry: 5–6 cm proximal to the final cone, depending on skin laxity.
(c) Exit point—1–1.5 cm distal to the last cone-closer to the lip.
(d) Anchoring side—mark the proximal exit point—6–6.5 cm proximal to the entry point. The anchoring point is recommended to be placed in more dense and less mobile tissue (Fig. 17.7).

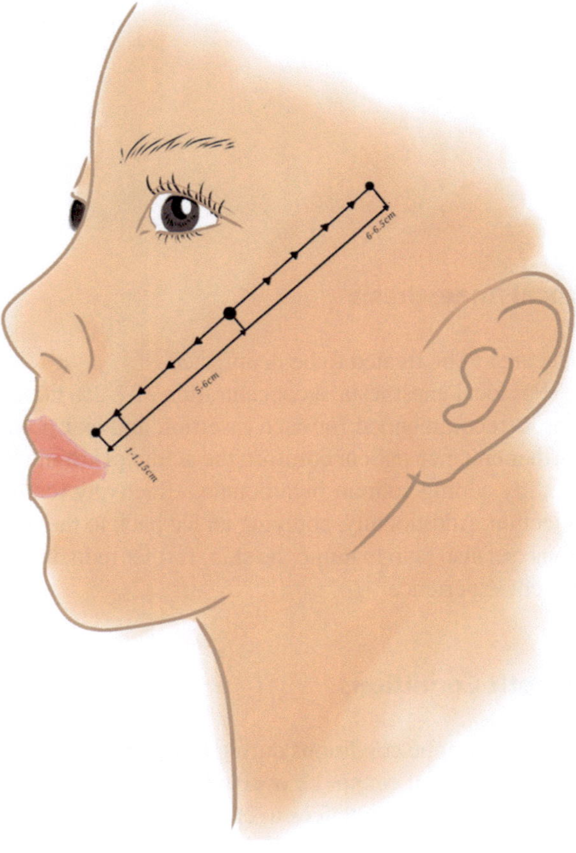

Fig. 17.6 For an eight-cone suture in midface treatment: Step 1. Define the position of the distal cone for targeted fat compartment repositioning. Step 2. Place the entry point 5–6 cm proximal to the final cone, adjusted for skin laxity. Step 3. Select the exit point 1–1.5 cm distal to the last cone, approximately 0.5 to 1 cm away from the upper lip. Step 4. Mark the proximal exit point for the anchoring side 6–6.5 cm proximal to the entry, choosing tissue that offers greater density and stability

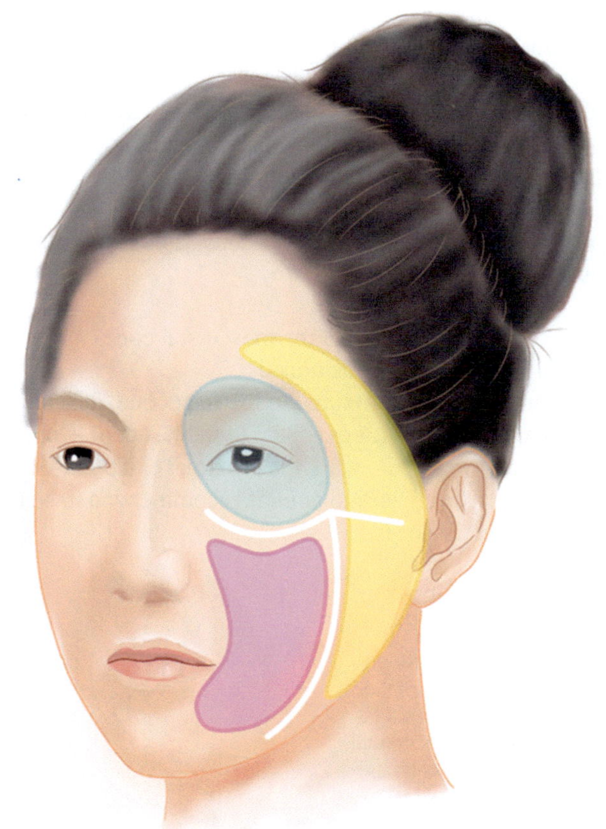

Fig. 17.7 Anchoring point is recommended to be placed in more dense and less mobile tissue. Posterior to the masseteric ligament and superior to the zygomatic ligament. The repositioning: anterior and mobile tissue. Pink: mobile zone Yellow: fixed zone

Local Anaesthesia

The area to be treated to be disinfected.

For local anesthesia, a concentration of 1-2% lidocaine with or without epinephrine is recommended for each insertion and exit point to minimize discomfort. To further enhance patient comfort, the acidic pH of the lidocaine solution can be buffered by adding sodium bicarbonate, effectively reducing the sting associated with injection. Additionally, applying an ice pack to the treatment area prior to the injections can also help to numb the skin, further reducing pain and enhancing the overall patient experience.

Aseptic Conditions

Ensuring aseptic conditions during thread placement and procedures is a fundamental principle that cannot be overstated. Aseptic technique for thread lifting encompasses several key practices to ensure the safety and effectiveness of the procedure. Here's a summary of the crucial points:

- Sterilization of Instruments: All surgical instruments involved in the thread lifting process must be thoroughly sterilized to eliminate any potential microbial contamination. Single-use, pre-sterilized instruments are recommended.
- Use of Sterile Consumables: This includes sterile gloves, drapes, and gowns to maintain a controlled environment free from pathogens.
- Skin Disinfection: The patient's skin at and around the insertion site should be meticulously cleaned and disinfected with appropriate antiseptic solutions to reduce the risk of infection.
- Sterile Field Maintenance: The surgical area must be isolated and protected with sterile barriers to prevent the entry of microbes during the procedure.
- Minimal Touch Technique: Limiting direct contact with the threads and the insertion site minimizes the chance of introducing contaminants.
- Proper Waste Disposal: Ensuring that all used materials are disposed of in a manner that prevents the spread of infectious agents.
- Post-Procedure Care: Applying antiseptic or antibiotic ointments as needed and providing the patient with instructions for maintaining the cleanliness of the treated area.

Insertion of Threads: [1] (Fig. 17.8)

The procedure for inserting Silhouette soft threads involves several precise steps to ensure effective and aesthetically pleasing results. Here's a description of the process:

Preparation of Sutures: Before insertion, ensure the knots on the sutures are securely tightened by applying firm tension to the PLLA/PLGA monofilament, ensuring the structure's integrity and function.

Entry/insertion point: Use an 18-gauge needle to carefully place an entry point into the subcutaneous layer, preparing the pathway for the suture's insertion. Only the tip of the needle should be used to prevent damage to underlying structures.

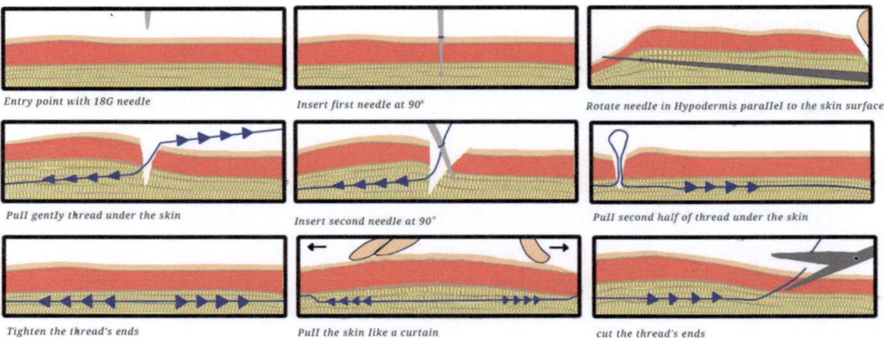

Fig. 17.8 Insertion of threads

Insertion Technique:
- Begin with the more anterior section targeting the mobile soft tissue. Insert the needle attached to the suture perpendicularly into the dilated site, adhering to a depth of up to 5mm, as indicated on the needle.
- Adjust the needle's angle to 90 degrees without withdrawing it, ensuring the depth remains less than 5mm for precise control.
- Advance the needle smoothly through the subcutaneous plane towards the designated exit site, maintaining even progression.

Thread Engagement:
- Gently pull the suture cones through the entry point, ensuring they engage effectively with the subcutaneous tissue. For the distal end, particularly in less mobile areas behind the masseteric ligament and above the zygomatic ligament, repeat the insertion steps, ensuring the suture lays correctly beneath the skin.Once positioned, apply tension to both ends of the suture to confirm engagement and correct placement, addressing any superficial placement issues like dimpling by adjusting the thread's depth.

Final Adjustments: With the suture in place, maneuver the ptotic tissue over the inferior cones to secure the lift, applying firm tension to the superior suture for a slight overcorrection, a common step that settles naturally post-treatment (Slight skin bunching or pleating is normal and resolves within 2-3 days post-treatment).

Reassess the lifted tissue, engaging the superior cones with a gentle massage to ensure the tissue settles over the cones correctly. Dimpling along the track indicates cones catching on the dermis due to too-superficial placement. Palpable and too superficial threads may need to be removed.

Conclude the procedure by trimming any excess suture ends after confirming the desired lift in an upright patient evaluation.

Post-Procedure Care: Apply an antiseptic and antibiotic ointment to the entry and exit points as a precaution against infection, and instruct the patient on aftercare to maintain the integrity of the lift and promote healing.

The procedure for inserting threads during a lifting process involves several precise steps to ensure effective and aesthetically pleasing results. Here's an enhanced description of the process:

Post-Procedure Care Instructions [1]

- Apply cold packs immediately following the operation (cold packs should be wrapped to avoid direct contact with skin and insertion points).
- Avoid applying makeup or face washing for 24 h; sleep with head raised for three to five nights using an aircraft pillow.
- Gently cleanse, shave, and dry the face without rubbing for 5 days.
- Abstain from excessive chewing, dramatic facial movements, and high-impact activity for 2 weeks.

- For 3 weeks, abstain from saunas and steam rooms, dental operations, and face-down massages.
- For 4 weeks, abstain from face and neck massages and facial aesthetic treatments.

Complications

PLLA has a long safety profile. Due to its exceptional biocompatibility, PLLA has been employed in a range of biomedical devices for over four decades as absorbable plates, screws, and suture materials. Additionally, it is licensed as a filling agent to manage HIV-associated face lipoatrophy [2, 3]. Subcutaneous nodules persisting up to 2 years after the injection has been observed in conjunction with PLLA injections and late-onset granulomas. Experienced practitioners with appropriate protocols (adequate hydration time, adequate product placement, sufficient intervals between treatments, and posttreatment massage) have reported long-term safety, longevity, and satisfaction [2, 4]. PLLA promotes the ingrowth of type I collagen, resulting in long-term tissue volumization [5]. Although uncommon, granulomatous responses (local and/or regional and/or systemic delayed and recurrent) can complicate PLLA gel injections [6]. Delayed inflammatory responses lasting up to 5 years have been reported with PLLA implant devices, and foreign-body reactions were with PLGA implants [7–10].

The safety and complications of absorbable threads made of PLLA and polylactide/glycolide were examined by two clinicians publishing their experience with 148 consecutive patients with a median follow-up period of 22 months [5]. They gathered published studies on complications of absorbable threads, including the data from their study (Table 17.1).

In their research, it is noteworthy that all patients were given oral antibiotics (amoxicillin-clavulanic acid) and topical antibiotics (mupirocin) for 5 days post-procedure. Exclusion criteria for the procedure included a previous history of auto-immune diseases, any known allergy or foreign body sensitivities to plastic biomaterial, permanent fillers, and active infection in suture areas. Reported complications were described as minimal or moderate without permanent sequela. Skin dimpling and irregularity were the most often seen complications, followed by ecchymosis, discomfort/pain, and suture extrusion. Except for one of their patients, skin dimpling disappeared spontaneously within 3–7 days. One patient required subcision after 7 days. Migration was noted in three patients. For the 22-month duration of their study, no acute hypersensitivity or delayed type foreign-body reactions were observed.

Skin dimpling and irregularity have been reported by multiple studies with various threads used for facial rejuvenation. [5, 11–15] There is consensus among authors and experts that this is due to incorrect patient selection or technique (incorrect placement or too superficial insertion of the threads). Dimpling at the exit site of the suture can be avoided by not exiting transcutaneously [15]. When employing coned sutures, a singular entry point accommodates the insertion of two needles, directing thread sections in opposing trajectories. Despite utilizing the same entry

Table 17.1 Complications of absorbable threads

Author, year	No	Material	Complications	Intervention for complications	Permanent sequela	Follow-up
Bisaccia et al. (2009) [5]	30	PDO	Swelling Ecchymosis Tenderness over malar eminences Extrusion (protrusion) 4 pts	2 patients with protrusion were treated with 2 small nick incision	NO	6 months
Savola et al. (2014) [2]	37	Caprolactone	7 (18.9%)% asymmetry Ecchymosis 23 (62%), mild erythema 15 (40%), small hemorrhage 9 (25%), mild transitory esthesia 2 (6%), mild swelling 15 (40%)	5 patients needed additional threads (30–45 days later) 2 just compression (2 weeks)	NO	12 months
Suh et al. (2015) [3]	31	PDO	Bruising 29 (93.5%) Mild swelling 23 (90.3%) Mild asymmetry 2 (6.5)	NO	NO	24 weeks
Kang et al. (2017) [4]	39	PDO	Overall 6 (15.4%) Dimpling 2 (5.1%) Bruising 1 (2.6%) Asymmetry 1 (2.6%) Extrusion 1 (2.6%) Malar eminence accentuation 1 (2.6%)	Dimpling, needed subcision	NO	6 months
Baek et al. (2017) [6]	61	PDO	Pustule formation, pain, swelling Subjective discomfort of tightness, skin dimpling	NO	NO	24 weeks
Kim et al. (2017) [7]	38	PDO	Edema Erythema	NO	NO	7 months
Present study	148	PLLA And PLGA	Overall 40 (27%) Dimpling $n = 17$ (11.4%) Ecchymosis 12 (8.1%) Pain and discomfort 4 (2.7) Extrusion 4 (2.7%) Migration and expulsion 2 (1.35%)	Dimpling was subcised in 1 patient Thread was cut in 2 patient	NO	Median 22 months (range; 6–36 months)

Reproduced with permission from Sarigul Guduk, S. and Karaca, N., 2018. Safety and complications of absorbable threads made of poly-L-lactic acid and poly lactide/glycolide: experience with 148 consecutive patients. *Journal of Cosmetic Dermatology*, 17(6), pp.1189–1193

point, variations in the depth and pathway of needle insertion can occur, potentially leading to uneven skin texture upon suture tensioning. This underscores the need for precise technique to ensure symmetrical depth and alignment during insertion, minimizing the risk of post-tightening irregularities.[5].

A meta-analysis and systematic review of the incidences of complications following facial thread-lifting was published in 2021. The complications were divided into five groups: [16]

1. Short-term symptoms
   (a) Bruising
   (b) Pain
   (c) Swelling
   (d) Bleeding
   (e) Hematoma
2. Aesthetic concerns
   (a) Skin dimpling
   (b) Irregularity
   (c) Abnormal facial contour
3. Neurosensory sequelae
   (a) Paresthesia
       (i) Tension
       (ii) Numbness
       (iii) Pruritus
4. Infection, inflammation, abscess, thread extrusion, subcutaneous induration, and granuloma.
5. Injury to surrounding structures
   (a) Facial nerves
   (b) Parotid gland
   (c) Parotid duct and vasculature

While most of these problems are minor and may resolve spontaneously or with nonsurgical techniques, some (e.g. thread exposure, subcutaneous nodule, and infection) may necessitate surgical approaches, including thread removal and debridement [16–18]. These issues invariably lengthen the recovery period and may undermine the cosmetic and functional outcomes [19, 20]. The analysis found that the longevity of the results may not be as expected previously. The most often seen complication was oedema, skin dimpling, paresthesia, thread visibility/palpability, infection, and thread exposure. Furthermore, it was found that complications are more likely to occur with non-absorbable threads and older individuals [16].The proficiency of practitioners plays a pivotal role in reducing the incidence of adverse effects and ensuring the safety and effectiveness of the treatment. This underscores the importance of a holistic approach to patient care, encompassing accurate patient selection, an informed selection of thread materials, technique, thorough aftercare, to optimize outcomes and minimize the risk of adverse effects.

References

1. Goldberg DJ. Stimulation of collagenesis by poly-L-lactic acid (PLLA) and-glycolide polymer (PLGA)-containing absorbable suspension suture and parallel sustained clinical benefit. J Cosmet Dermatol. 2020;19(5):1172–8.
2. Mest DR, Humble GM. Retreatment with injectable poly-l-lactic acid for HIV-associated facial lipoatrophy: 24-month extension of the blue Pacific study. Dermatol Surg. 2009;35(s1):350–9.
3. Siemionow MZ. Plastic and reconstructive surgery: experimental models and research designs. Springer; 2015.
4. Kates LC, Fitzgerald R. Poly-L-lactic acid injection for HIV-associated facial lipoatrophy: treatment principles, case studies, and literature review. Aesthet Surg J. 2008;28(4):397–403.
5. Sarigul Guduk S, Karaca N. Safety and complications of absorbable threads made of poly-L-lactic acid and poly lactide/glycolide: experience with 148 consecutive patients. J Cosmet Dermatol. 2018;17(6):1189–93.
6. Alijotas-Reig J, Garcia-Gimenez V, Vilardell-Tarres M. Late-onset immune-mediated adverse effects after poly-L-lactic acid injection in non-HIV patients: clinical findings and long-term follow-up. Dermatology. 2009;219(4):303–8.
7. Mosier-LaClair S, Pike H, Pomeroy G. Intraosseous bioabsorbable poly-L-lactic acid screw presenting as a late foreign-body reaction: a case report. Foot Ankle Int. 2001;22(3):247–51.
8. Chen C-Y, Chang C-H, Lu Y-C, Chang C-H, Tsai C-C, Huang C-H. Late foreign-body reaction after treatment of distal radial fractures with poly-L-lactic acid bioabsorbable implants: a report of three cases. JBJS. 2010;92(16):2719–24.
9. Böstman O. Osteoarthritis of the ankle after foreign-body reaction to absorbable pins and screws: a three-to nine-year follow-up study. J Bone Joint Surg. 1998;80(2):333–8.
10. Landes CA, Ballon A, Roth C. Maxillary and mandibular osteosyntheses with PLGA and P (L/DL) LA implants: a 5-year inpatient biocompatibility and degradation experience. Plast Reconstr Surg. 2006;117(7):2347–60.
11. Kang SH, Byun EJ, Kim HS. Vertical lifting: a new optimal thread lifting technique for Asians. Dermatol Surg. 2017;43(10):1263–70.
12. Suh DH, Jang HW, Lee SJ, Lee WS, Ryu HJ. Outcomes of polydioxanone knotless thread lifting for facial rejuvenation. Dermatol Surg. 2015;41(6):720–5.
13. Baek WI, Kim WS, Suh JH, Kim BJ. Lower facial rejuvenation using absorbable casting barbed thread. Dermatol Surg. 2017;43(6):884–7.
14. Eremia S, Willoughby MA. Novel face-lift suspension suture and inserting instrument: use of large anchors knotted into a suture with attached needle and inserting device allowing for single entry point placement of suspension suture. Preliminary report of 20 cases with 6-to 12-month follow-up. Dermatol Surg. 2006;32(3):335–45.
15. Hochman M. Midface barbed suture lift. Facial Plast Surg Clin North Am. 2007;15(2):201–7.
16. Niu Z, Zhang K, Yao W, Li Y, Jiang W, Zhang Q, et al. A meta-analysis and systematic review of the incidences of complications following facial thread-lifting. Aesthet Plast Surg. 2021;1-11:2148–58.
17. Rezaee Khiabanloo S, Jebreili R, Aalipour E, Saljoughi N, Shahidi A. Outcomes in thread lift for face and neck: a study performed with silhouette soft and promo happy lift double needle, innovative and classic techniques. J Cosmet Dermatol. 2019;18(1):84–93.
18. Unal M, İslamoğlu GK, Ürün Unal G, Köylü N. Experiences of barbed polydioxanone (PDO) cog thread for facial rejuvenation and our technique to prevent thread migration. J Dermatol Treat. 2021;32(2):227–30.
19. Bertossi D, Botti G, Gualdi A, Fundarò P, Nocini R, Pirayesh A, et al. Effectiveness, longevity, and complications of facelift by barbed suture insertion. Aesthet Surg J. 2019;39(3):241–7.
20. Bae KI, Han DG, Kim S-E, Lee YB. Minimally invasive facial rejuvenation combining thread lifting with liposuction: a clinical comparison with thread lifting alone. Arch Aesthetic Plast Surg. 2019;25(2):52–8.

Non-surgical Rejuvenation of the Face Using Threads

18

Haiyan Cui and Souphiyeh Samizadeh

Abstract

This chapter presents Dr. Cui's innovative facial assessment and rejuvenation techniques, "未来" (meaning "future"), based on Chinese calligraphy. "Double-plane 'Continuous Multi-Z Method'" and the "Double-plane Tightening and Lifting with Threads with a single insertion point," methods are explained, both of which are meticulously designed to address the complexities of facial aging. These techniques leverage strategic thread placement in dual planes to optimize soft tissue elevation and contouring, particularly focusing on the mid and lower facial regions prone to ptosis. Utilizing materials such as PPDO, PDO, and PLCL, these methods aim to achieve a harmonious, natural lift, effectively blending the principles of traditional facelifts with minimally invasive thread lifting.

Keywords

East Asian beauty · Asian beauty · Facial rejuvenation · Thread lifting · Non-surgical facial rejuvenation · Asian thread lifting · Facial contouring · Facelift · Non-surgical facelift · PDO · PCL · PLA · PLACL · 'Future' assessment and treatment planning technique · Dr. Cui 'Future' technique

H. Cui (✉)
Department of Plastic and Cosmetic Surgery, Tongji Hospital of Tongji University, Shanghai, China

S. Samizadeh
King's College London, London, UK

University College London, London, UK

Great British Academy of Aesthetic Medicine, London, UK

The Great Shift

In recent years, as living standards have elevated and societal attitudes have evolved, there's been a discernible increase in the pursuit of aesthetic enhancement and youth preservation. This evolution within the field of aesthetic medicine mirrors a broader transition: from extensive and invasive procedures to those that are minimally invasive or entirely non-invasive; from isolated treatments to comprehensive, holistic care strategies. Concurrently, our medical paradigm has shifted from a purely biomedical approach to one that embraces a bio-psycho-social perspective, recognizing the intricate interplay between biological, psychological, and social factors in patient care.

This paradigm shift underscores a movement within both medical and aesthetic disciplines towards a more integrated and holistic approach to health and beauty. Aesthetic medicine, inherently blending art and science, advocates for a balanced, harmonious, and rejuvenated appearance, achievable not through singular interventions but through a meticulously planned, holistic strategy. This approach not only addresses physical aspects but also considers the psychological and social impacts on an individual's well-being.

As such, the field is progressively favoring non-surgical and minimally invasive procedures that offer effective results with minimal recovery time, reflecting a significant transformation in how aesthetic enhancements are perceived and implemented. This evolution signifies a comprehensive approach to beauty, prioritizing patient safety, comfort, and satisfaction while fostering a deeper understanding of the multifaceted nature of aesthetic medicine [1–4].

Differences Between East and West

The aesthetic ideals between Eastern and Western cultures diverge significantly due to distinct racial and cultural influences. 1 [1, 2, 5]. For example, Caucasians usually have clear facial contours, narrow cheekbones, three-dimensional facial structures, and obvious light and shadow effects with very firm skin. East Asians have a full face, wide cheekbones, lack of clear contours, less distinct light and shadow contrasts, and delicate skin texture. Consequently, Western aesthetic requests frequently center on facial rejuvenation and anti-aging treatments aimed at volumizing and lifting. In contrast, Eastern preferences tend towards enhancing facial filling and contouring to accentuate three-dimensional facial features. Notably, East Asians tend to seek cosmetic interventions at a younger age, primarily focusing on altering their facial shape and contours [6, 7].

Despite these differences, the foundational principles of aesthetics, such as symmetry, balance, proportions, harmony, and functionality, remain universally applicable across all cultures and ethnicities.[6, 8–10].

Training and Education

Aspiring aesthetic doctors should receive further training after their primary medical training on concepts of beauty, anatomy, physiology, pharmacology, patient assessment, patient management, and various facets of aesthetic medicine including techniques and technologies. Nonetheless, a multidisciplinary approach among professionals is recommended to address various patient concerns. In addition to taking medical history and history of previous cosmetic procedures, the psychological state of the patients should be assessed as part of the consultation and their expectations understood. Treatment planning should be carried out with the patient to reach a mutually agreeable plan with a complete understanding of all treatment options, risks, benefits, details of the procedure (what to expect without the use of medical jargon), and pre- and aftercare of the proposed procedure. This forms the foundation of a successful aesthetic practise, complications prevention, complications prevention, and optimal patient outcomes. Thread lifting procedures should be carried out in a clinical or surgical room under strict aseptic technique.

Thread Lifting: Definition and Concept

Definition

The thread lifting techniques aim to volumize by compressing the soft tissues (Fig. 18.1), repositioning the soft tissues and hence the lifting effect. Local volumization, contouring, and skin rejuvenation can be achieved by implantation of threads into the dermis, subcutaneous layer, SMAS layer, muscle layer, or periosteum. It is a minimally invasive procedure for rejuvenation and recontouring of the face and body.

There is a shift internationally towards minimally invasive and non-invasive procedures and hence thread lifting has become more popular.

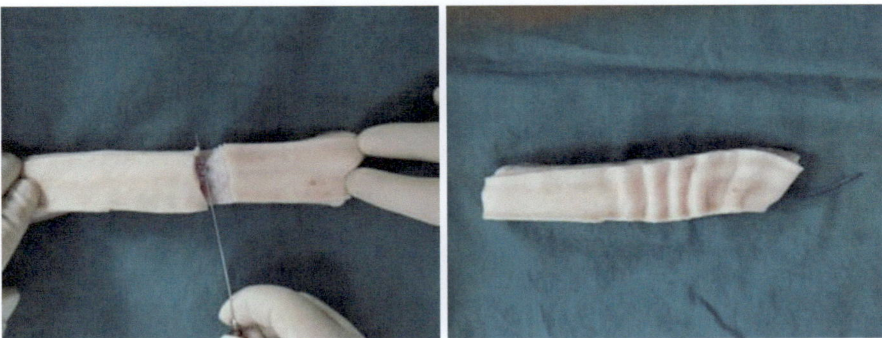

Fig. 18.1 Example of compression of the soft tissues using threads

Thread Lifting Vs Rejuvenation Using Threads

The principle of thread lifting is to tighten, lift, and rejuvenate the skin and to fill and change the contours of the target area. Skin tightening is the most important factor as a youthful face is characterized by firm, smooth, and elastic skin with minimal to no pigmentation and undisturbed contours. This rejuvenating effect of the threads on the skin is achieved through their bio-stimulatory characteristic. The thread material plays a key role in this bio-stimulation and directly influences short-term and long-term results.

The term "thread lifting" can lead to misconceptions among both patients and healthcare professionals. Patients may erroneously equate the results of a thread lifting procedure with those of a traditional surgical facelift, leading to unrealistic expectations. Similarly, among healthcare providers, especially those who are less experienced or not specialized in surgery, there can be an overemphasis on the transformative potential of threads. This optimistic view may lead to an oversight of the threads' inherent limitations and a deviation from the principles of minimally invasive aesthetic medicine, potentially causing issues such as skin irregularities, distorted facial contours, and unnatural expressions.

A more accurate descriptor for these procedures could be "Rejuvenation with Threads." This terminology better aligns with the outcomes achievable through proper thread application—when threads are placed precisely within the correct anatomical layers, the risks of complications such as skin indentations, irregularities, prolonged recovery, and unnatural appearances are minimized. The strategic use of threads for the 'tightening' and 'compression' of soft tissues facilitates realignment and contouring, culminating in a rejuvenated and more youthful facial silhouette without misleading expectations.

The application of threads in aesthetic medicine is undergoing rapid evolution, with continuous advancements in technologies and methodologies. Clinicians are in pursuit of materials and tools that are safe, straightforward, and user-friendly. The ideal threads for use in aesthetic procedures should possess the following characteristics:

- Excellent biocompatibility
- Resistance to bacterial adhesion
- Have sufficient 'holding' power
- Relative durability
- Have a certain degree of flexibility
- It can be degraded or easily taken out
- Bio-stimulatory stimulates collagen regeneration
- Easy to handle

Various thread compositions are available in the market, and these are discussed in other chapters in this book. In a summary:

- Polydioxanone (PDO)
- Polylactic acid (PLA)
- Poly-caprolactone (PCL)

- Polypropylene (non-absorbable)
- Silicone (solid and from medical grade)
- Polyester (polyethylene terephthalate—PET)
- Polylactic acid-caprolactone (PLACL)
- Polylactic-co-glycolic acid (PLGA)
- Poly(lactic acid/caprolactone acid) hyaluronic acid P(LA/CL)HA

Relevant Anatomy Pearls

A profound comprehension of the diverse physical and chemical properties of threads, coupled with an in-depth knowledge of facial and neck anatomy, is indispensable for practitioners offering thread lift treatments. Understanding the nuances of facial aging is foundational for employing threads in facial rejuvenation and contouring effectively. This knowledge not only equips physicians to devise safer and more efficient treatment strategies, significantly reducing the risk of complications but also enhances the ability to sculpt the face and neck, yielding results that are both natural-looking and harmonious.

Facial Compartments [11–13]

In aesthetic medicine, the face is often divided into three sections: upper, middle, and lower. This division method is practical, but it is not a division method based on the function of the face. The face can be divided into two parts: the anterior part and the lateral part. The anterior part is highly evolved, complex, and functionally responsible for facial expressions and communication, while the lateral part is relatively immobile and houses important structures. The two are roughly bounded by a vertical line passing through the lateral border of the bony orbit. Along this vertical line, many restrictive ligaments are distributed, separating the anterior and lateral portions. In the anterior portion, the eye and mouth fissures are surrounded by abundant muscles of expression, most of which are superficially located. The soft tissues in this area are highly mobile and can produce finer movements under the action of the muscles of expression, which are also more prone to laxity and sagging with ageing. In contrast, the lateral cheeks, which cover the masticatory muscles (masseter and temporalis) and the parotid gland, are relatively immobile areas. Several critical anatomical considerations are paramount for ensuring procedural success and patient safety. Detailed below are essential anatomical insights that practitioners must be well-versed in:

Facial Layers [14]

For placing threads, it is important to be familiar with the anatomical layers of the face. Depending on the location and purpose, different threads may be embedded in the subcutaneous fat layer, within the muscles, in the interstitial space, and on the periosteum. Without considering the specific variations that exist in many areas, the face can be divided from superficial to deep into the classic five layers: skin, subcutaneous fat layer, SMAS layer, lax reticular layer (interstitial and ligamentous), and periosteum.

Fascial Spaces [15, 16]

Fascial spaces have firm borders formed by supporting ligaments. These spaces are relatively anatomically 'safe' areas, with no significant structures crossing them and all facial nerve branches running outside the spaces. The superior border of the spaces are the weakest area compared to the ligament-reinforced edges and are susceptible to laxity due to ageing. Differences in the degree of laxity in these areas are the main cause of the characteristic ageing facial appearance.

Facial Nerve and Its Branches [17]

The facial nerve's branching pattern within the parotid gland, extending into the temporal, zygomatic, buccal, mandibular margin, and cervical branches, is essential knowledge for avoiding nerve injury. These branches are especially vulnerable during thread placement, necessitating a thorough understanding of their trajectories to prevent complications such as muscle paralysis. Upon entering the parotid gland, the facial nerve bifurcates into upper and lower trunks before further dividing into five principal branches: temporal, zygomatic, buccal, mandibular margin, and cervical. These branches emerge from the parotid gland and navigate beneath the deep fascia within the lateral aspect of the face. As the nerve transitions to the anterior facial region, it descends into a more superficial layer, closely interacting with the expressive muscles. This transition zone, from the deeper fifth layer to the more superficial fourth layer, is particularly susceptible to nerve injury, often compounded by the proximity to supporting ligaments that confer stability and protection to the nerve pathways.

In general, of all the branches of the facial nerve, the temporal and mandibular marginal branches of the facial nerve are more likely to experience paralysis of the innervated muscles after an injury because of the lack of compensatory branches. During thread placement, when the guide needle passes through the surface of the zygomatic arch, the temporal branch of the facial nerve may be damaged and unilateral paralysis of the frontalis muscle may occur, which can be recovered mostly within 3 months; when the guide needle passes through the midface, a nerve short circuit may be formed between the zygomatic and buccal branches. In addition, the injection of local anaesthetic may also cause temporary paralysis of the temporal branch, zygomatic branch, and mandibular margin branch, resulting in the appearance of drooping eyebrows, poor eye closure, oblique corners of the mouth and other manifestations, which recovers after the effect of local anaesthetic is eliminated.

The 'Future/未来' Aesthetic Evaluation Method for the Overall Facial Rejuvenation [18, 19]

The first author, Dr. Cui has developed a unique facial assessment and treatment planning method known as the "Future" technique, deeply inspired by the principles of Chinese calligraphy. This method employs the two Chinese characters '未来', translating to 'Future' in English, to outline a comprehensive approach to the art of

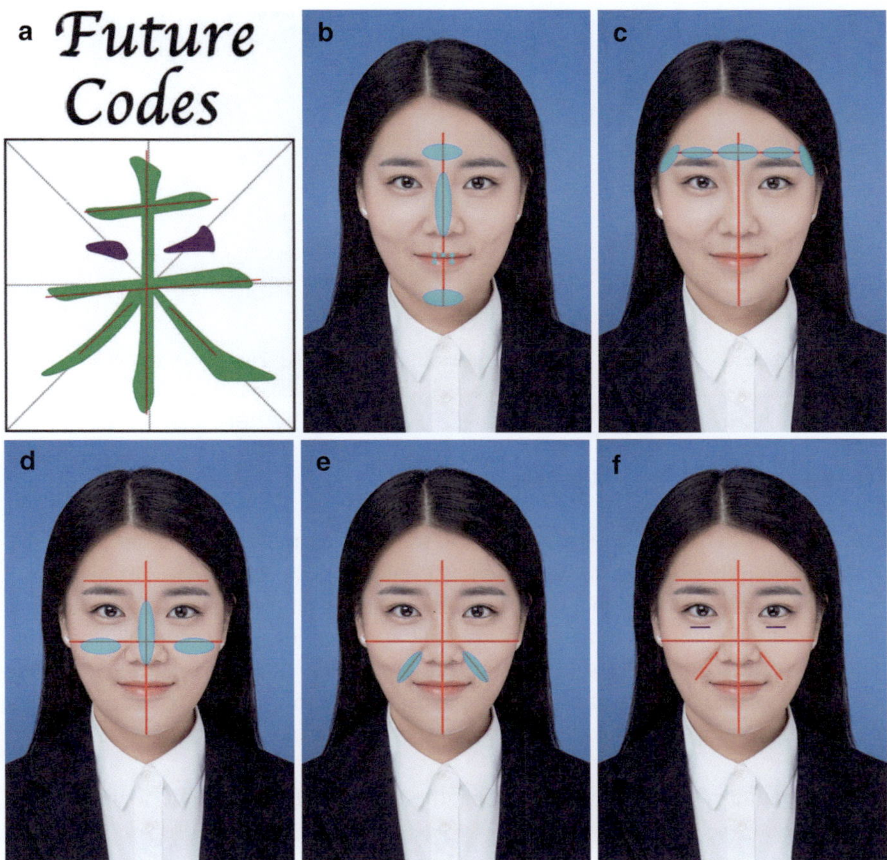

Fig. 18.2 Dr. Cui's facial assessment and treatment planning method is based on Chinese calligraphy. (**a**) 2 Chinese characters '未来', which means 'Future' in English. The concept encompasses the systematic overall design for the art of facial injections in Asians. (**b**) The middle line of the face (a 26-year-old female) passes through the forehead, the glabella complex, the nose, the lips, and the chin. (**c**) The first horizontal line passes the arch of the temple region, the eyebrow, and the glabella complex. (**d**) The second horizontal line passes through medial cheeks. (**e**) The other 2 oblique lines run along the nasolabial folds. (**f**) Finally, 2 lines for nasojugal folds/tear troughs are added. These lines can be used as a guide for facial rejuvenation and contouring using injectables and threads

facial injections, particularly tailored for Asian patients. The "Future" technique is characterized by its strategic use of lines across the face, serving as guides for rejuvenation and contouring through injectables and threads (Fig. 18.2).

The facial midline, encompassing the forehead, eyebrows, nose, lips, and chin, plays a pivotal role in defining the three-dimensionality, symmetry, balance, and interplay of light and shadow on an individual's face. Additionally, the horizontal

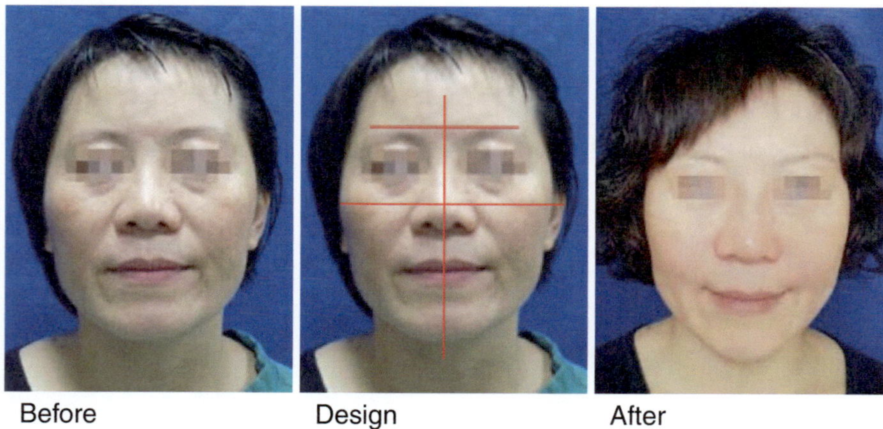

Fig. 18.3 Example of treatment with this concept

lines extending from the eyebrow arches to the temples and across the midface serve as crucial markers for evaluating the signs of aging.

Aging manifests through a combination of soft tissue ptosis displacement of tissue structures, emergence of skin folds, textural changes, and volume loss. These phenomena are encapsulated in the Chinese concept of 'future', (Fig. 18.3) with the deepening of facial lines and tear troughs being notable indicators of aging. For clarity, refer to Fig. 18.2 and the description below for clarification:

1. An imaginary horizontal line along the arch of the eyebrows including the temples.
2. A second horizontal line that traces the medial cheeks, often referred to as the 'apples of the cheeks' in Chinese.
3. A central line that runs from the forehead, between the eyebrows, across the nose, lips, and down to the chin.
4. Finally, the two 'strokes' on either side of the line in the middle correspond to the tear troughs.

With regards to the use of threads for rejuvenation, this technique can be used to:

1. The objective of treatment—whether it's rejuvenation or recontouring, skin tightening, enhancing skin quality, lipolysis, lifting, or a combination thereof.
2. The preoperative planning process, including the selection of specific landmarks and threads.
3. The identification of the correct anatomical sites and layers for thread placement.
4. The integration of additional modalities, such as botulinum toxins, dermal fillers, and various devices. The significance of adopting a combination therapy approach to achieve the best possible outcomes cannot be overstated, ensuring a holistic and nuanced approach to facial rejuvenation.

Thread Placement

The first author has come up with two simple designs:

1. The double-plane 'two-point three-sector method'
2. The double-plane 'continuous multi-Z method'

A vertical line is drawn 1 cm outside the level of the lateral canthus, and double plane thread placement is performed inside and outside this vertical line. Outside the vertical line, the thread can run in the SMAS fascia layer; inside the vertical line, the thread must run in the superficial layer of the SMAS. This conforms to the principles of anatomy and rejuvenation, and at the same time strengthens the effect of tightening and lifting.

SMAS Layer Tightening Is the Key to Ptosis Reduction and Facial Rejuvenation

Facial rejuvenation techniques have undergone substantial evolution, moving from traditional facelifts to more advanced procedures involving SMAS (Superficial Muscular Aponeurotic System) tightening and combined SMAS and subperiosteal lifts. Initially, facelifts had a high risk of complications such as suboptimal outcomes, skin necrosis, and scarring due to incision tension. The discovery of the SMAS anatomical layer represented a significant breakthrough in facial cosmetic surgery. Tightening the SMAS layer has become a cornerstone of modern facelift techniques, effectively reducing tension at the skin incision while enhancing the lifting effect. This dual action of tightening both the SMAS and the skin contributes to a more elevated and youthful facial contour.

The principles of SMAS facelift can be used in thread-lifting techniques. Achieving effective soft-tissue tightening through thread implantation in merely the subcutaneous and dermal layers is challenging; over-tightening can lead to wrinkles, indentations, and skin irregularities. However, by intricately weaving and tightening the SMAS layer with threads, the procedure aligns with the essential principles and anatomical considerations necessary for facial rejuvenation.

The SMAS layer is anatomically divided into frontal and lateral segments, allowing for nuanced manipulation during procedures like surgical canthoplasty. Thread placement navigates through and around the SMAS fascia—above, below, and within the lateral section, while maintaining superficial engagement in the medial section. This strategic dual-plane approach enhances both the safety and efficacy of the procedure, offering a structured and anatomically informed method for achieving facial rejuvenation.

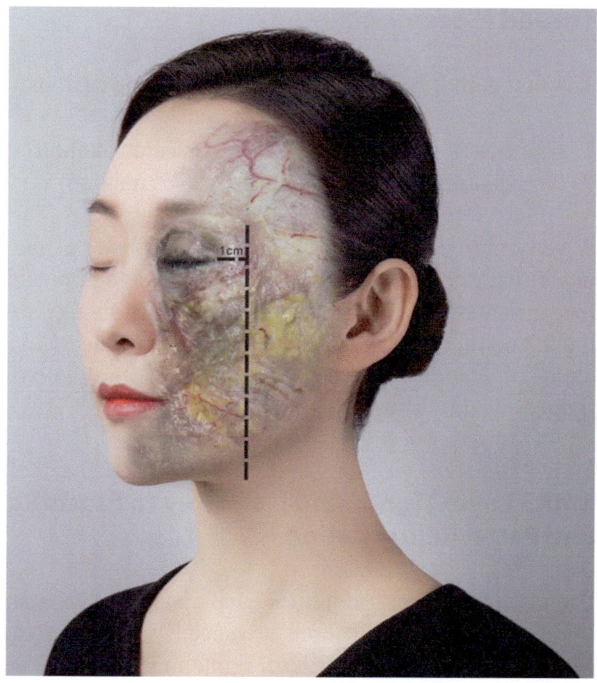

Fig. 18.4 Double-plane tightening and lifting with threads guided by anatomical landmarks

Double-plane Tightening and Lifting with Threads

A vertical line is drawn 1 cm lateral to the lateral canthus for guidance. In the region lateral to this line, the Superficial Muscular Aponeurotic System (SMAS) and subcutaneous fat layers are notably dense, and the facial nerve descends to a deeper plane, making SMAS elevation in this zone relatively safe during traditional facelift surgeries. The technique involves elevating the SMAS, removing any excess, and then suturing it to achieve a tighter SMAS layer. A 'tongue-shaped' fascial flap of the SMAS, located anterior to the ear, can be created and repositioned towards the posterior mastoid area. This maneuver tightens the lower middle portion of the face. Additionally, folding and securing the SMAS fascia in front of the ear further tightens this layer. This approach informs the thread implantation process, suggesting that threads can be positioned within the mid-SMAS fascia, lateral to the vertical line and 1 cm beyond the level of the external canthus. By weaving threads through the SMAS in this region, it is possible to reinforce, secure, and tighten the SMAS layer. The subsequent scar formation and inflammatory response to thread implantation promote adhesion of the SMAS fascia, thereby enhancing and prolonging the face's tightening and lifting effects achieved with threads(Fig. 18.4). Various threads, including PPDO, PDO, and PLCL, are suitable for this purpose, offering a nuanced approach to achieving a lifted and rejuvenated facial appearance.

Two-plane 'Continuous Multi-Z Method'

This technique is optimally designed for individuals experiencing sagging or ptosis of the soft tissues in the mid to lower facial regions. Utilizing a single insertion point for the entire face minimizes trauma, with the primary goal being to achieve a natural-looking lift. For this approach, threads of either 45 cm or 35 cm in length can be selected, allowing for comprehensive treatment of the middle and lower face through just one entry point and a single, elongated thread. The outcome of this procedure is consistently natural and reliably replicable, offering a subtle yet effective rejuvenation (Fig. 18.5).

An insertion point, strategically located above the zygomatic arch and just anterior to the hairline, serves as the starting point from which the needle is directed toward the infraorbital and medial cheek regions. For the lateral cheeks, positioned outside the lateral canthal line and 3–5 cm anterior to the ear, the thread is guided through the SMAS layer in a wavelike pattern; whereas, within the region demarcated by the lateral canthal line, the thread traverses the superficial layer of the SMAS. This technique ensures a precise and tailored approach to lifting and rejuvenating the facial contours.

For the lower eyelid region (distinct from the medial cheek area), thread implantation employs a back-and-forth motion approximately 2–3 times without

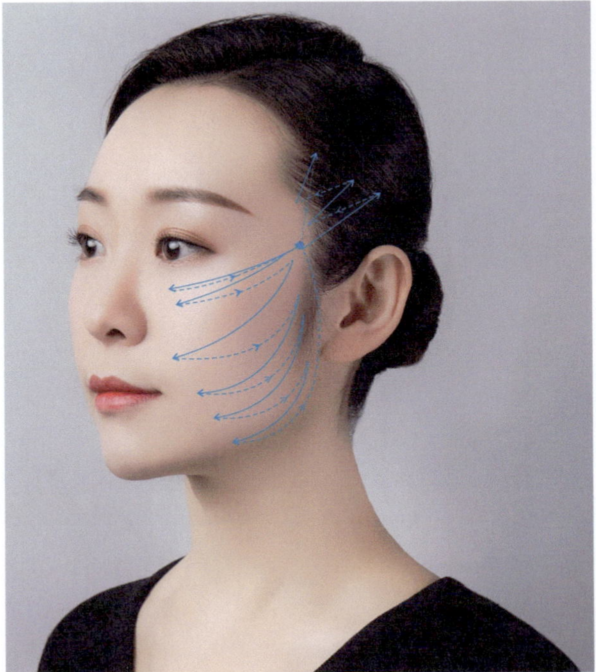

Fig. 18.5 Bi-layer continuous thread implantation with Multiple Z sharped technique. The continuous arrow indicates placement of the thread, dotted line indicates reversal of the cannula towards the insertion point and without exiting, re-insertion in the new path. The threads are placed in the midface and jawline and then redirected towards the temple

retracting the needle from the insertion point. Subsequently, the direction is adjusted downward to navigate across the zygomatic arch, weaving back and forth around 3 times towards the external aspect of the nasolabial fold and the outer corner of the mouth. The process then extends towards the lower jaw, anterior to the ear, and down to the earlobe. The placement of the thread proceeds in reverse, heading back towards the initial insertion point. Importantly, the thread is not withdrawn from the insertion point; instead, it is routed in reverse towards the temporal hairline, employing subcutaneous wiring 2–3 times to utilize the remainder of the thread. Any excess thread can be trimmed and removed as needed, ensuring a clean and precise application (Figs. 18.6, 18.7, 18.8, 18.9, 18.10, 18.11, 18.12, 18.13, 18.14).

After the procedure, a gentle massage of the face may be performed with two pieces of gauze to ensure the absence of dents, depressions, or any unevenness. Subsequently, compression garments for the face, neck, and jawline are applied to support and secure the treated areas. These compression garments should be removed within 2 hours post-procedure. Patients are advised to minimize facial expressions, movements, and avoid excessive chewing for a period of 3–5 days to ensure optimal healing and results.

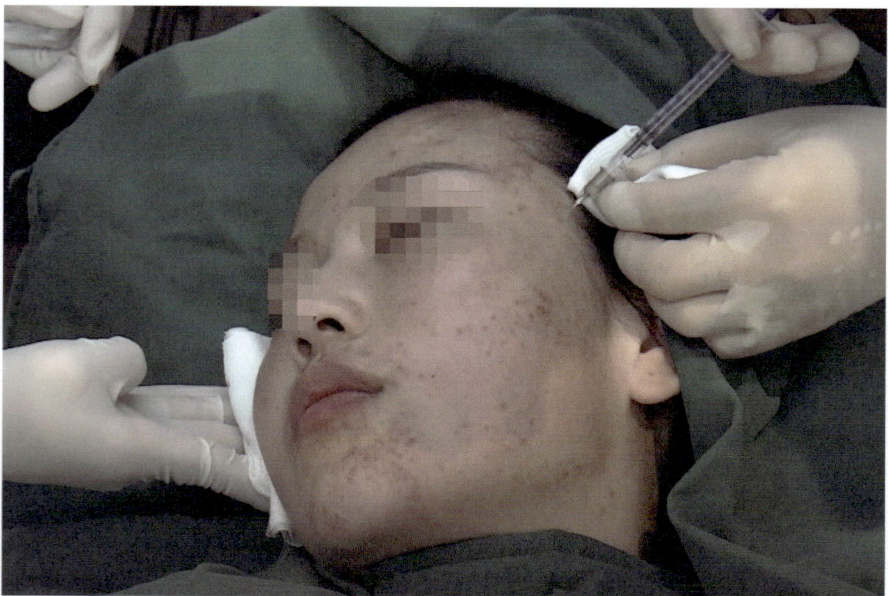

Fig. 18.6 Anaesthesia

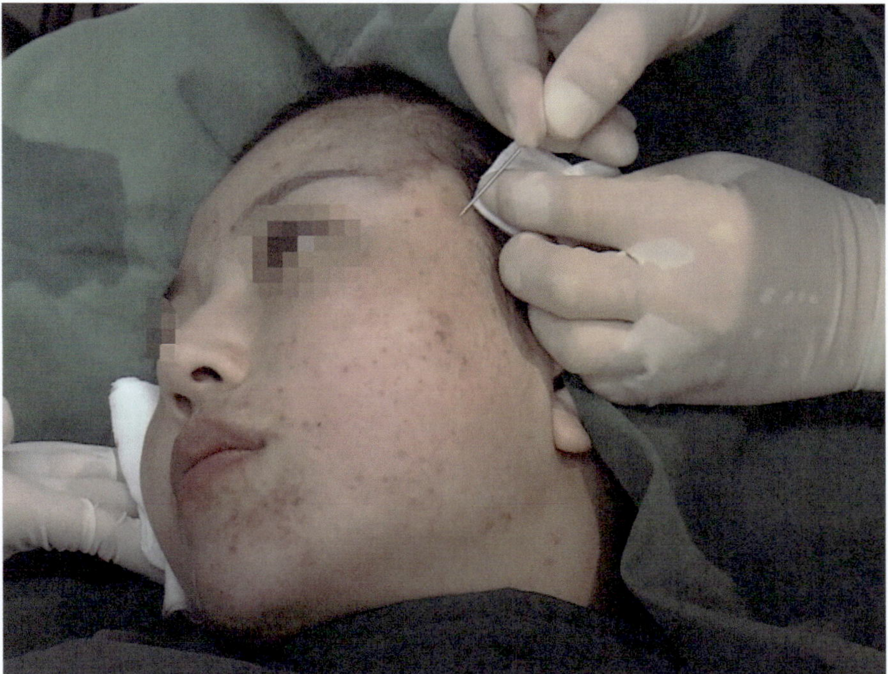

Fig. 18.7 Insertion point with 18G needle

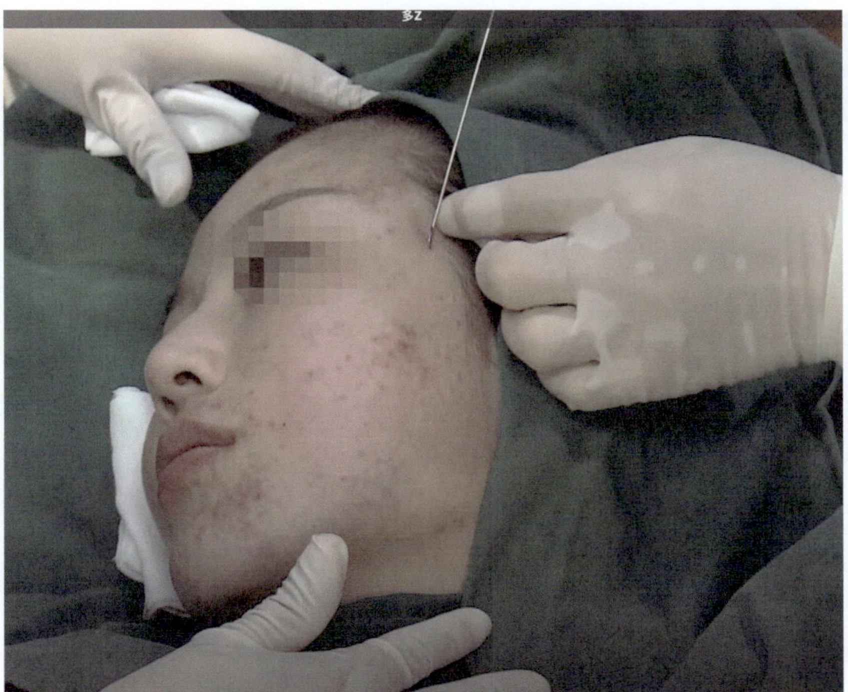

Fig. 18.8 Placement of thread with a cannula

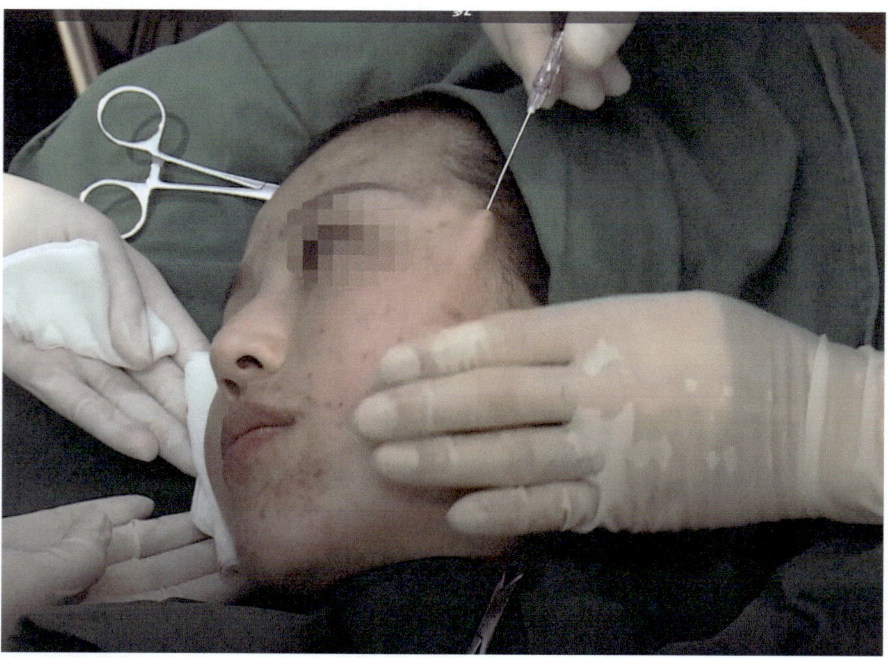

Fig. 18.9 The pattern shown in Fig. 18.5 is followed starting superiorly medially to laterally inferiorly

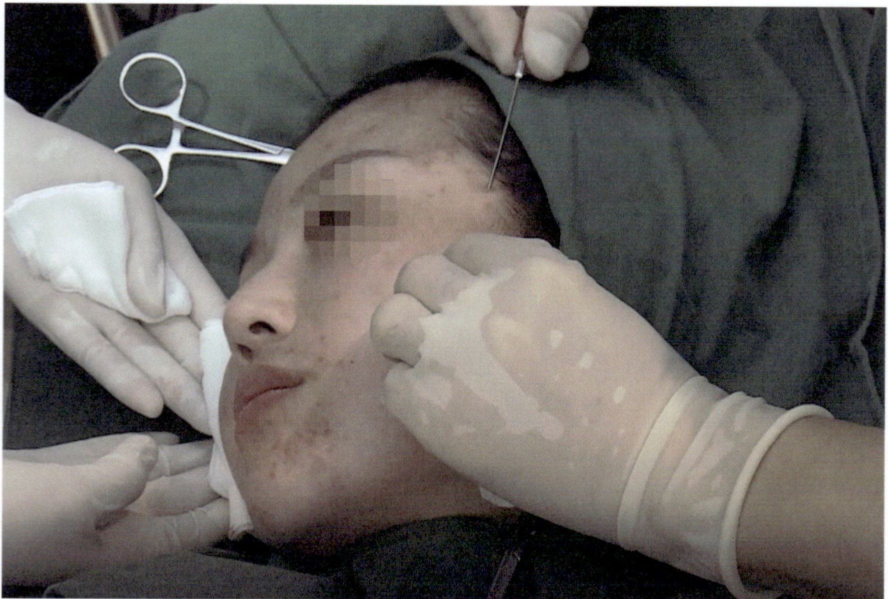

Fig. 18.10 The non-dominant hand helps guide the cannula and ensure placement in the correct layer

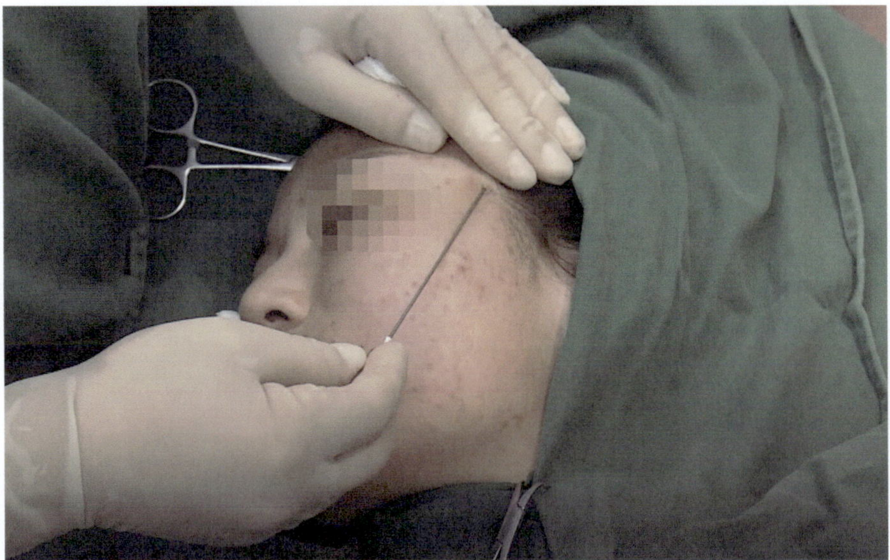

Fig. 18.11 Re-direction of the cannula after completion of placement of the thread for the mid- and lower face and placement of thread in the temple area

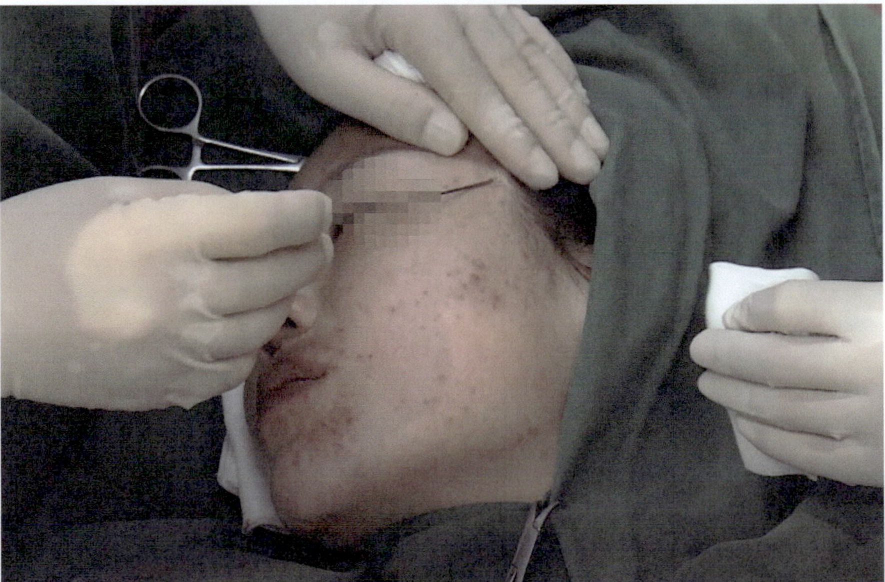

Fig. 18.12 Placement of thread in the temple area

                                           H. Cui and S. Samizadeh

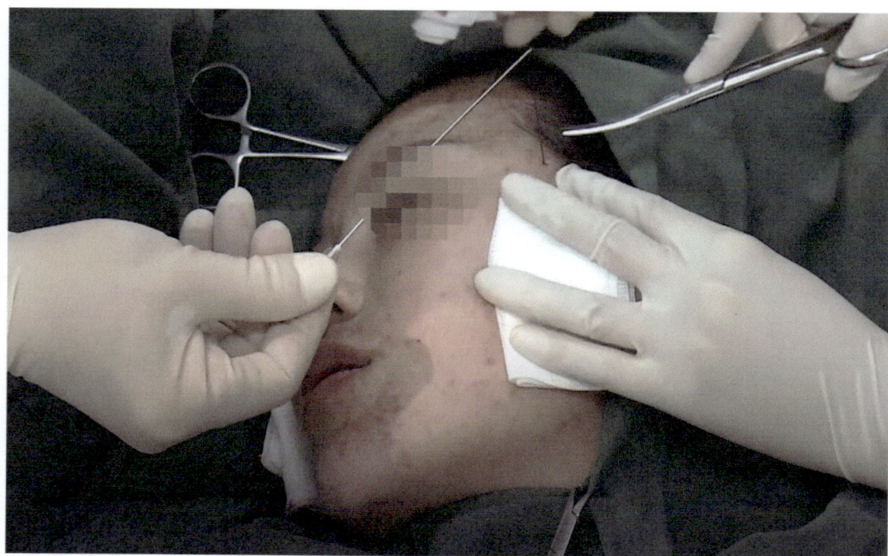

Fig. 18.13 At the end of the procedure, the remaining thread is either placed in the temporal area or removed and cut off

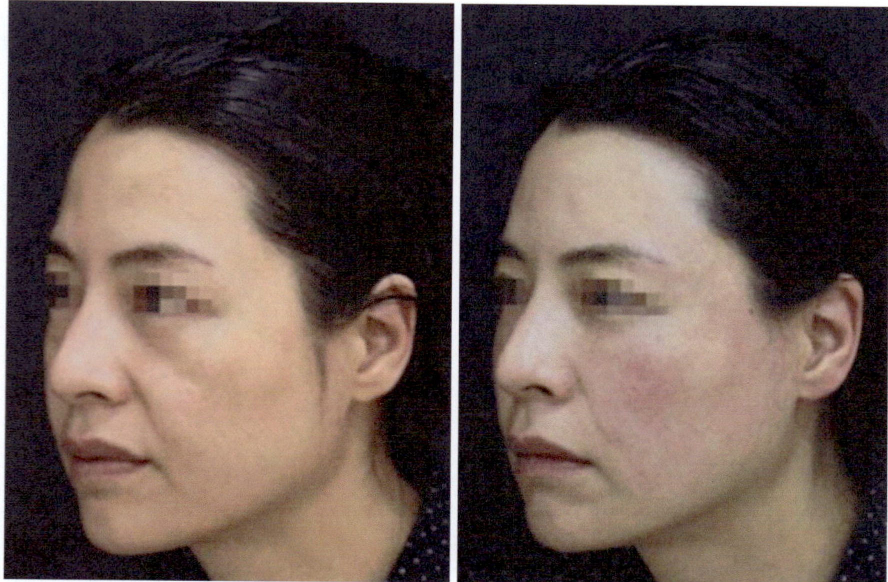

Fig. 18.14 Before and after picture using two-plane 'Continuous Multi-Z Method'

Two Planes, Two Insertion Points Method

This technique is specifically designed for individuals experiencing loss of volume and ptosis of the soft tissues in the mid- and lower face. Employing two insertion points simplifies the procedure by facilitating navigation around the zygomatic arch and mitigating the risk of postoperative distortions that could lead to unnatural appearance.

Procedure Details: First Insertion Point (E1): Positioned in front of the hairline, just above the zygomatic arch, the needle is directed from this point towards the infraorbital area. For the lateral cheek area, external to the lateral canthus and 3–5 cm anterior to the ear, the thread follows a wave-like pattern within the SMAS layer. In the region internal to the lateral canthal line, the thread placement in the superficial SMAS layer aids in tightening the lower eyelid and medial cheek areas. The insertion trajectory aims towards the medial cheek and nasolabial fold in an inferiomedial direction. Additionally, a vertical downward insertion through this point extends to the posterior third of the mandibular margin, enhancing the lift in the subzygomatic and posterior mandibular areas.

Second Insertion Point (E2): Located below the zygomatic arch and in front of the hairline, this point allows for thread placement in the lateral cheek, outside the lateral canthal line and 3–5 cm anterior to the ear, in a wave-like pattern within the SMAS. Inside the lateral canthal line, the thread navigates the superficial layer of the SMAS. This arc-shaped wiring targets the lower nasolabial fold, the outer corner of the mouth, and the anterior mandibular margin, effectively addressing nasolabial folds, marionette lines, and enhancing the contour of the mandibular margin.

By utilizing three to five threads in each specified direction, this method achieves a comprehensive rejuvenation and contouring effect, focusing on elevating and refining the facial features for a more youthful and harmonious appearance. The first insertion point (E1) is located in front of the hairline above the zygomatic arch, and the needle is directed towards the infraorbital area from this point. (Figs. 18.15, 18.16, 18.17, 18.18, 18.19, 18.20, 18.21, 18.22, 18.23, 18.24).

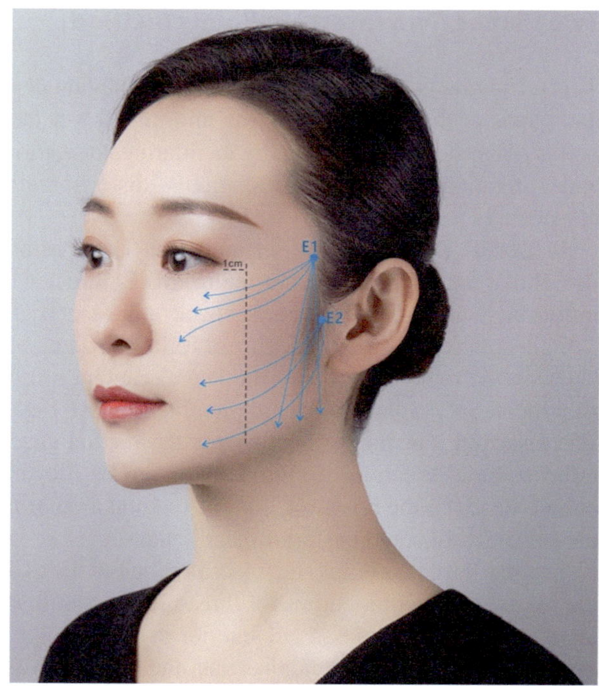

Fig. 18.15 Bi-layer, two entry points, three fan-shaped thread implantation technique

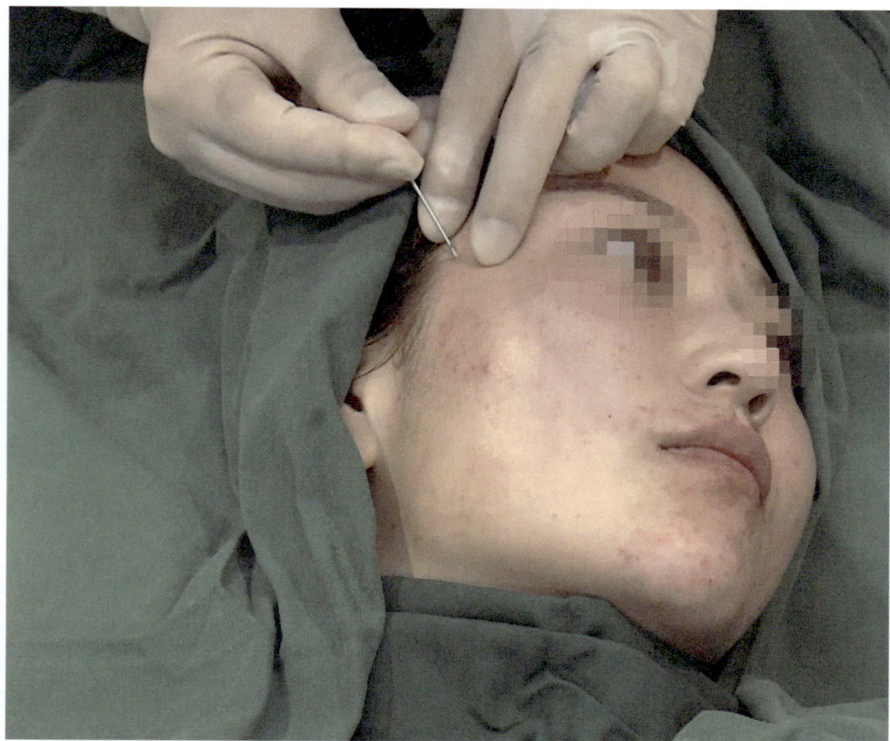

Fig. 18.16 First insertion point-E1

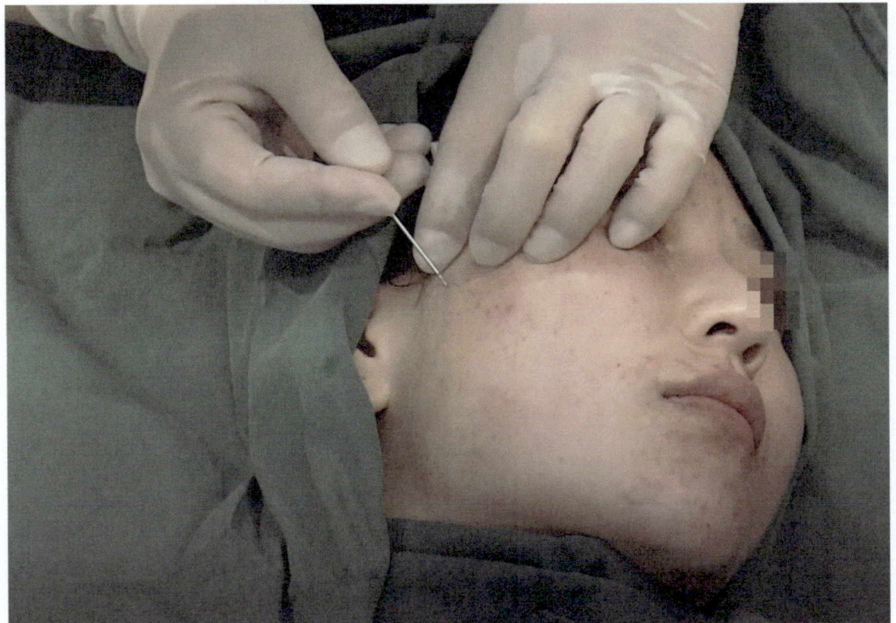

Fig. 18.17 Second insertion point (E2)

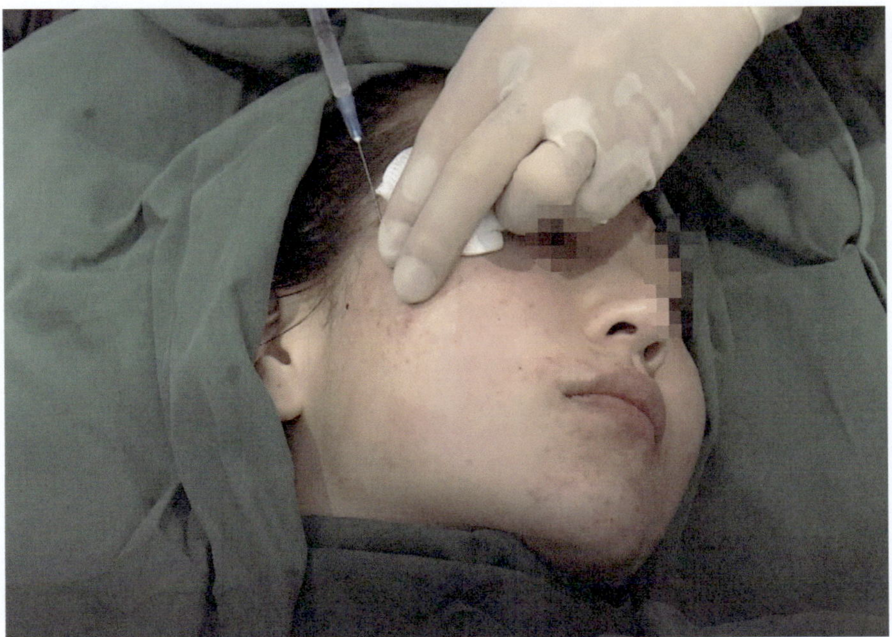

Fig. 18.18 Anaesthesia

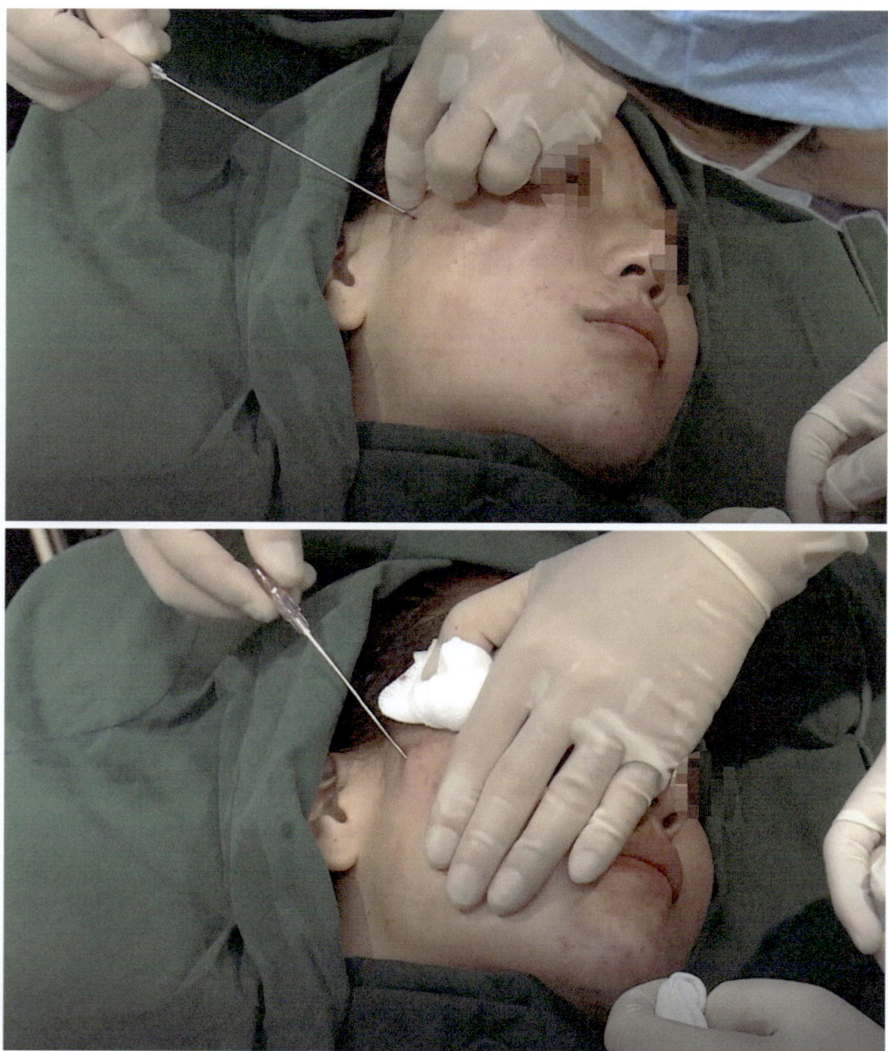

Fig. 18.19 Insertion of the first thread. Note the use of the non-dominant hand

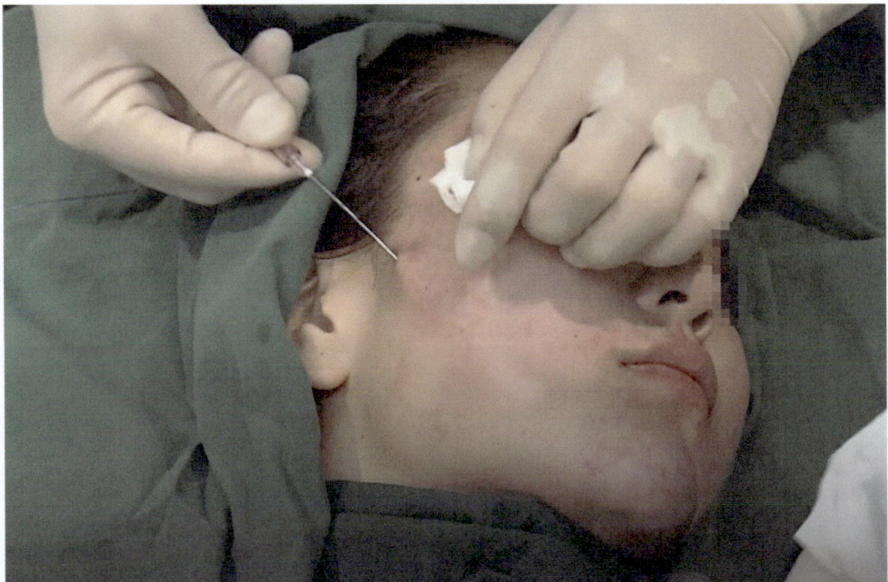

Fig. 18.20   Check the depth of the cannula prior to placing the thread. This can be done by lifting the cannula

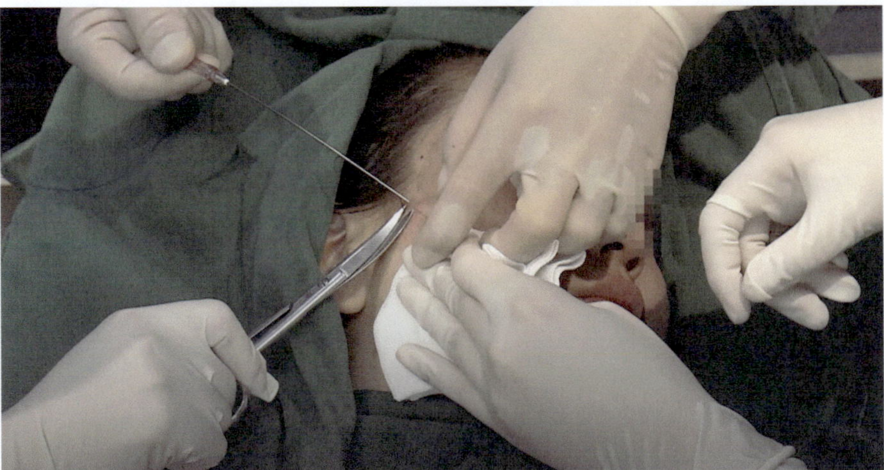

Fig. 18.21   Once the placement is complete, the cannula is removed from the insertion point, and the extra thread is cut

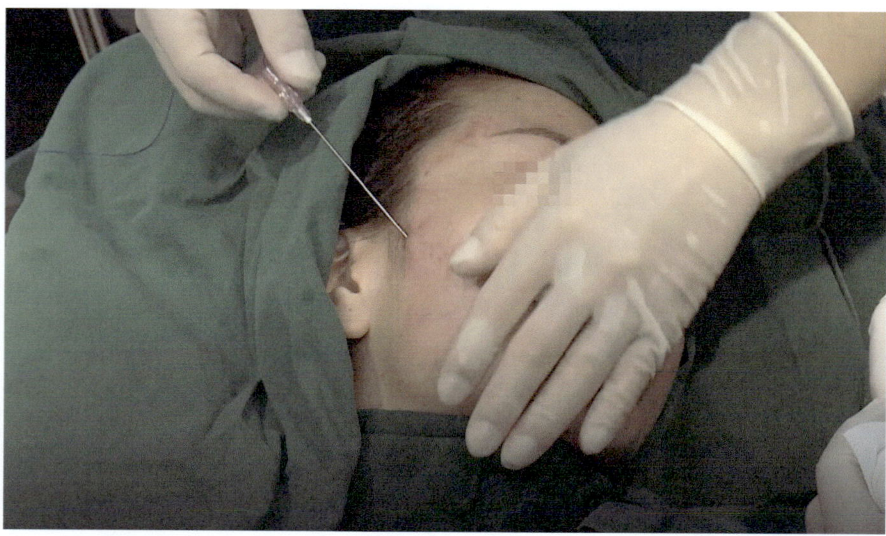

Fig. 18.22 The cannula is then re-inserted from the same insertion point and advanced in a different path. This is done for all three lines drawn from E2 in the illustration

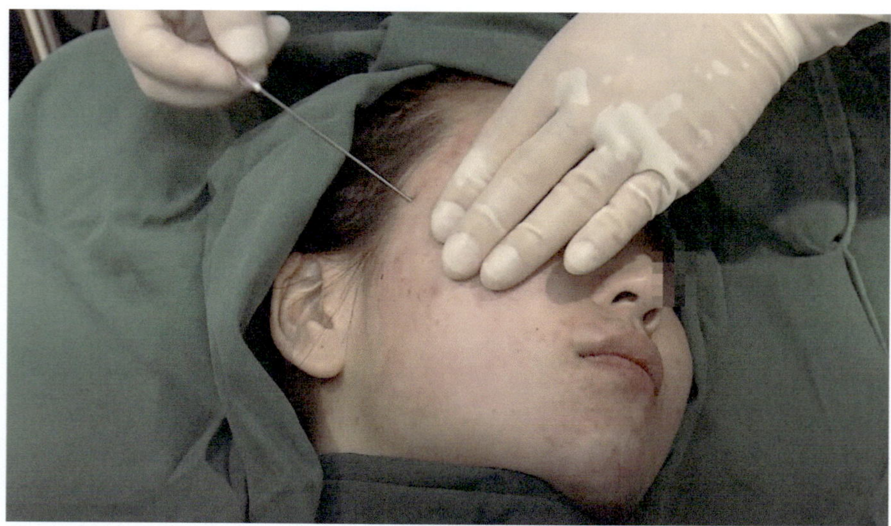

Fig. 18.23 Same process is repeated from insertion point E1

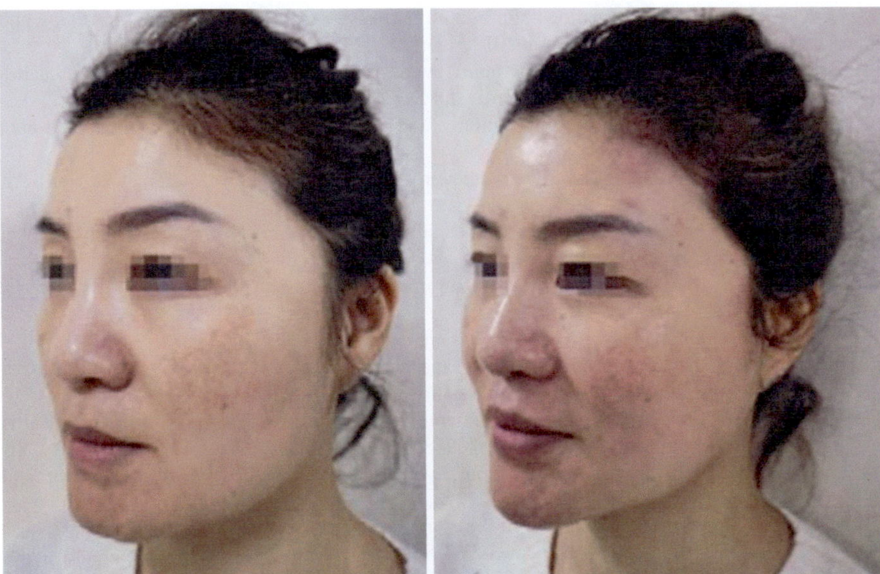

Fig. 18.24 Before and after picture

Conclusion

In conclusion, the advancement and refinement of thread lifting techniques represent a significant leap forward in the field of aesthetic medicine, offering a minimally invasive alternative for facial rejuvenation and contouring. By understanding the intricate anatomy of the facial structure and employing strategic insertion points and thread materials, practitioners can achieve natural-looking, harmonious results that address soft tissue ptosis in the mid-face and beyond. The judicious selection of barbed threads and materials such as PPDO, PDO, and PLCL, coupled with a precise approach to thread distribution, allows for customized treatment plans that cater to the unique anatomical and aesthetic needs of each patient. This chapter underscores the importance of a deep anatomical knowledge, meticulous technique, and the artistry inherent in aesthetic medicine, paving the way for innovative solutions to facial aging that prioritize patient safety, comfort, and satisfaction.

References

1. Samizadeh S. The ideals of facial beauty among Chinese aesthetic practitioners: results from a large national survey. Aesthet Plast Surg. 2018;43:1–13.
2. Samizadeh S, Wu W. Ideals of facial beauty amongst the Chinese population: results from a large national survey. Aesthet Plast Surg. 2018;43:1–11.

3. Levy LL, Emer JJ. Complications of minimally invasive cosmetic procedures: prevention and management. J Cutan Aesthet Surg. 2012;5(2):121–32.
4. Cohen BE, Bashey S, Wysong A. Literature review of cosmetic procedures in men: approaches and techniques are gender specific. Am J Clin Dermatol. 2017;18(1):87–96.
5. Samizadeh S. Chinese facial physiognomy and modern day aesthetic practice. J Cosmet Dermatol. 2019;19:161–6.
6. Samizadeh S. Beauty standards in Asia. In: Non-surgical rejuvenation of Asian faces. Springer, pp. 21–32; 2022.
7. Liew S, et al. Consensus on changing trends, attitudes, and concepts of Asian beauty. Aesthet Plast Surg. 2016;40(2):193–201.
8. Samizadeh S. Facial beauty. In: Non-surgical rejuvenation of Asian faces. Springer, pp. 3–20; 2022.
9. Langlois JH, Roggman LA. Attractive faces are only average. Psychol Sci. 1990;1(2):115–21.
10. Rhodes G, et al. Attractiveness of facial averageness and symmetry in non-Western cultures: in search of biologically based standards of beauty. Perception. 2001;30(5):611–25.
11. Alghoul M, Codner MA. Retaining ligaments of the face: review of anatomy and clinical applications. Aesthet Surg J. 2013;33(6):769–82.
12. Luo S-K, et al. Clinical anatomy for minimally invasive cosmetic treatments. In: Non-surgical rejuvenation of Asian faces. Springer; 2022. p. 59–82.
13. Mendelson B, Wong C-H. Anatomy of the aging face. Plast Surg. 2013;2:78–92.
14. Mendelson BC, Muzaffar AR, Adams JW. Surgical anatomy of the midcheek and malar mounds. Plast Reconstr Surg. 2002;110(3):885–96; discussion 897–911.
15. Kitamura S. Anatomy of the fasciae and fascial spaces of the maxillofacial and the anterior neck regions. Anat Sci Int. 2018;93(1):1–13.
16. Pessa JE. SMAS fusion zones determine the subfascial and subcutaneous anatomy of the human face: fascial spaces, fat compartments, and models of facial aging. Aesthet Surg J. 2016;36(5):515–26.
17. Gosain AK. Surgical anatomy of the facial nerve. Clin Plast Surg. 1995;22(2):241–51.
18. Cui H-Y. Aesthetic facial injection in Asians. Beijing, China: Peking University Medical Press; 2017.
19. Cui H, et al. An innovative approach for facial rejuvenation and contouring injections in Asian patients. In: Aesthetic Surgery Journal Open Forum. Oxford University Press US; 2021.

Deep Plane Thread Lift of the Buccal Fat Pad

19

Yun-Ta Tsai and Chao-Huei Wang

Abstract

Skin, subcutaneous tissue, muscle, and bone all undergo changes as we age. The relationship between the facial space and surrounding tissue is not similar to a youthful face due to volumetric alterations. Buccal fat pad displacement (pseudoherniation) may cause a puffy cheek mass. With upward displacement into the buccal region, pseudoherniation of the buccal fat pad can be easily minimized. With a thorough understanding of facial anatomy and surgical proficiency, the deep plane thread lift is a safe, practical, and simple procedure for repositioning the buccal fat pads. Buccal fat pad repositioning to improve the aesthetic contour of the lower face may be a viable treatment for patients with buccal fat pad pseudoherniation.

Keywords

Facial rejuvenation · Thread lift · Deep plane thread lift · Buccal fat repositioning · Thread lift for buccal fat repositioning · Asian facial rejuvenation · Asian thread lift

Facial Ageing

Facial ageing is inevitably and continually progressing. With time, the youthful, inverted triangular face becomes saggy and volume-depleted. Age-related changes are not due to problems in a single layer but in a whole layer [1–4]. Ageing changes

Y.-T. Tsai (✉)
Dr. Shine Clinic, Kaohsiung, Taiwan

C.-H. Wang
Dr. Shine Clinic, New Taipei City, Taiwan

© Springer Nature Switzerland AG 2024
S. Samizadeh (ed.), *Thread Lifting Techniques for Facial Rejuvenation and Recontouring*, https://doi.org/10.1007/978-3-031-47954-0_19

can be seen in skin, subcutaneous tissue, muscle, and bones [1, 3–9]. Moreover, with a better understanding of the anatomical structures, we can identify that facial fat pads and retaining ligaments also play crucial roles in facial ageing [10–14]. All these factors must be considered when a plastic surgeon attempts to perform facial rejuvenation procedures in patients. To address the problem of ageing, a comprehensive understanding of facial ageing on an anatomical basis is essential.

The face can be divided into the highly mobile anterior and the less mobile/fixed lateral part. The primary function of the anterior face is to show facial expressions using the active facial muscles, whereas the function of the lateral face is mastication using the deep muscles. Because of the dynamic movement of the muscles of facial expression, repetitive motions can cause pressure on the soft tissues, resulting in facial fat atrophy. However, the main problem in the lateral face is the inferior displacement of the superficial tissue. Therefore, the concepts of facial rejuvenation for treating the anterior and lateral face are different. Usually, deflation occurs in the anterior face, while sagging takes place in the lateral face.

Facial Fat Compartments

Patients with midface hollowing and facial atrophy show preservation of the nasolabial fold and jowl fat. This suggests that regions of fat behave differently during the ageing process. Rohrich introduced the concept of facial fat compartments in 2007 [10]. Superficial cheek compartments include infraorbital fat, nasolabial fat, medial cheek fat, middle cheek fat, lateral cheek fat, and superior and inferior jowl fat (Fig. 19.1a). All of them are distinct and separated from each other by septa. The deep cheek compartments comprise the medial suborbicularis oculi fat (SOOF), the

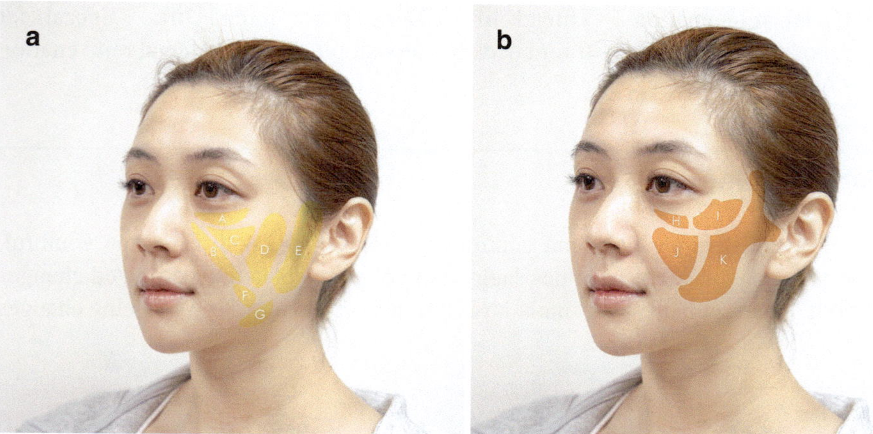

Fig. 19.1 (**a**) Superficial cheek fat compartments: (A) Infraorbital fat, (B) Nasolabial fat, (C) Medial cheek fat, (D) Middle cheek fat, (E) Lateral cheek fat, (F) Superior jowl fat, (G) Inferior jowl fat. (**b**) Deep cheek fat compartments: (H) Medial sub-orbicularis oculi fat, (I) Lateral sub-orbicularis oculi fat, (J) Deep medial cheek fat, (K) Buccal fat

lateral SOOF, the deep medial cheek fat (DMCF), and the buccal fat (Fig. 19.1b). Facial ageing is characterized by how these compartments change with age.

Several anatomical studies on the description of facial compartments have increased our understanding of age-related changes (Fig. 19.1). Schenck et al. [15] proved that the superficial cheek compartments behave differently when fillers are placed: injection of volumizing material leads to an inferior displacement of the superficial nasolabial, middle cheek, and jowl compartments. Injection into the medial cheek, lateral cheek, and superficial temporal compartments increases volume without causing inferior displacement. Cotofana et al. [16] concluded that inferior displacement of the deep facial fat compartments does not occur with increasing age. The increasing volume did not cause an inferior displacement of the injected material. This also emphasized the importance of the deep facial fat compartments in supporting the overlying structures.

Buccal Fat Pad

The buccal fat pad was first mentioned by Heister in 1732 and is considered to be glandular in nature. In 1802, Bichat recognized the buccal fat pad's anatomical structure, comprising the main body and the buccal, pterygoid, and temporal extensions. The functions of the buccal fat pad include protection and cushioning and separation of the cheek muscles. It also supports the facial tissue to prevent depression during sucking in infants. With ageing, the function of the buccal fat pad becomes less critical.

The buccal fat pad is a part of the deep facial fat compartment. Volumetric changes of the buccal space during ageing result in pseudoherniation of the buccal fat pad. Matarasso [17] advocated for removing the buccal fat pad to improve facial aesthetics. The buccal fat pad could be removed smoothly without damaging Stenson's duct or the facial nerve through an intraoral incision with meticulous dissection into the buccal space.

Although pseudoherniation of the buccal fat pad could result in a puffy cheek mass, other reasons may also develop a perioral mass. An accurate diagnosis should be made in advance to treat the puffy cheek mass. Differential diagnoses of the perioral mass include pseudoherniation of the buccal fat pad, thickening of the modiolus, superficial jowl fat hypertrophy, and inferior displacement of the superficial jowl fat.

The method to ensure the patient has pseudoherniation of the buccal fat is to ask the patient to look up, with the chin and forehead on the same horizontal plane. If the puffy cheek mass disappears, pseudoherniation of the buccal fat pad can be diagnosed. Modiolus or superficial jowl fat should be suspected if the mass does not disappear. Performing the pinch test could be helpful in diagnosing the presence of superficial jowl fat.

After the diagnosis of pseudoherniation of the buccal fat pad is confirmed, buccal fat pad management is considered. Although Matarasso advocated excision of the buccal fat pad, the removal procedure alone does not always provide a promising

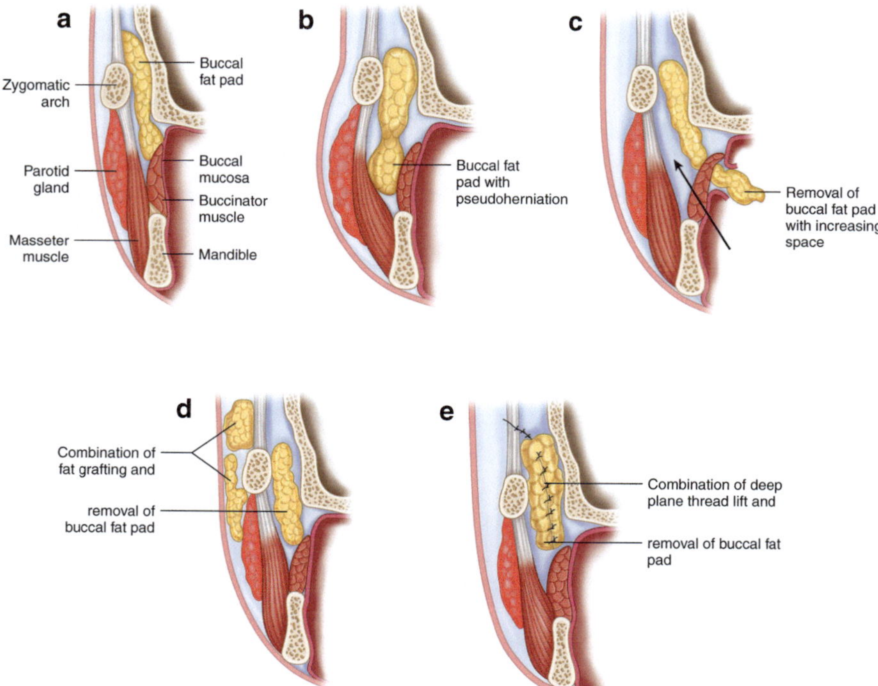

Fig. 19.2 (**a**) Young face with content-to-space ratio ≈ 1. (**b**) Ageing face with buccal fat pad pseudoherniation and smaller content-to-space ratio. (**c**) Removal of the buccal fat pad with smaller content-to-space ratio. (**d**) Combined removal of the buccal fat pad with face fat grafting. (**e**) Combined removal of the buccal fat pad with thread lift

aesthetic result. A probable explanation is a relationship between the contents and the space (Fig. 19.2a, b). Removing the buccal fat pad might help decrease the perioral mass volume, but it could also lead to a smaller content-to-space ratio (Fig. 19.2c). However, the satisfaction rate is usually higher if the procedure is combined with thread lift or face fat grafting. Combining buccal fat pad removal with face fat transfer (Fig. 19.2d) or thread lift (Fig. 19.2e) could increase the content-to-space ratio. A higher content-to-space ratio increases the facial structures' fullness or tightness; therefore, the aesthetic result is usually satisfactory.

Concept of the Buccal Fat Pad Repositioning

Since the buccal fat pad is a deep facial fat compartment, its role in supporting the overlying structures should not be ignored. Although pseudoherniation of the buccal fat pad could result in an unsightly puffy cheek mass, excision of the buccal fat pad might not be the only way to improve aesthetic appearance. Pseudoherniation of the buccal fat pad is caused by volumetric changes in the buccal space, with the buccal fat pad 'falling' into a wider space. In this case, 'repositioning' the falling buccal fat pad rather than removing it would be an even better way to restore the youthful, inverted triangle of the face. Repositioning the buccal fat pad allows facial fullness with underlying support by deep fat pads and prevents sagging caused by the over-resection of the buccal fat pad. Allows some extent of 're-distribution' of contents in the space. The content-to-space ratio does not decrease after the procedure; therefore, the patient's facial fullness is preserved (Fig. 19.2).

Thread Lifting for Repositioning of the Buccal Fat Pad

Over the past few years, thread lifting for facial rejuvenation has been increasingly advocated. Although thread lift maintenance is not as long-lasting as facelift surgery, its minimally invasive feature remains popular. As the thread-lifting procedure evolves, the meticulous design of the route on an anatomical basis is suggested. The latest critical points of thread lifting include vector design, the relationship between the thread and the movable tissue, three-dimensional lifting rather than two-dimensional lifting, anchor point selection, the plane of suspension, and target tissue lifting.

Selecting the appropriate target tissue to be lifted is essential to achieving good thread lift results. With a better understanding of facial fat compartments, passing through them with inferior displacement could be helpful for facial reshaping. According to Schenck [15], injecting a volumizing material leads to an inferior displacement of the superficial nasolabial, middle cheek, and jowl compartments. It indicates that the superficial nasolabial, middle cheek, and jowl compartments are the target tissues that benefit from a thread lift.

The deep facial fat compartments provide support to the overlying structures. Inferior displacement of the deep facial fat compartments does not occur with increasing age. Since the buccal fat pads are located at the junction of the anterior and lateral aspect of the face, volumetric change of the buccal space causes pseudoherniation of the buccal fat pad. Capsular thickening of the buccal fat pad provides its upper anchoring point so that the buccal fat pad is 'reducible' into the masticator space. Therefore, it is called pseudoherniation. Therefore, reducing the 'herniated' buccal fat pad through thread lifting is another option to improve facial contour.

The deep plane thread-lift technique was proposed in the thread-looping method advocated by Wang et al. [18]. The so-called 'deep plane thread lift' involves the passage of the thread deeper than the zygomatic arch [19]; in this case, the thread passes through the masticator space smoothly, with the involvement of the buccal fat pad.

Deep Plane Thread Lift Surgical Technique for Repositioning of the Buccal Fat Pad

The STRATAFIX™ Symmetric size 2-0 or 3-0 suture device (Ethicon, Somerville, NJ) was used in our practice. The recommended barbed suture should be adequately strong and secure for high tension. The inlet point of the thread is 1.5 cm above the zygomatic arch, just along the sideburn (Fig. 19.3a). The inlet point at this location is selected to avoid injuring the course of the middle temporal vein. The direction of the cannula is positioned 0.5–1 cm lateral to the modiolus (Fig. 19.3b). Once the cannula passes deeper than the zygomatic arch, the tip of the cannula is kept sliding along the deep surface of the zygomatic arch to prevent the cannula from going outside the masticator space. The other hand is used to press against the buccal mucosa (Fig. 19.3c) to feel the cannula moving next to the buccinator muscle; this way, the cannula could pass through the masticator space with the involvement of the buccal fat pad and cause no vessel or nerve injuries. When the cannula passes over the horizontal level of the labial commissure, the thread is inserted until there is no space for the tip of the thread to move further forward. The thread is pulled back with the other hand, compressing the cheek to secure the involvement of the buccal fat pad with the thread. After pulling the thread back, tying, or hiding, the thread in the deeper tissue is suggested; this way, loosening of the thread lift could be prevented.

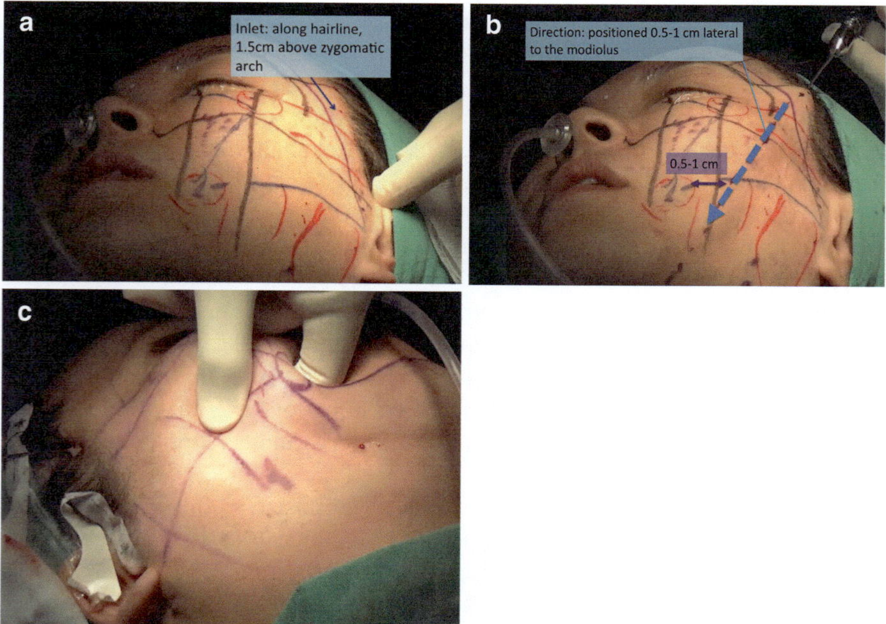

Fig. 19.3 Surgical technique of the deep plane thread lift. (**a**) Inlet point: 1.5 cm above the zygomatic arch, along hairline (**b**). Direction: position 0.5–1 cm lateral to the modiolus. (**c**) Using left hand to press buccal mucosa and feel the location of the cannula

After the procedure, the mouth should be opened to check whether there are penetrating buccal mucosa injuries. If any part of the thread is left exposed in the buccal mucosa, the thread should be removed irrespective of size.

Post-operative Care

An antibiotic ointment may be applied to the inlet point of the thread. Patients are advised to avoid vigorous mouth opening, sleep with an elevated head for several days postoperatively, and apply ice packs during the first three days. Ecchymosis and oedema are minimal if the procedure is performed correctly. Facial massage should be avoided during the first two months.

Summary

Appropriate management of the puffy cheek mass depends on accurate differential diagnosis. Pseudoherniation of the buccal fat pad, thickening of the modiolus, superficial jowl fat hypertrophy, and inferior displacement of the superficial jowl fat must be considered prior to treatment selection. Once the diagnosis of pseudoherniation of the buccal fat pad is confirmed, a deep plane thread lift for the repositioning of the buccal fat pad is a good option for achieving good aesthetic results (Fig. 19.4). The procedure could be performed smoothly, with meticulous design and a comprehensive understanding of the anatomy without critical soft tissue injuries.

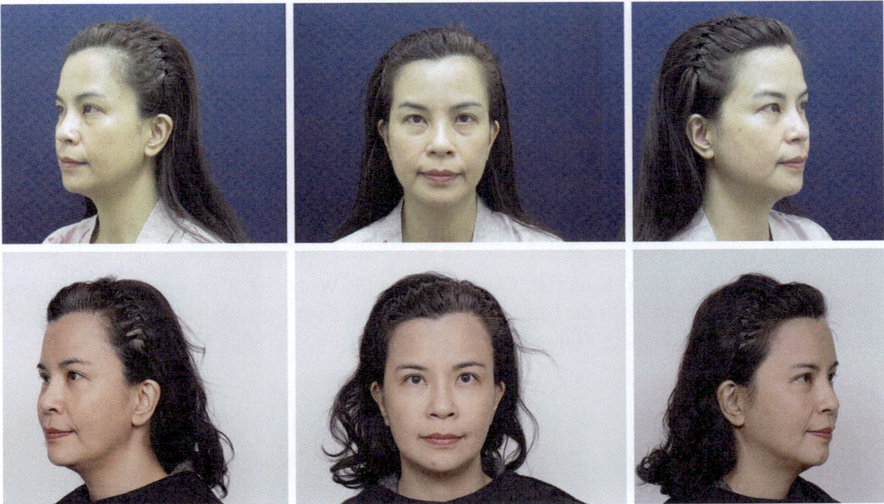

Fig. 19.4 Before and After

References

1. Pessa JE, Zadoo VP, Mutimer KL, et al. Relative maxillary retrusion as a natural consequence of aging: combining skeletal and soft-tissue changes into an integrated model of midfacial aging. Plast Reconstr Surg. 1998;102:205–12.
2. Pessa JE. An algorithm of facial aging: verification of Lambros's theory by three-dimensional stereolithography, with reference to the pathogenesis of midfacial aging, scleral show, and the lateral suborbital trough deformity. Plast Reconstr Surg. 2000;106:479–88.
3. Kahn DM, Shaw RB Jr. Aging of the bony orbit: a three-dimensional computed tomographic study. Aesthet Surg J. 2008;28:258–64.
4. Pessa JE, Chen Y. Curve analysis of the aging orbital aperture. Plast Reconstr Surg. 2002;109:751–5.
5. Kahn JL, Wolfram-Gabel R, Bourjat P. Anatomy and imaging of the deep fat of the face. Clin Anat. 2000;13:373–82.
6. Lambros V. Observations on periorbital and midface aging. Plast Reconstr Surg. 2007;120:1367–76.
7. Montagna W, Carlisle K. Structural changes in the aging skin. Br J Dermatol. 1990;122(suppl 35):61–70.
8. Wulf HC, Sandby-Moller J, Kobayashi T, et al. Skin aging and natural photoprotection. Micron. 2004;35:185–91.
9. Gosain AK, Klein MH, Sudhakar PV, et al. A volumetric analysis of soft-tissue changes in the aging midface using high-resolution MRI: implications for facial rejuvenation. Plast Reconstr Surg. 2005;115:1143–1152, discussion 1153–5
10. Rohrich RJ, Pessa JE. The fat compartments of the face: anatomy and clinical implications for cosmetic surgery. Plast Reconstr Surg. 2007;119:2219–27.
11. Rohrich RJ, Pessa JE. The retaining system of the face: histologic evaluation of the septal boundaries of the subcutaneous fat compartments. Plast Reconstr Surg. 2008;121:1804–9.
12. Wong CH, Hsieh MK, Mendelson B. The tear trough ligament: anatomical basis for the tear trough deformity. Plast Reconstr Surg. 2012;129:1392–402.
13. Furnas DW. The retaining ligaments of the cheek. Plast Reconstr Surg. 1989;83:11–6.
14. Wong CH, Mendelson B. Facial soft-tissue spaces and retaining ligaments of the midcheek: defining the premaxillary space. Plast Reconstr Surg. 2013;132:49–56.
15. Schenck TL, Koban KC, Schlattau A, et al. The functional anatomy of the superficial fat compartments of the face: a detailed imaging study. Plast Reconstr Surg. 2018;141:1351–9.
16. Cotofana S, Gotkin RH, Frank K, et al. The functional anatomy of the deep facial fat compartments: a detailed imaging-based investigation. Plast Reconstr Surg. 2019;143:53–63.
17. Matarasso A. Buccal fat pad excision: Aesthetic improvement of the midface. Ann Plast Surg. 1991;26:413–8.
18. Wang CH, Liu HJ, Tsai YT, Lin HI, Wu PY, Lin JW. An innovative thread-looping method for facial rejuvenation:minimal access multiple plane suspension. Plast Reconstr Surg Glob Open. 2019;7:e2045.
19. Tsai YT, Zhang Y, Wu Y, Yang HH, Chen L, Huang PP, Wang CH. The surgical anatomy and the deep plane thread lift of the buccal fat pad. Plast Reconstr Surg Glob Open. 2020;8:e2839.

Non-surgical Nose Modification Using Threads

20

Non-surgical Rhinoplasty

Konstantin Sulamanidze, George Sulamanidze, Marlen Sulamanidze, and Souphiyeh Samizadeh

Abstract

Surgical rhinoplasty is one of the most common cosmetic surgeries worldwide and can help increase quality of life and self-esteem. With the increased interest and request for non-surgical and minimally invasive procedures, options for treatment of the nose have been limited. With the advancement of knowledge and technology, dermal fillers and threads can be used to reshape the nose, elevate the tip of the nose, reduce appearance of the prominence of the bump on the nose bridge, eliminate some deformities and irregularities, and smooth the contour of the nose profile. Dermal fillers carry the risk of vascular compromise in this high-risk zone, embolism, and blindness. In this chapter, modification of the nose using P (LA / CL) is explained.

Keywords

Thread lift · Threads rhinoplasty · Rhinoplasty · Non-surgical rhinoplasty · Thread lifting · Non-surgical facial rejuvenation · Facelift · Non-surgical facelift · APTOS

K. Sulamanidze · G. Sulamanidze (✉) · M. Sulamanidze
Total Charm Clinic, APTOS, Tbilisi, Georgia
e-mail: const@aptos.ru; aptos@aptos.ge; gracia@aptos.ru

S. Samizadeh
King's College London, London, UK

University College London, London, UK

Great British Academy of Aesthetic Medicine, London, UK
e-mail: info@baamed.co.uk

S. Samizadeh (ed.), *Thread Lifting Techniques for Facial Rejuvenation and Recontouring*, https://doi.org/10.1007/978-3-031-47954-0_20

Introduction

Rhinoplasty ranks among the most frequently performed cosmetic surgeries globally, catering to individuals across all genders. This procedure not only augments self-esteem but also significantly enhances the quality of life by aligning the nose's appearance with the patient's desired aesthetic, given its central position on the human face [1–3].

Plastic surgeons are increasingly challenged by patients to refine their surgical techniques, aiming for minimal scarring, shortened operative times, and expedited recovery periods. This demand aligns with the notable surge in the popularity of minimally invasive aesthetic interventions over the past two decades. Among these, thread lifting has gained considerable attention for its dual benefits of rejuvenation and lifting when executed proficiently.

The thread lift market is diverse, with numerous manufacturers, innovators, and surgeons across the globe holding patents for a wide array of threads, each differing in composition, type, and application technique. This chapter focuses on APTOS threads, renowned for their efficacy in facial and body lifting, contouring, and rejuvenation. Originating in 1996 by the Georgian plastic surgeon Marlen Sulamanidze, the APTOS thread lifting technique has been refined and advanced by George and Constantin Sulamanidze.

APTOS

Over 25 years have elapsed since the introduction of the APTOS thread and technique, during which APTOS has innovated the 'Sole rhinoplasty method'—a unique approach and thread design for non-surgical modification of the nose.

Patient selection is key. Understanding anatomy is paramount. Indications include:

- Concave/under projected nasal dorsum (Low nasal bone)
- A droopy/downward rotated nasal tip—nasal tip ptosis
- A droopy/downward rotated columella
- Naso-labial angle (tip-lip) correction
- Nasal valve problems
- Nasal tip deviation (only if septoplasty is not necessary)
- Wide nostrils
- Wide tip

Differences in different ethnic facial features and beauty ideals should be considered before treatment planning.

Thread Composition

P (LA/CL) – L-polylactide-Σ-caprolactone [4].

This suture material has been used in surgery for over 30 years.

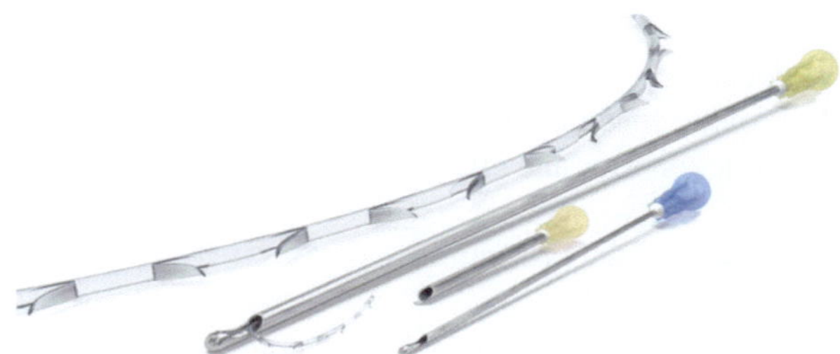

Fig. 20.1 The thread itself is preinstalled into the round tip cannula. The surface characteristics of the thread can be appreciated in this figure

Thread Characterization

Thread is composed of P (LA/CL), which has multidirectional barbs along the whole length of the thread. One of the most important parts of the thread is the fixator which is intended to fix thread in tissue and allows to reposition the skin and tissues in an aesthetically favourable position.

APTOS has developed uniquely designed barbed threads, crafted through specialized cutting techniques to ensure robust and immediate anchorage within soft tissues. This innovation facilitates the instant repositioning of fat compartments, leading to immediate aesthetic enhancements.

The threads are preloaded into a round-tip cannula, designed to be atraumatic, significantly minimizing the risk of injury to vessels, nerves, and surrounding tissue. The distinctive arrangement of the barbs, positioned opposite one another, allows for independent operation of each barb segment. This configuration guarantees that upon thread insertion, the barbs engage with the tissue instantaneously, securing a robust fixation. Importantly, the design ensures that the accidental breakage of any barb does not compromise the overall stability of the thread within the tissue, maintaining the integrity of the aesthetic correction (Fig. 20.1).

APTOS Thread Package Contents (for Non-surgical Rhinoplasty)
- P(LA/CL) thread with barbs USP 2/0, EP3, 120 mm—5 pieces
- Round tip hollow needle 20G × 120 mm, straight—5 pcs
- Round tip hollow needle 23G × 80 mm, straight—1 pcs
- Lancet point needle 18G × 40 mm, straight—1 pcs
- Lancet point needle 30G, straight—1 pcs

Patient Preparation for the Procedure

1. Begin with a comprehensive consultation that covers the various treatment options, alongside their associated risks and benefits. Discuss all potential complications and adverse effects, the expected recovery timeline, and the healing process in detail. Collect the patient's medical history, including any chronic conditions affecting the lungs or cardiovascular system, systemic and endocrine disorders, previous surgical and cosmetic procedures, known allergies, current medications, pregnancy/breastfeeding and relevant menstrual cycle information.

2. Allow a cooling-off period for the patient to reflect and make an informed decision.
3. Provide specific pre-procedure instructions, such as abstaining from alcohol for 24 hours prior and arriving without makeup on the day of the procedure.

On the day of the procedure:

4. Before proceeding, reconfirm the procedure details, risks, benefits, and recovery expectations, and obtain informed consent.
5. Ensure all makeup is removed before documentation and the procedure itself.
6. Take standardized pre-procedure photographs for accurate before-and-after comparisons.
7. Finalize the treatment plan and the placement of thread vectors.

Medical Photography

For comprehensive evaluation and documentation, photograph the patient before the procedure, immediately afterwards, and then at intervals of 2 weeks, 1 month, 3 months, and 6 months against a monochromatic, contrasting background. Maintain an optimal distance of 1—1.5 meters between the patient's face and the camera lens. General Tips for Consistent Clinical Photography:

- Use a monochromatic background to avoid distractions and ensure focus on the facial features.
- Maintain a standardized distance between the camera and the patient, ideally around 1 to 1.5 meters, to avoid distortion.
- Consistent lighting is key; use soft, diffused lighting to minimize shadows and highlight facial contours.
- Ensure the camera is at eye level with the patient for all views to maintain consistency across different photo sessions.

These standardized photographic positions and settings provide a reliable basis for evaluating pre- and post-procedure outcomes, facilitating a clear, objective comparison over time.

Standard positions for face photography

1. Full-Face View: The patient should face the camera directly, with eyes looking forward. Ensure the line between the pupils (interpupillary line) is horizontal and parallel to the camera's horizon. This ensures a symmetrical frontal view for accurate assessment.
2. Profile View: The patient turns to the side, presenting a direct profile of one side of the face to the camera. Align the patient so that the ear closest to the camera is visible and the nose profile is clearly defined against the background. The profile view is crucial for evaluating the lateral aspects of facial structures, including the nose, lips, and chin projection.
3. Side (Oblique) View: The patient should be positioned at a 45-degree angle to the camera, showcasing a blend of the frontal and profile features. This view

provides a comprehensive perspective on the contours and asymmetries of the face, particularly useful for assessing the mid-face area, nasal tip, and cheek definition.

Instruments and Consumables for the Procedure

- Procedure Environment: A designated procedure room or operating room that meets clinical standards for sterility and equipment.
- Medical Utility/Procedure Table: A clean, organized table for arranging necessary instruments and consumables.
- Sterile Instruments: Essential tools including forceps, scissors, and skin procedure clips. For specific needs, consider adding two mosquito-type forceps and hats to the kit, or opt for the specialized APTOS Medical Kit (Fig. 20.2).
- Syringes and Needles: A minimum of two 5- or 10-mL syringes, along with 30G and 18G needles, unless these are already included with the threads.
- Antiseptics: A selection of hydrochloride-based antiseptics (such as Octenisept, with hydrochloride (1 mg/mL) and phenoxyethanol (20 mg/mL)), Clinisept, Betadine, or Chlorhexidine for skin preparation.
- Anaesthetic: An adrenaline-containing anaesthetic, ranging in concentration from 1:100,000 to 1:200,000, including options like ultracaine, Ubistesin, or Septanest, for patient comfort during the procedure.
- Personal Protective Equipment (PPE) for the Practitioner: Sterile gloves, gown, cap, and mask to maintain a sterile environment and protect both the practitioner and the patient.
- Procedure Gown/Cover and Cap for the Patient: To ensure patient safety and maintain sterility throughout the procedure.

▶ **Important** Since thread lift is a minimally invasive procedure, all aseptic and antiseptic rules must be strictly observed.

Fig. 20.2 APTOS medical kit with sterile content

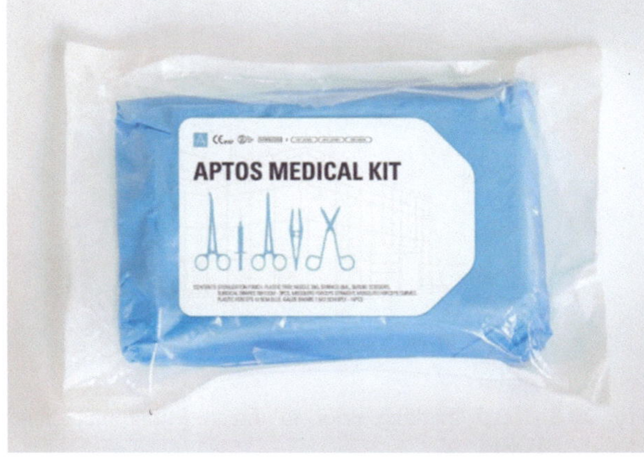

Marking

Utilize a medical marking pen for precision, with a preference for red ink, to ensure visibility. The objective of these markings is to establish symmetry in thread placement and fixation points. It's essential to perform these markings while the patient is in an upright position to accurately assess facial contours and symmetry.

- Dorsal Line Marking: Begin at the nasal tip, drawing a line along the dorsum up to the radix. This serves as a guide for the thread's trajectory and fixation along the nose's length (Fig. 20.3a). Columellar Line Marking: From the nasal tip, extend a vertical line down to the columella, ending at the columellar base (Fig. 20.3b). This marking is critical for precise columellar adjustment.
- Columella Correction with Tip Elevation: Start marking from the columellar base, drawing a vertical line upwards to the nasal tip (see Fig. 20.3c). This approach is used for elevating the tip while adjusting the columella. (Fig. 20.3c).

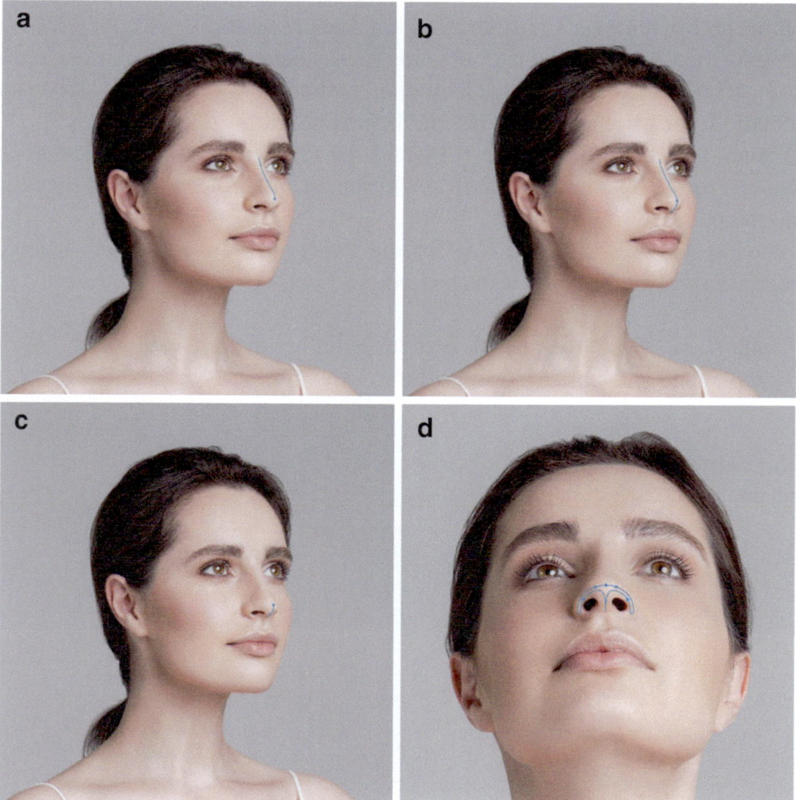

Fig. 20.3 Nasal marking prior to thread lifting including insertion and fixation. (Image credit: APTOS)

– Correcting Small Deformities and Tip Elevation: Mark from the initial entry point to the nasal tip, then extend lines along the alar rims to the alar base and down the mid-columella to the columellar base. For isolated nostril corrections without tip elevation, the entry point begins at the lateral part of the nostril, extending a line to the nasolabial angle and then laterally towards the tip. This technique provides structural support similar to a rim graft (Fig. 20.3d).

In these procedures, threads act as a structural columellar graft, offering support and contouring to the columella and surrounding nasal structures.

Dorsum Correction and Tip Elevation: Initiate the marking from the nasal tip, drawing a vertical line up to the radix for dorsal correction (Fig. 20.3a). For tip elevation, extend another vertical line from the tip down to the nasolabial angle (Fig. 20.3b).

Nasal Valve Deformation: For corrections involving the nasal valve, mark a line from the nasal tip following the lateral contour of the alar down to the alar base (Fig. 20.3c). Nostril Correction: When focusing solely on nostril adjustments, the marking should mimic the approach of a rim graft for targeted enhancement (Fig. 20.3d).

Anaesthesia

- Tissue Infiltration: Perform anesthesia infiltration at the procedure's entry points to prepare the tissue.
- Cannula Selection: For safety and ease, opt for 23G × 80 mm cannulas (available in some APTOS kits or separately) or 25–27G cannulas for the infiltration process.
- Anesthetic with Adrenaline: Utilize an anesthetic solution that includes adrenaline for its vasoconstrictive properties, which also extends the anesthetic effect, barring any individual contraindications.
- Anesthetic Agent Options: Recommended agents include Ultracain, Ubistesin (forte), Septanest, Scandonest, or a 0.25% lidocaine solution with adrenaline in ratios of 1:100,000 or 1:200,000.
- Adjusting the Anesthetic Solution: If necessary, dilute the anesthetic with an equal part saline solution and incorporate a small quantity of sodium bicarbonate (0.2 mL per 2 mL of anesthetic solution) for optimal pH balance.
- Cannula Insertion: Gently insert the cannula into the subcutaneous tissue, following the pre-marked lines.
- Optimal Anesthetic Volume: Administer an appropriate volume of anesthetic, typically between 2-4 mL, depending on the procedure's extent.
- Anesthesia Exposure Time: Allow 1–2 minutes for the anesthetic to take full effect before proceeding with the procedure.

Technique

1. Initiating the Procedure: Begin by creating an entry point at the tip of the nose using an 18-gauge needle, facilitating the insertion of a round-tip cannula.
2. Cannula Insertion Technique: Insert the cannula perpendicularly into the superficial fatty layer of the nasal tip. Adjust the cannula to a horizontal position and, while pulling the tip with your finger, guide it along the dorsum towards the radix. Then, retract it back to the tip, distributing the thread through the dorsum's superficial fatty layer. Without removing the cannula, rotate it from the tip and vertically align it along the columella down to its base, repeating this manoeuvre 2–3 times before withdrawing (Fig. 20.4).

Fig. 20.4 (**a**) surface anatomy of the nose, (**b**) layered anatomy: Skin and soft tissue envelope (skin, superficial fatty layer, fibro-muscular layer, deep fatty layer, and perichondrium or periosteum). Nasal skin characteristics vary significantly in a different portion of the nose. Ethnic differences should be understood. For example, the Asian nasal envelope is different from Caucasians. It has a thick subcutaneous fat layer which is oilier and denser than the fibro-fatty layer [5].

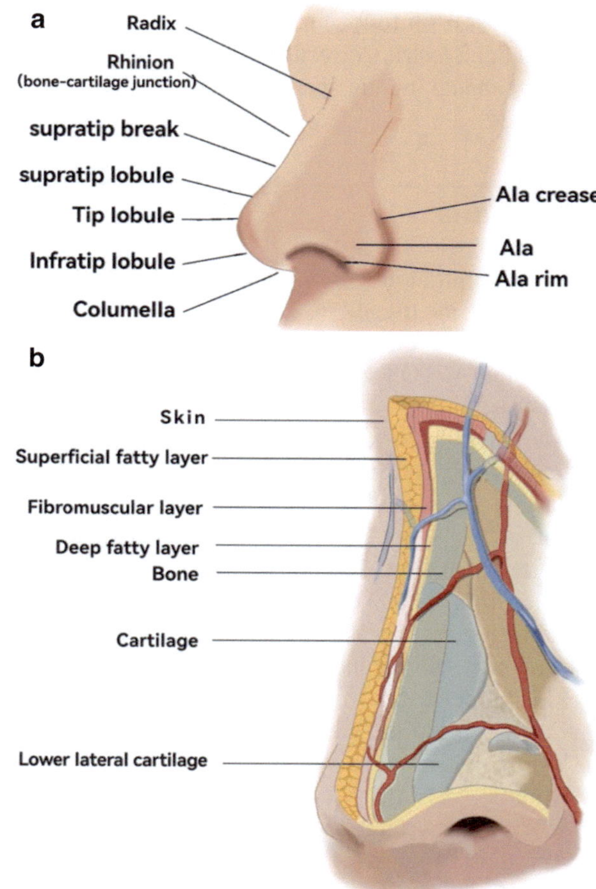

3. Addressing Nasal Valve Deformities: For nasal valve corrections, start from the nasal tip, moving the cannula to the lateral alar sides, reaching the alar base. Then, proceed from the tip through the columella to the nasolabial angle, ensuring even thread distribution. The thread length is 12 cm, there is the possibility to repeat this manoeuvre 3–4 times with one thread.
4. Columella and Alar Corrections: Similar to surgical rhinoplasty techniques, threads serve as columellar grafts for structure and support. The entry point for columella corrections is from its base, moving vertically through to the tip, touching the maxilla. For deformations and external valve issues, initiate from the nasal tip, maneuvering the cannula along the lateral alars to the alar base and back, akin to a rim graft technique.

The placement of threads on the columellar is similar to the columellar graft used during surgical rhinoplasty.

The placement of threads on the Alar is similar to the rim graft used during surgical rhinoplasty.

Recommendations After Procedure

- Avoid exercising for 48 h after treatment
- Refrain from wearing heavy glasses for 1 week
- Avoid sun exposure and head (e.g. sauna/hot bath) for 2 weeks
- Massaging or pressing the nose, including facials and skin extractions, should be avoided
- Consider taping the nose to aid lift stabilization and swelling reduction.
- Follow the prescribed postoperative medication regimen (antibiotics, painkillers).
- Post-procedural regenerating cream or gel, e.g. Recowell post-procedural regenerating cream-gel.

Possible Side Effects and Complications

- Discomfort, pain, bruising, swelling, and soreness.
- Risk of hematoma, dimpling, and irregularities.
- Visibility of sutures.
- Dimpling and irregularities.
- Infection.
- The potential for thread protrusion, extrusion, or migration.

Possible Combinations with Other Cosmetic Techniques

- Botulinum toxins: 2 weeks before the procedure.
- Filler injection in the same region: after 2–3 weeks.
- Chemical peeling can be concurrent with the procedure.

The Technique of Removing Installed Threads

After implantation, threads remain in the patient's body for an indefinite period: they do not need to be removed without a specific need. In case of some complications, the threads may need to be removed. To remove the thread, the following instruments, medications, and consumables are required:

- Adrenaline-containing anaesthetic (Ultracaine DS, etc.)
- 5 mL syringe
- 27G injection needle
- 'Mosquito' forceps
- Cooper's scissors
- Glover's hook, 1–1.5 mm thick
- 18G Injection Needle (or scalpel No. 11)

Begin by accurately marking the puncture point on the skin while the patient stands upright. This mark indicates where the thread lies within the subcutaneous tissue. Following the administration of local anesthesia, puncture the skin at the marked location using either an 18G needle or a No. 11 scalpel, ensuring the incision is about 1 mm in length. Subsequently, insert Glover's hook through the puncture into the subcutaneous layer to latch onto the thread and gently draw it out to the surface. The thread may then be extracted either in part or in full, depending on the requirement. Should the thread prove challenging to remove with the hook alone, the incision may need to be slightly enlarged to 2 mm to facilitate removal, preferably with a mosquito-type clip for ease. Once the thread has been successfully removed, immediately secure the puncture site with a sterile adhesive patch to promote healing and prevent infection.

Case Studies

See Figs. 20.5, 20.6, 20.7, 20.8

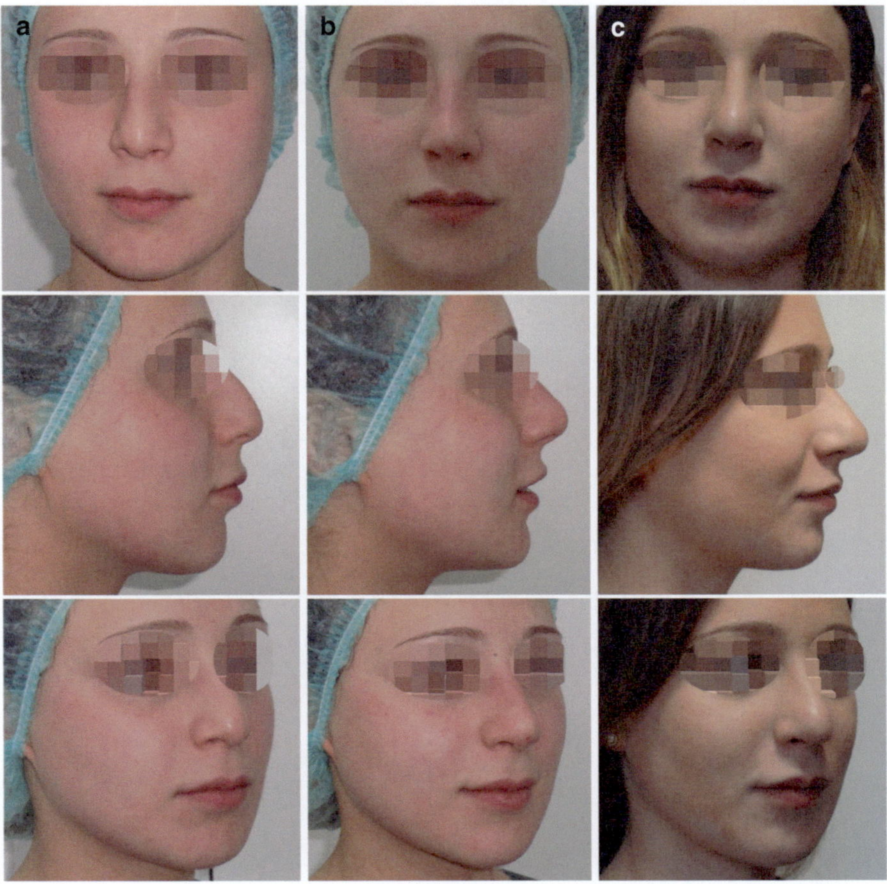

Fig. 20.5 Patient with droopy nasal tip (**a**) Image before sole rhinoplasty method. (**b**) Immediately after procedure (**c**) 1.5 years after the procedure. (Image credit: APTOS)

Fig. 20.6 Patient with downward rotated nasal tip (**a**) Image before sole rhinoplasty method. (**b**) Immediately after procedure. (Image credit: APTOS)

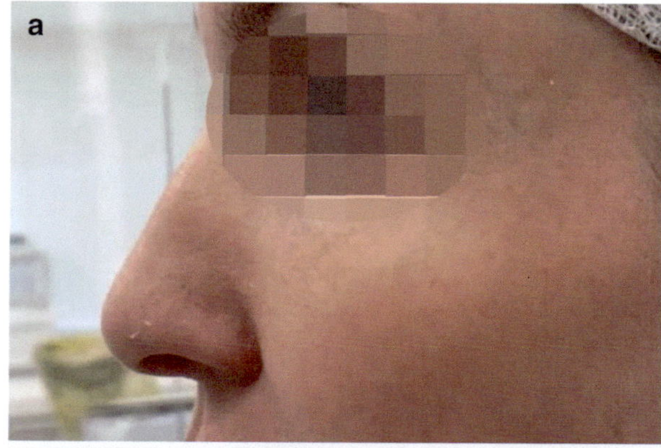

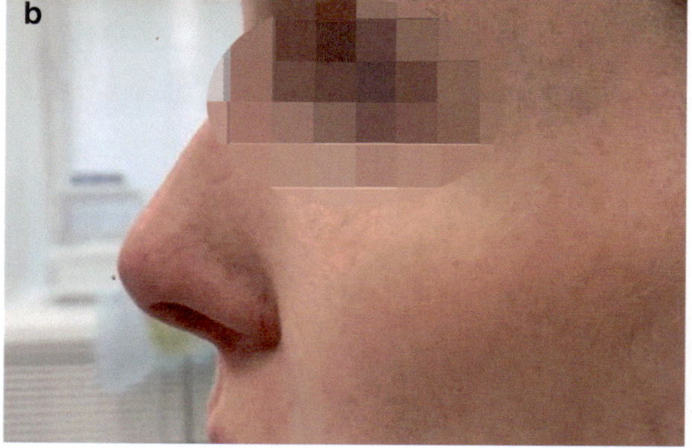

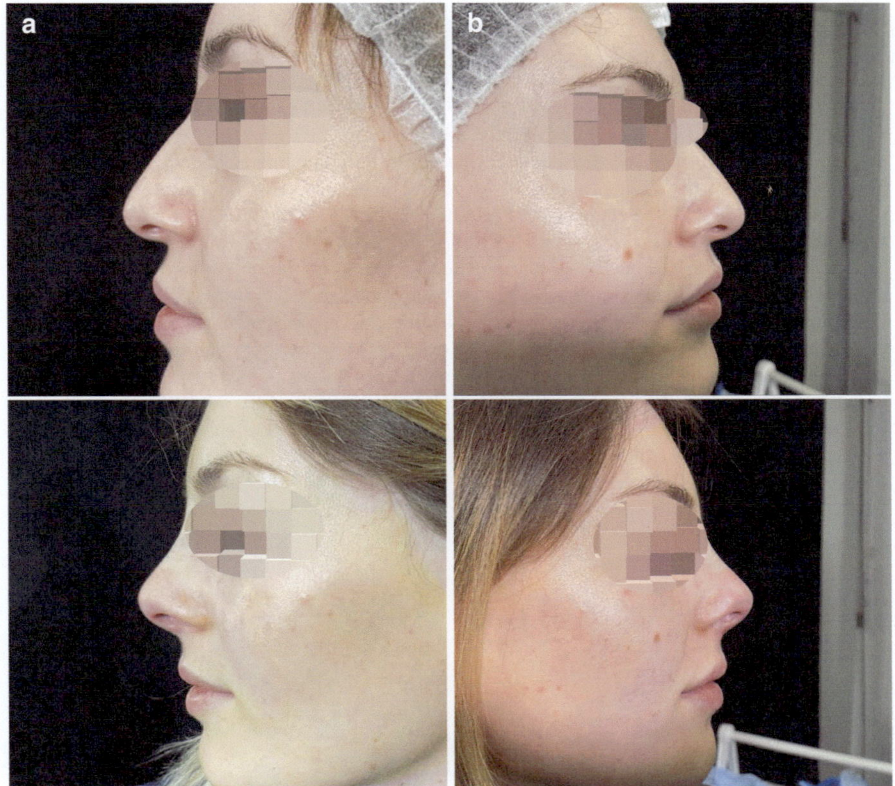

Fig. 20.7 (**a**) Image before sole rhinoplasty method. (**b**) Immediately after procedure. (Image credit: APTOS)

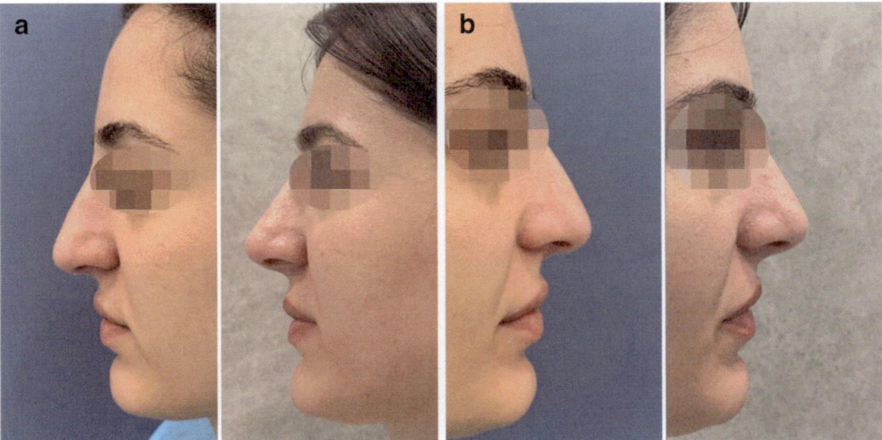

Fig. 20.8 (**a**) Image before sole rhinoplasty method. (**b**) Immediately after procedure. (Image credit: APTOS)

References

1. Rezaee Khiabanloo S, Nabie R, Aalipour E. Outcomes in thread lift for face, neck, and nose, a prospective chart review study with APTOS. J Cosmet Dermatol. 2020;19(11):2867–76. https://doi.org/10.1111/jocd.13397. Epub 2020 Apr 8.
2. Borujeni LA, Pourmotabed S, Abdoli Z, Ghaderi H, Mahmoodnia L, Sedehi M, et al. A comparative analysis of patients' quality of life, body image and self-confidence before and after aesthetic rhinoplasty surgery. Aesthet Plast Surg. 2020;44(2):483–90.
3. Yang F, Liu Y, Xiao H, Li Y, Cun H, Zhao Y. Evaluation of preoperative and postoperative patient satisfaction and quality of life in patients undergoing rhinoplasty: a systematic review and meta-analysis. Plast Reconstr Surg. 2018;141(3):603–11.
4. Wong V. The science of absorbable poly(L-lactide-co-ε-caprolactone) threads for soft tissue repositioning of the face: an evidence-based evaluation of their physical properties and clinical application. Clin Cosmet Investig Dermatol. 2021;14:45–54. https://doi.org/10.2147/CCID.S274160.
5. Khaliq A, Daniel Z, Javed N. Rhinoplasty, a powerful tool to boost patient's self-confidence. Ann Punjab Medical College (APMC). 2020;14(2):149–52.

Combination Treatment: Threads and Dermal Fillers

With Special Emphasis on Restoring Lower Face Curvature in East Asians

Chao-Chin Wang

Abstract

The process of facial ageing includes skin laxity, tissue sagging, and depression of facial contours caused by loss of bony support and volume of soft tissue. A natural, rejuvenated look can be achieved through a balanced improvement in each aspect of ageing—the loose skin tightened, the sagged tissue lifted, and the depression of facial contour restored. It is often necessary to combine different modalities to achieve this goal non-surgical. Until recently, some injectable fillers and their original indication for correcting volume loss have also been advocated for 'lifting'. Injecting the fillers into the bases of the retaining ligaments reinforced the ligaments, weakening and tilting because of age and resulting in a 'lifted' appearance. As a non-surgical option for lifting, thread lifts are faster than energy-based devices in the onset of action, while their longevity remains in debate. The author proposed the 'The Dual Lift technique' to improve the tissue sagging and facial contour with the optimal combination of bi-directional cog threads and injectable fillers. The filler-reinforced ligaments synergistically enhance the effect of lifting by threads, and the longevity of fillers complements the threads and leads to a longer-lasting result of the procedure.

Keywords

Threads · Thread lifts · Injectable filler · Dual lift · Skin ageing

C.-C. Wang (✉)
Tainan Vigor Clinic, Tainan, Taiwan

Liberal Vigor Clinic, Kaohsiung, Taiwan

© Springer Nature Switzerland AG 2024
S. Samizadeh (ed.), *Thread Lifting Techniques for Facial Rejuvenation and Recontouring*, https://doi.org/10.1007/978-3-031-47954-0_21

Characteristics of Skin Ageing in Asians

Skin ageing in Asians is heralded by the formation of pigmented spots, while wrinkles and tissue sagging occur slower in Asians than in Caucasians [1]. However, the lower third of the Asian face is often square-shaped with greater mandibular width and retruded chin [2] (Fig. 21.1), which commonly leads to a wrong impression of sagging, albeit the sagging is mild. Therefore, this group will benefit from thread lift systems with a balanced profile of efficacy and downtime rather than systems with robust lifting but much more extended downtime.

The ideal facial shape for Asian females is an oval shape with smaller bizygomatic width and a pointy chin (Fig. 21.2). High cheekbones and prominent sub-zygomatic depressions are considered less attractive in Asian faces.

Combining thread and injectable fillers for non-surgical rejuvenation in Asians has several advantages: ethnic Asians have dense fat and fibrous connection between the superficial muscular aponeurotic system (SMAS) and the deep fascia, which not only reduce midfacial sagging for longer but also serve as a good framework for the

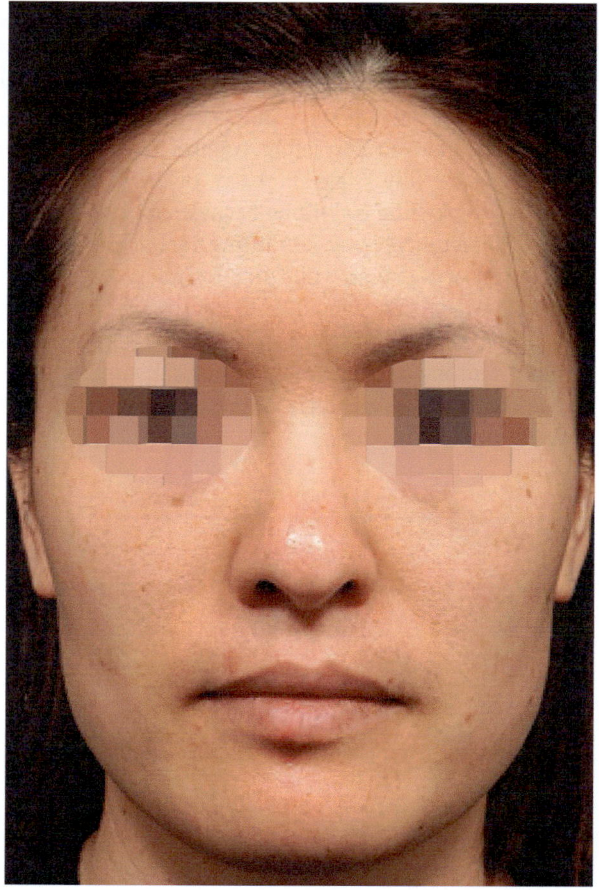

Fig. 21.1 Lower third of the Asian face is often square-shaped with greater mandibular width and retruded chin [2]. Reproduced with permissions from Liew, S. et al. Consensus on Changing Trends, Attitudes, and Concepts of Asian Beauty. *Aesth Plast Surg* **40**, 193–201 (2016). (http://creativecommons. org/licenses/by/4.0/)

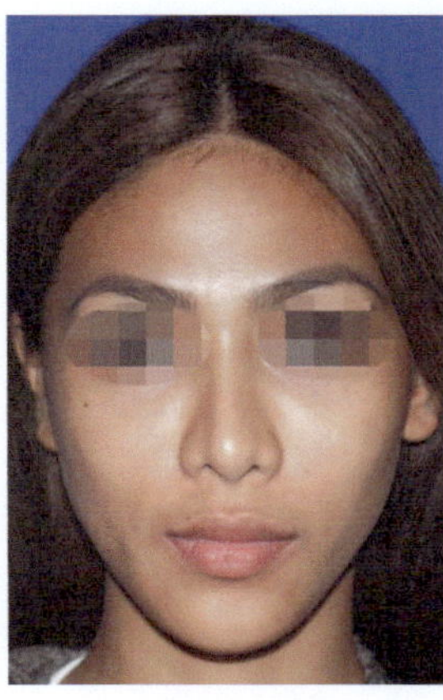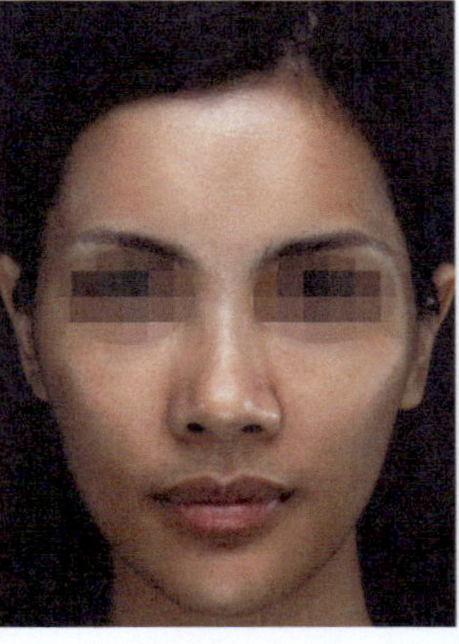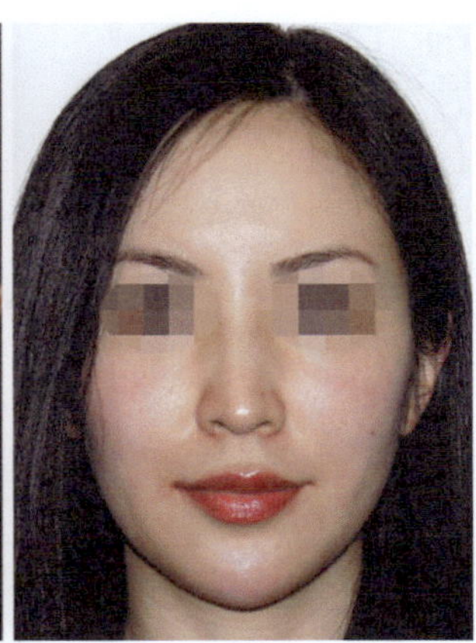

Fig. 21.2 Ideal facial shape for Asian females: oval shape with smaller bi-zygomatic width and pointy chin [2]. Reproduced with permissions from Liew, S. et al. Consensus on Changing Trends, Attitudes, and Concepts of Asian Beauty. *Aesth Plast Surg* **40**, 193–201 (2016). (http://creative-commons.org/licenses/by/4.0/)

threads to work on; Asians have thicker skin than age-matched Caucasians [3] which is less likely to encounter 'thread show' when the threads implanted become palpable or visible in thinner skin; the ligaments reinforced by fillers further strengthen the framework; and finally, the facial contour and proportion may be fine-tuned by fillers.

Ageing with Particular Emphasis on Jowl Problem

Changes in the Fat Compartments

During the ageing process, the superficial fat compartments of the face droop with time while the deep fat compartments relocate and become atrophy [4] (Fig. 21.3). And drooping of the superficial fat compartments [5] is related to the deepening of the nasolabial folds and jowl formation.

Ligaments and Bone

The ageing changes associated with the retaining ligaments are biphasic. Initially, their firm, bone-to-skin attachments help support the adjacent tissues against droop-ing. Meanwhile, the tethering and folds of skin look deeper due to the firm attach-ments, especially near the boundary of the fat compartments. However, with further ageing, the retaining ligaments gradually lose elasticity and precipitate to further fat protrusion and drooping. In the example of jowl formation, the mandible and alveo-lar bone also resorb in the advanced stage, leading to worsening of jowling [4].

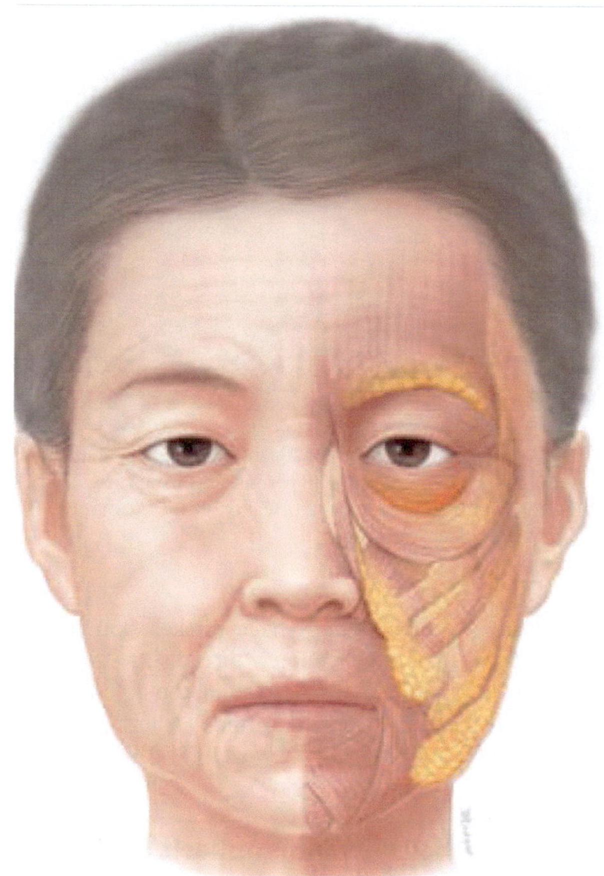

Fig. 21.3 The superficial fat compartments of the face droop during facial ageing. Reproduced with permissions from *HJ Kim et al, Clinical Anatomy of the Face for Filler and Botulinum Toxin Injection*

In cases with mild jowling accompanied by concurrent volume loss in the cheeks, restoring the volume deficiency in the deep fat compartment of the cheeks may rebalance the mildly sagged superficial fat compartments and produce a skin tenting effect to pull up the descended jowl (Fig. 21.4). For cases with prominent jowl problem, it is necessary to manage all the contributing factors to deliver the optimal result, while thread lifts being an option of management for sagginess.

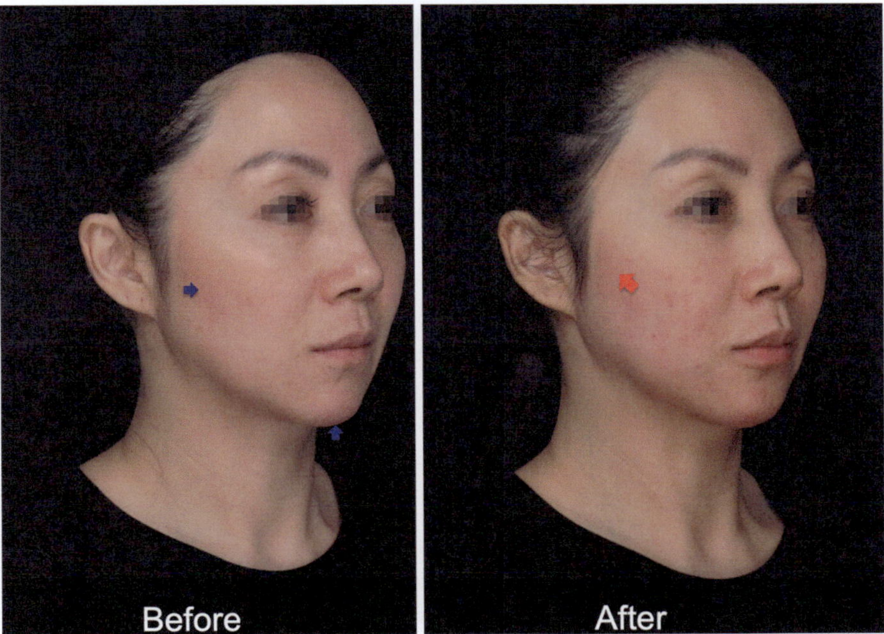

Fig. 21.4 In mild jowl problem, filling up the volume deficiency in the deep fat layer of the cheeks may rebalance the mildly sagged superficial fat compartments and produce skin tenting effect to pull up the descended jowl

Anatomical Consideration for Safe Thread Insertion

The primary concern of safety for injectable fillers is to avoid intravascular injection. Likewise, thread lifts are to prevent nerve damage. As the trunks of motor nerves passing through the facial area run deep to the SMAS layer [6], keeping the depth of thread constantly above the SMAS layer is generally safe (Fig. 21.5). It is worth noticing that the frontal branch of the facial nerve travels superficially over the zygomatic arch and most of its path falls within the range of the middle third of the arch. Therefore, it is safe to direct the thread across the posterior third of the zygomatic arch and keep the plane of treatment above the SMAS (Fig. 21.6).

The depth of thread implantation is adjustable, either superficial or deep, as long as it is within the safe range. The retinacular cutis, or the fibrous extensions of SMAS anchoring to the dermis [4], could serve as a nice target for the cogs of the threads to integrate within the superficial plane (Fig. 21.7). However, placing threads in the superficial plane in thin-skinned cases should be cautious, as the tracts of the threads might be visible or palpable from the skin surface.

The immobile SMAS is an important landmark for thread lifts on mid-to-lower face. SMAS over the lateral face is thick where it is relatively immobile and fused with the parotid capsule. Yet over the highly mobile cheek, the aponeurotic layer is

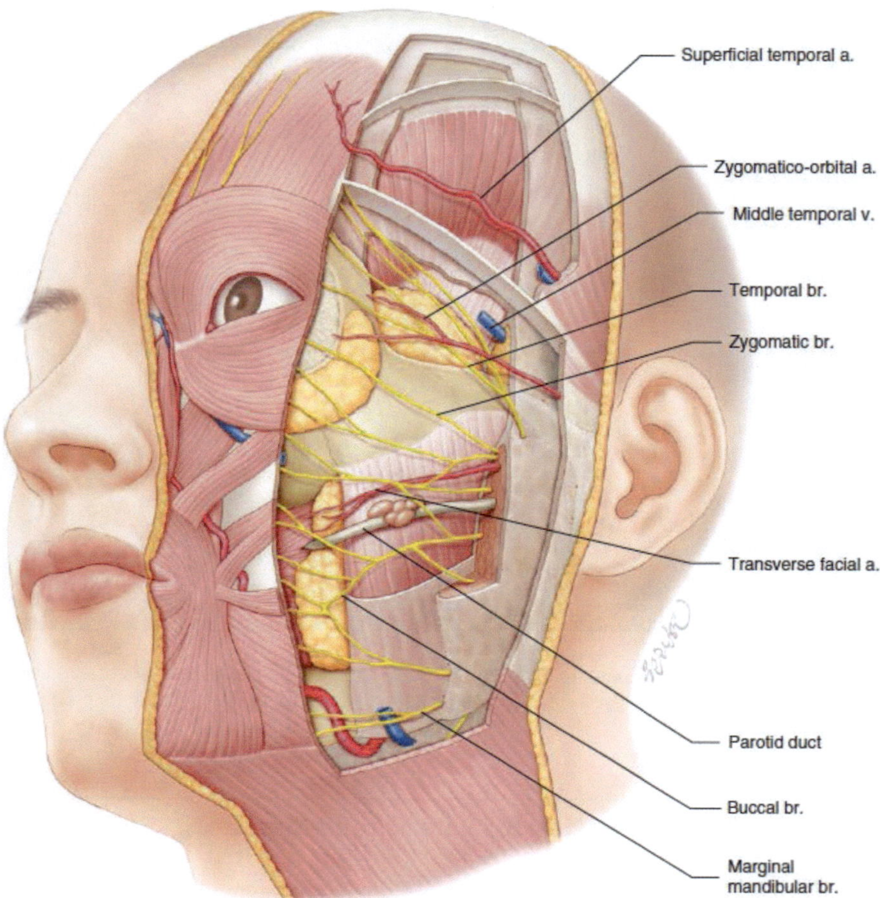

Fig. 21.5 The facial nerve branches travel deep to the SMAS layer. Reproduced with permissions from Kim, B., Oh, S., Jung, W. (2019). Anatomy for Absorbable Thread Lifting. In: The Art and Science of Thread Lifting. Springer, Singapore

so thin as to be difficult to define [7]. Once the soft tissue over the immobile SMAS is caught by the cogs of the threads and uplifted, the adjacent tissue overlying the mobile SMAS on the cheek will also be pulled up. Therefore, the threads stay over the relatively immobile tissue without interfering with the contraction of the mimetic musculature, which ensures natural improvement and little chance of thread migration during facial movement. Moreover, lifting or plication of the SMAS is possible in this deep subcutaneous plane.

Fig. 21.6 The frontal branch of the facial nerve travels within the range of the middle third of the arch. Reproduced with permissions from Kim, B., Oh, S., Jung, W. (2019). Anatomy for Absorbable Thread Lifting. In: The Art and Science of Thread Lifting. Springer, Singapore

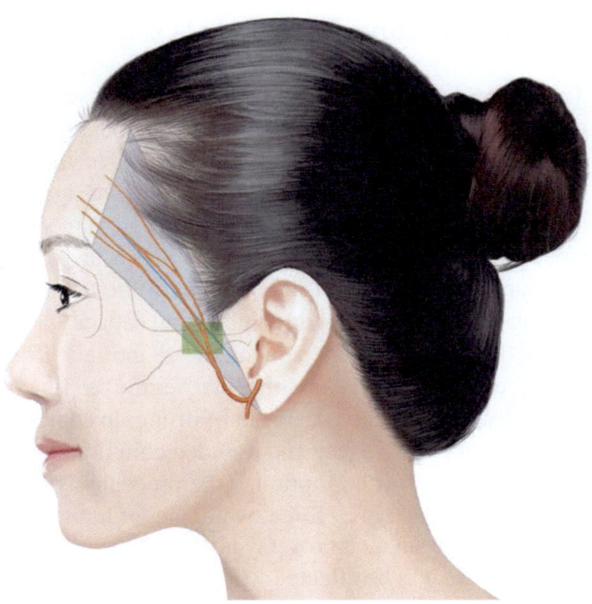

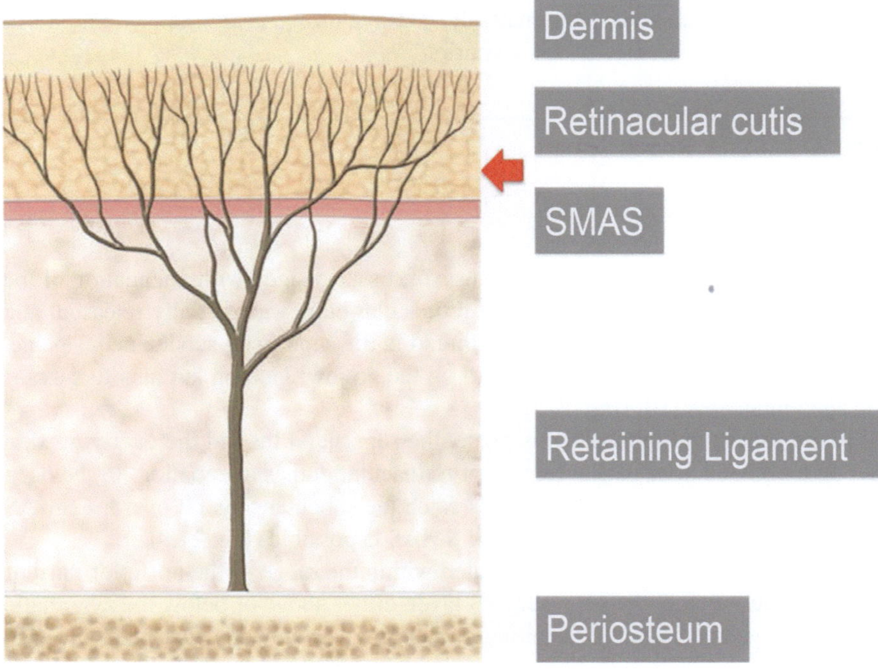

Fig. 21.7 The retinacular cutis is the fibrous extension of SMAS through the adipose layer anchoring to the dermis. Reproduced with permissions from Kim, Hee-Jin & Seo, Kyle & Lee, Hong & Kim, Jisoo. (2016). Clinical Anatomy of the Face for Filler and Botulinum Toxin Injection: General Anatomy of the Face and Neck. 10.1007/978-981-10-0240-3

Anatomical Consideration for Combining Filler Injection

The SMAS layer is attached to the underlying facial skeleton by retaining ligaments of the face. These connect the musculoaponeurotic layer to the underlying periosteum at specific fixation points in relation to the bony cavities, e.g. orbicularis retaining ligament, zygomatic, and mandibular ligaments [7].

During the ageing process, the retaining ligaments lose their elasticity and elongate, leading to the descending of the SMAS layer and the associated soft tissue. A non-surgical technique of retightening of the retaining ligaments was proposed by placing injectable fillers with high lifting capacity at the base of the ligaments, providing direct support of ligaments and an indirect lifting of the SMAS layer, a 'cantilever' effect [8]. Therefore, the filler-reinforced ligaments could act synergistically with threads to enhance the result of lifting. In addition, combining injectable fillers to reshape the square face and retruded chin in Asian faces and rebalance the facial asymmetry may further optimize the procedure's outcome. Therefore, fillers with high lifting capacity (G′ force) would better fit the situation.

There has been a controversy about whether the longevity of the polydioxanone (PDO) suture will be affected when used in conjugation with hyaluronic acid filler. A non-controlled in vitro observation showed that polydioxanone (PDO) suture immersed in non-crosslinked hyaluronic acid seemed to develop hydrolytic degradation microscopically within 72 h [9]. However, it is too preliminary to conclude this without further studies. Alternatively, non-hyaluronic acid fillers with high lifting capacity could be used in this scenario.

The 'Dual Lift' Procedure

The Principle

For cases with prominent jowl problems, soft tissue sagged with attenuation of the retaining ligament. The attenuation of retinacular cutis was partially released, and the tissue was then dragged up by the thread in the superficial subcutaneous plane. The fillers were injected not only to fill up the prejowl haloing but also to support the aged ligaments [10] (Fig. 21.8).

In the superficial subcutaneous plane, the superficial fat and the overlying skin can be mobilized after partial release of retinacular cutis's attenuation. In the deep subcutaneous plane, having the threads catch the subcutaneous fat over the SMAS layer, lifting or plicating the underlying SMAS is possible (Fig. 21.9).

The preferred insertion point is located within the range of the posterior third of the zygomatic arch in the supra-SMAS layer, either above or below the zygomatic arch, to avoid trauma to the facial nerve running over the bony surface of the arch (Fig. 21.10).

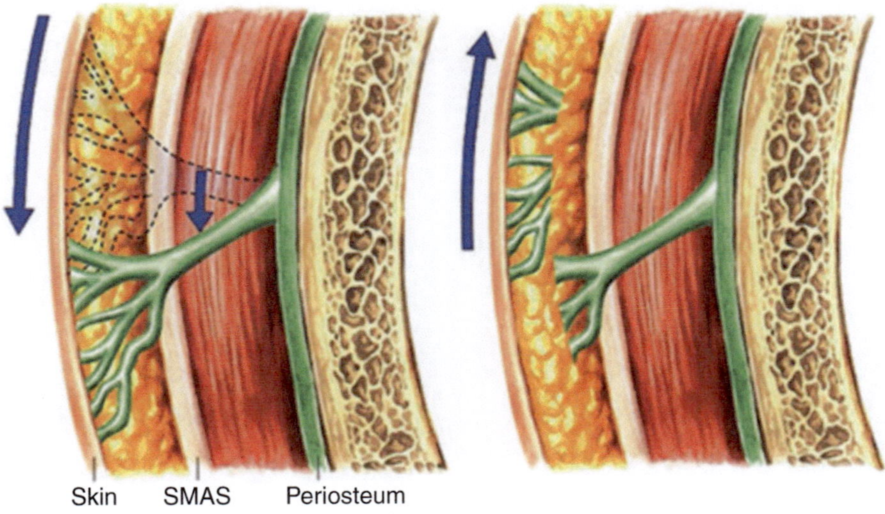

Fig. 21.8 The attenuation of retinacular cutis was partially released, and the fillers were injected to support the aged ligaments. Reproduced with permissions from Kim BJ, Choi JH, Lee Y. Development of Facial Rejuvenation Procedures: Thirty Years of Clinical Experience with Face Lifts. *Arch Plast Surg.* 2015 Sep;42(5):521–31

Fig. 21.9 The superficial subcutaneous plane and the deep subcutaneous plane of lifting. Reproduced with permission from Mendelson, B.C. (2008). Advances in Understanding the Surgical Anatomy of the Face. In: Eisenmann-Klein, M., Neuhann-Lorenz, C. (eds) Innovations in Plastic and Aesthetic Surgery. Springer, Berlin, Heidelberg

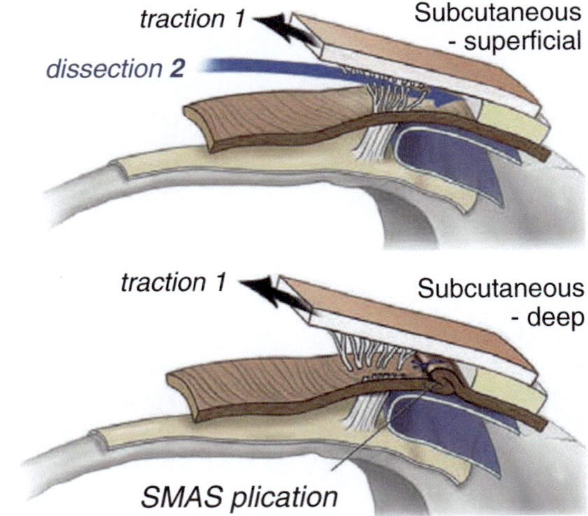

Scheme of the Thread-Lift Design

The superficial part of the mandibular ligament is partially released, and filler is placed deeply to support the ligament. Volumization of subzygomatic area tents up the tissue, and additional strengthening of platysma auricular fascia can also contribute to a different lifting vector if necessary. Bi-directional cog threads are chosen over other robust types of threads owing to the nice balance between

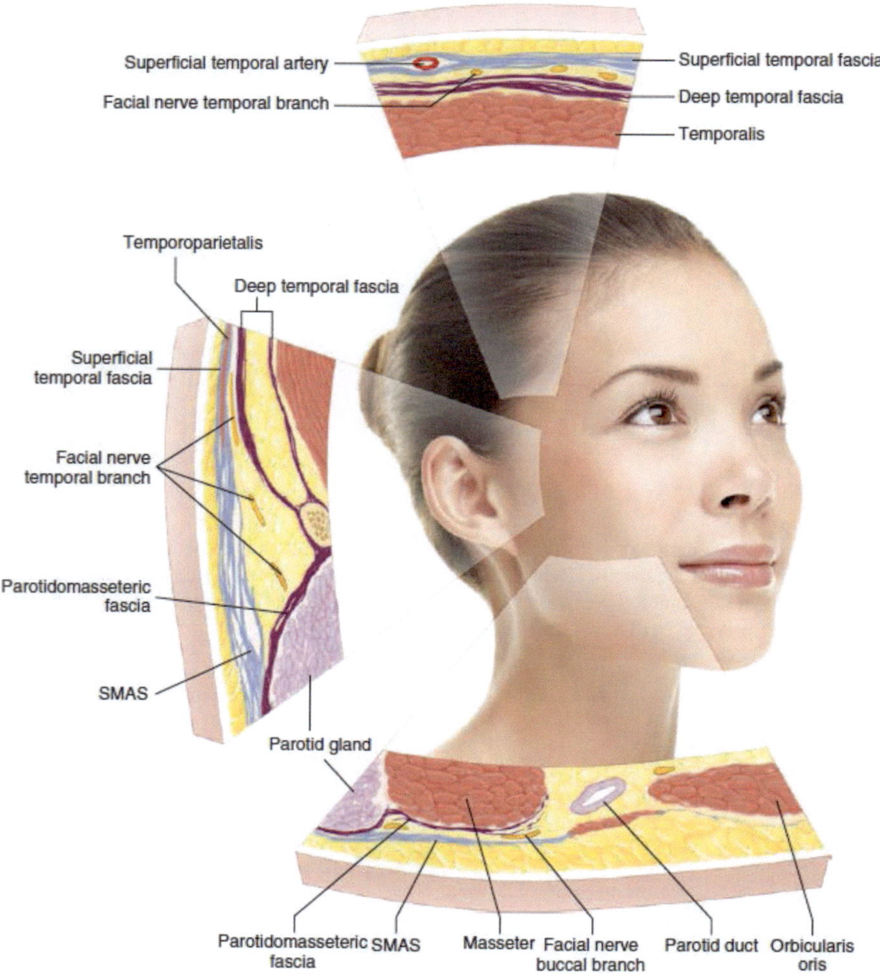

Fig. 21.10 The preferred insertion point of thread is located in the posterior third of the zygomatic arch in the supra-SMAS layer, either above or below the zygomatic arch. Reproduced with permissions from Kim, B., Oh, S., Jung, W. (2019). Anatomy for Absorbable Thread Lifting. In: The Art and Science of Thread Lifting. Springer, Singapore

efficacy and downtime. The fibrous extensions of retinacular cutis serve as the fixation point of the threads. The preferred insertion point is located within the range of the posterior third of the zygomatic arch in the supra-SMAS layer (Fig. 21.11).

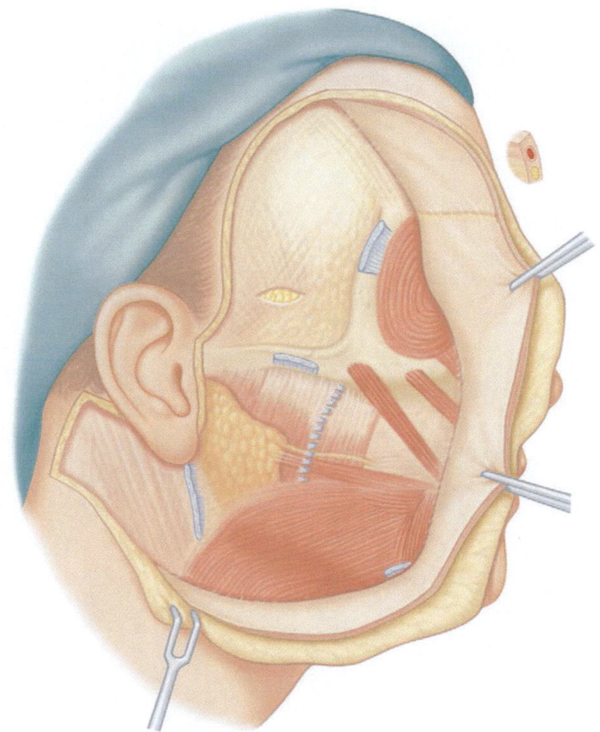

Fig. 21.11 The scheme of the Dual Lift technique. (Reproduced with permissions from Facial Rejuvenation Surgery, BM Jones et al., Page 19, Copyright Elsevier 2008)

Step-by-Step

1. 23G blunt cannula was used for dissection with anterograde infusion of diluted lidocaine 0.2% at the plane of supra-SMAS.
2. Some superficial attaching fibres of the mandibular retaining ligaments were released by cannula before the further step of lifting. And the prejowl concavity was filled up from this point of entry if necessary. Tethering of the fibres could be seen in this view.
3. The first step of lifting started with injectable fillers. The ligaments were strengthened by injecting fillers with high G' force at their bases. The concavity could be filled up at the same time if necessary.
4. The second step of lifting was by bi-directional cog threads. The thread was introduced by cannula through the superficial fibres of the zygomatic retaining ligament and slowly advanced above the SMAS layer. The cannula can be bent first before insertion to fit the curve of the cheek better.
5. The traction of the thread mobilized the subcutaneous fat and the underlying SMAS.
6. The mobilized tissue was reposed close to the superficial portion of the zygomatic ligament.
7. The final step of fine-tuning comprised refinement of facial contour and asymmetry by filler.

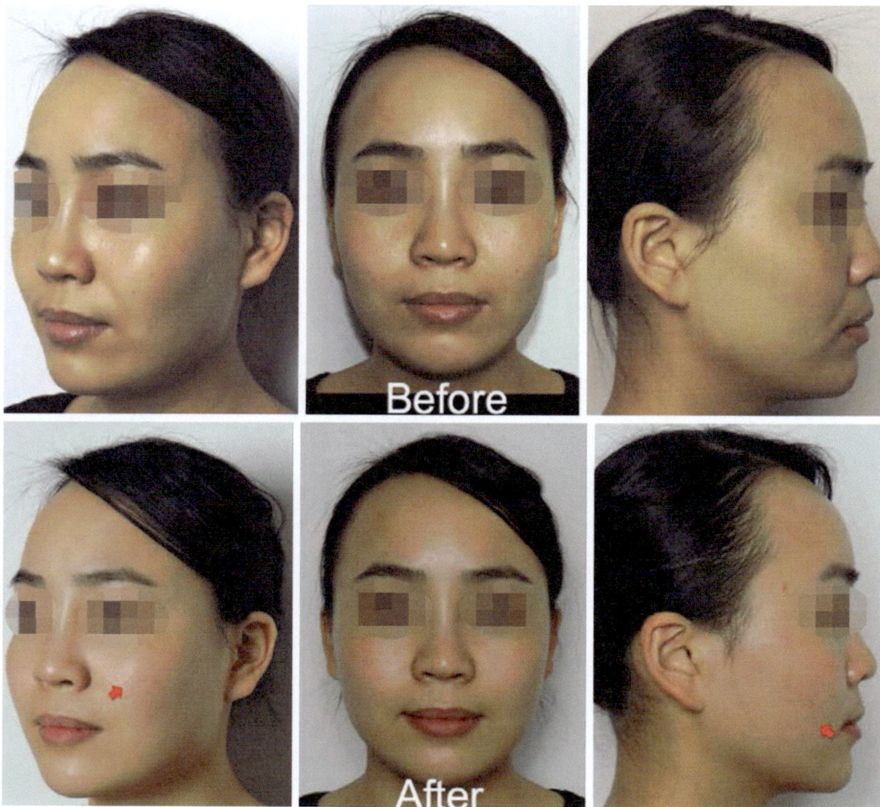

Fig. 21.12 Thread lift in cases of facial asymmetry. At baseline, this case had facial asymmetry and was more drooping on the left side (*left*). She received thread lifts for the mid and lower face on her left side first (*middle*). This showed the immediate result after both sides of the face were treated with thread lifts (*right*). In this case, injectable fillers' fine-tuning facial proportion and asymmetry are mandatory

Indication

Like most thread lift techniques, the Dual Lift technique is best indicated for cases with mild to moderate sagging and moderate tissue quantity (Fig. 21.12).

Limitation

The limitations of the technique are patients with barely any volume loss or heavy face.

Complication

There are some possible but rare complications of this procedure.

Migration and protrusion of threads: if this occurs within days after the procedure, it mostly comes from technical problems like an inaccurate plane of thread insertion. If this develops months after the procedure, it likely results from the weakening of the cogs, especially if the threads are placed through an area of facial expression. It is easy to make a puncture near the tip of protruded thread and remove the fragment.

Skin dimpling: usually results from the superficial placement of the thread, especially in the sunken area like the lateral cheeks. Subcision with or without injectable fillers typically helps in this situation.

References

1. Sykes JM. Management of the aging face in the Asian patient. Facial Plast Surg Clin North Am. 2007;15:353–60.
2. Liew S, et al. Consensus on changing trends, attitudes, and concepts of Asian beauty. Aesth Plast Surg. 2016;40:193–201.
3. Querleux B, et al. Skin from various ethnic origins and aging: an *in vivo* cross-sectional multimodality imaging study. Skin Res Technol. 2009;15:306–13.
4. Kim H-J, Seo KK, Lee H-K, Kim J. Clinical anatomy of the face for filler and botulinum toxin injection. Springer Singapore; 2016. https://doi.org/10.1007/978-981-10-0240-3.
5. Donofrio LM. Fat distribution: a morphologic study of the aging face. Dermatol Surg. 2000;26:1107–12.
6. Kim, B., Oh, S. & Jung, W. The art and science of thread lifting based on pinch anatomy. (2019).
7. Burrows AM, Rogers-Vizena CR, Li L, Mendelson B. The mobility of the human face: more than just the musculature: SMAS and facial mobility in primates. Anat Rec. 2016;299:1779–88.
8. Huang P. The true lift technique™: facial ligament retightening, an anatomical approach. PMFA J. 2018;5
9. Suárez-Vega D, Velazco de Maldonado G, García-Guevara V, Miller-Kobisher B, Morena-López K. Microscopic and clinical evidence of the degradation of polydioxanone lifting threads in the presence of hyaluronic acid: a case report. Medwave. 2019;19:e7575.
10. Kim BJ, Choi JH, Lee Y. Development of facial rejuvenation procedures: thirty years of clinical experience with face lifts. Arch Plast Surg. 2015;42:521–31.

Thread Lifting: Complications and Management

22

Chia-Hsien Hsieh, Chung-Pin Liang, Peter Hsien-Li Peng, and Souphiyeh Samizadeh

C.-H. Hsieh
Diamond Cosmetic Clinic, Taipei, Taiwan, ROC

Diamond-Biotechnology Co., Ltd., Taipei, Taiwan, ROC

C.-P. Liang
Dr Shine Clinic, Taipei, Taiwan, ROC

Dermatologic Department of Cho Hospital, Changhua, Taiwan, ROC

Bestway International Medical Group, Shanghai, China

P. H.-L. Peng (✉)
P-Skin Professional Clinic & Hair Restoration Center, Kaohsiung, Taiwan, ROC

Department of Dermatology, Tri-Service General Hospital, National Defense Medical Center, Taipei, Taiwan, ROC

Laser and Photonics Medicine Society of Taiwan (LMSTW), Taipei, Taiwan, ROC

Taiwanese Dermatological Association (TDA), Taipei, Taiwan, ROC

Taiwanese Society for Dermatological & Aesthetic Surgery (TSDAS), Taipei, Taiwan, ROC

Taiwan Society of Hair Restoration Surgery (TSHRS), Taipei, Taiwan, ROC

Chinese Across the Strait Association of Plastic and Aesthetic (CASAPA), Beijing, China

ISDS, Darmstadt, Germany

DASIL, Milwaukee, WI, USA

International Medicine Affairs Committee, Kaohsiung City Medical Association, Kaohsiung, Taiwan, ROC

S. Samizadeh
King's College London, London, UK

University College London, London, UK

Great British Academy of Aesthetic Medicine, London, UK
e-mail: info@baamed.co.uk

© Springer Nature Switzerland AG 2024
S. Samizadeh (ed.), *Thread Lifting Techniques for Facial Rejuvenation and Recontouring*, https://doi.org/10.1007/978-3-031-47954-0_22

Abstract

Thread lifting encompasses a range of techniques that involve the insertion of absorbable or non-absorbable sutures to achieve facial rejuvenation and recontouring. This method is gaining renewed international popularity as a sought-after procedure for those seeking minimally invasive options for aesthetic enhancements. Absorbable threads, particularly those equipped with cogs, barbs, or cones, are the primary types of sutures utilized in thread lifting. These specialized threads are designed to provide optimal lift and support for the tissue, making them a popular choice among practitioners for achieving the desired aesthetic outcomes. While the procedure is generally safe for rejuvenation purposes, it is not without potential complications. These complications primarily arise from the technical execution of the procedure and, occasionally, patient-specific factors. Pain, swelling, and bruising are expected sequelae of this procedure. Complications can include infection, nerve injury, temporary facial stiffness, hair loss, skin dimpling, post-inflammatory hypo or hyperpigmentation, keloid formation, facial asymmetry, thread extrusion, thread visibility, thread migration, transient paresthesias, and change in facial expressions. Most are self-limiting and can be easily treated. However, surgical treatment and suture removal are sometimes necessary, and practitioners should have the knowledge and expertise to address these complications effectively.

Keywords

Thread lift · Thread lifting · Thread-lift method · Thread-lift technique · Thread-lift procedure · Threading · Facial rejuvenation · Complications

Polydioxanone (PDO) threads, widely available in the market, are fully absorbable and serve as potent stimulants for collagen production, gradually degrading over a period of 4–6 months. The efficacy of PDO threads is attributed to a combination of mechanical action, which facilitates tissue realignment, and the stimulation of collagen production. Despite the significant benefits and safety profile of PDO threads, as with all aesthetic interventions, potential complications or adverse effects can arise. In this chapter, potential complications associated with the use of PDO threads are discussed, emphasizing the need for a comprehensive medical history and a detailed account of any previous cosmetic procedures before proceeding with treatment planning and thread placement.

There are expected sequelae and possible complications/adverse effects like all aesthetic treatments. Comprehensive medical history and history of previous cosmetic treatments should be taken before treatment planning for thread placement. Contraindications include (not limited to) bleeding disorders (Haemophilia), active infection, active cancer treatment, anticoagulants, antiaggregant, body dysmorphic disorder, pregnancy, lactation, previous non-biodegradable injection materials or implants in the area, susceptibility to keloid scars, and any other acute disease or infection. The risk of complications normally increases with an increase number of threads placed [1].

Careful consideration and clinical judgment are essential when treating patients with atopic conditions and autoimmune diseases.

The procedure involves injections, insertion point of various sizes, insertion of threads, and anchorage of the threads. Hence in-depth knowledge of anatomy is crucial, and previous surgical training is recommended.

Post-procedure sequelae include:

- Pain and tenderness
- Swelling
- Bruising

Possible complications:
Early:

- Hematoma
- Skin dimpling
- Over-correction
- Facial asymmetry
- Nerve injury
- Parotid gland injury
- Thread exposure
- Irregularities
- Infection
- Impairment of facial movement

Late:

- Infection
- Chronic inflammatory reactions
- Post-inflammatory hyperpigmentation or hypopigmentation
- Protrusion or extrusion of threads
- Thread migration
- Alopecia or hair loss

A meta-analysis and systematic review of the incidences of complications following facial thread-lifting was published in April 2021. This included a total of 26 studies, and the findings were as follows [2]:

- Swelling (35%), most common
- Skin dimpling (10%)
- Paresthesia (6%)
- Thread visibility/palpability (4%)
- Infection (2%)
- Thread extrusion (2%).

I compared to non-absorbable threads, absorbable threads have been associated with a significantly reduced risk of paresthesia (3.1% vs. 11.7%) and thread extrusion (1.6% vs. 7.6%). Age also influences the risk of complications, with individuals older than 50 years experiencing higher rates of dimpling (16% vs. 5.6%) and infection (5.9% vs. 0.7%) compared to their younger counterparts, potentially due to increased skin laxity and diminished subcutaneous fat. Furthermore, a lower rate of long-term satisfaction has been observed.

A comprehensive pre-operative consultation is essential, during which patients' expectations and wishes and possible unrealistic expectations are discussed. The importance of aftercare, longevity of the results and the potential need for maintenance or complementary treatments should also be addressed. Patients should be made aware of potential complications, their management, and the associated costs involved. This structured approach ensures a comprehensive understanding for the patient and sets a professional and scientifically sound standard of care.

Pain

Pain relief medication can be taken as required. However, symptoms such as unmanageable pain, tingling sensations, numbness, or abnormal sensations in areas of the face or ear should not be dismissed as normal post-procedural effects. These are indicative of potential nerve damage and warrant immediate attention.

Hematoma

Hematoma formation following the procedure is not uncommon, with certain patients being more prone to it than others. The technique employed during the procedure significantly influences this risk. A comprehensive understanding of facial anatomy and the precise location of blood vessels is crucial to minimize the occurrence of hematomas. Pre-treatment precautions include abstaining from alcohol and NSAIDs, as well as avoiding specific vitamins and supplements known to elevate hematoma risk. Topical and systemic arnica may offer benefits. Post-treatment strategies to reduce hematoma risk include refraining from alcohol consumption, avoiding exercise, regular application of ice packs, and certain vitamins. Employing a blunt cannula and ensuring its placement at the correct depth during the operation significantly lowers the likelihood of bruising and hematoma formation.

Swelling

Swelling is a common postoperative response in most patients undergoing thread lifting procedures, with resolution generally occurring within two weeks post-procedure. To mitigate this swelling and enhance patient comfort during the recovery phase, applying cold compresses and administering oral non-steroidal anti-inflammatory drugs (NSAIDs) can be beneficial [2]. Additionally, ensuring patients maintain an elevated head position while resting can further aid in reducing swelling. Implementing these measures, alongside a tailored postoperative care plan that includes close monitoring and patient education on proper care techniques, can significantly improve the recovery experience and outcomes of thread lifting procedures for patients.

Infection

Infection ranks among the more prevalent complications, particularly at the needle insertion sites (Fig. 22.1). Such occurrences are typically attributed to inadequate disinfection practices and lapses in maintaining aseptic operational procedures [2]. Additionally, these complications can be linked to suboptimal adherence to aftercare instructions and the selection of unsuitable candidates for the procedure. Specifically, individuals with active infections or acne present a heightened risk, highlighting the critical importance of thorough patient screening and comprehensive education on post-procedure care to minimize the occurrence of such adverse outcomes.

Given that the needle insertion sites are frequently situated on the scalp—a region characterized by dense hair, making it challenging to maintain cleanliness post-procedure—patient diligence in following aftercare instructions is paramount. It is essential to keep the wound dry for the first 48 hours following the operation and to apply a topical antibiotic as prescribed. In certain cases, the administration of oral antibiotics may also be necessary to prevent infection and ensure optimal healing.

Cases of Mycobacterium abscessus infection and abscess have also been reported [3, 4].

Additionally, instances of abscesses and multiple ulcers have been documented. Such complications are often associated with the use of non-approved/unlicensed threads and breaches in aseptic technique [5, 6].

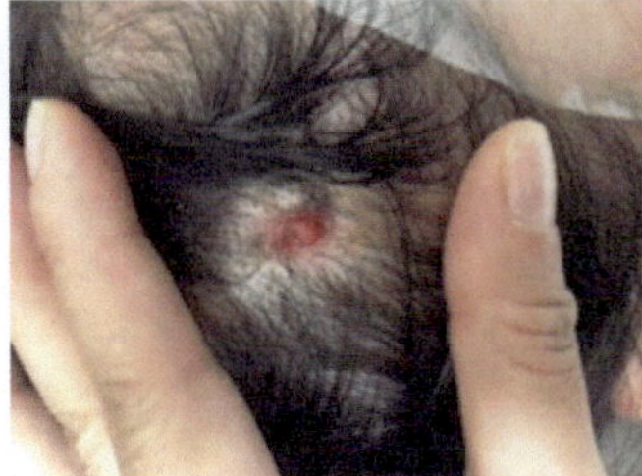
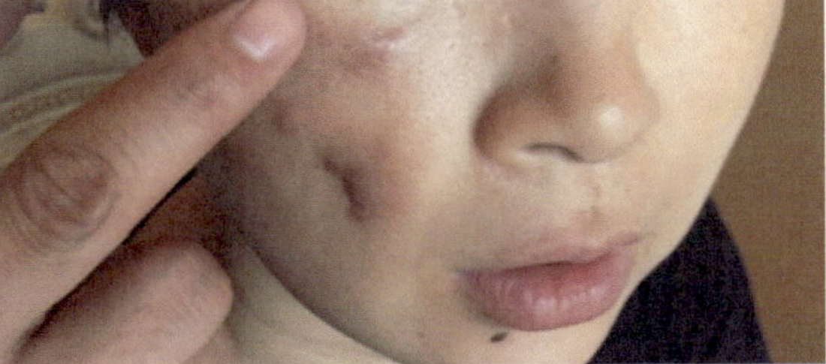

Fig. 22.1 A 40-year-old lady had a skin infection at the insertion point and along the route of threads after thread lifting

Tips [7]

- Thoroughly disinfect all treatment areas, including manipulated regions and entry points.
- Clean, disinfect, and remove hair from the insertion areas to ensure a clear field.
- Take care to prevent the entanglement and insertion of hair with the threads.
- Remove any hair that has entered the entry points meticulously post-procedure.
- Educate the patient on post-procedure infection prevention measures.

Treatment Options [2]

1. Administration of both local and systemic antibiotics.
2. For persistent infections, thread removal and extensive debridement may be required.
3. Mycobacterium infections necessitate prolonged treatment involving intravenous antibiotics and adequate drainage.

Skin Dimpling or Depression

Skin dimpling or depression (Figs. 22.2, 22.3, 22.4) is one of the most common complications of thread lifting. The causes include too superficial placement of the threads, the barbs penetrating the skin, or uneven tension. Too superficial thread insertion at the dermis rather than the superficial muscular aponeurotic system [2]. It has also been proposed that dimpling can happen due to subcutaneous scarring due to previous procedures such as liposuction that is not visible [8].

Mild depressions typically resolve spontaneously within a few days, while moderate depressions can persist for several weeks. Severe depressions may last for several months. Consequently, addressing moderate to severe depressions promptly post-treatment is advisable for optimal recovery.

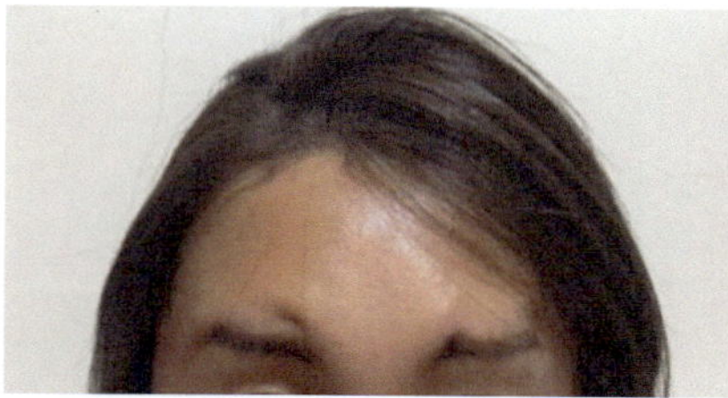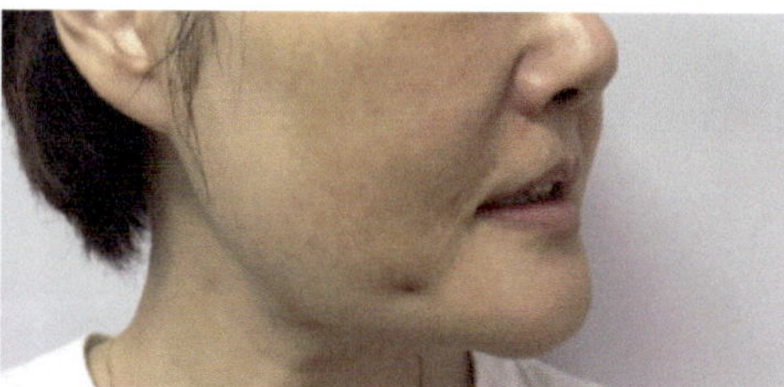

Fig. 22.2 Left: A 30-year-old lady had PDO thread lifting for bilateral eyebrow lifting. Skin dimpling was apparent immediately after the procedure and persisted for more than 1 week. Right: skin dimpling on the right marionette line area after PDO thread lifting, present at 1-week follow-up

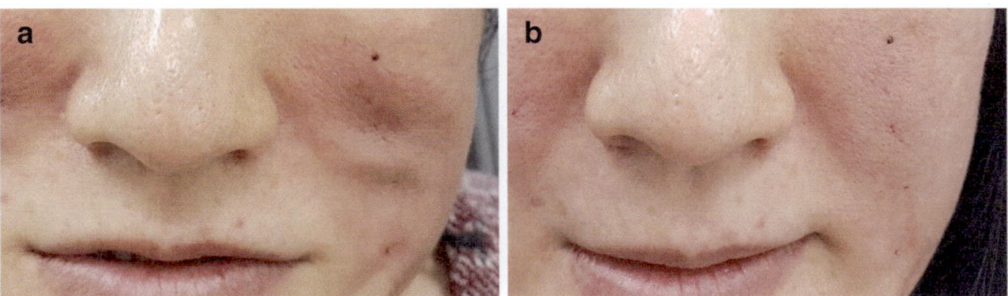

Fig. 22.3 (**a**) Skin dimpling after thread lift. (**b**) Manual therapy releases the tension of cog threads in the direction opposite that of placement. Reproduced with permission from Wang, C.K. Complications of thread lift about skin dimpling and thread extrusion. *Dermatologic Therapy* 2020; 33(4). Reproduced under a CC BY license [9]

Fig. 22.4 Treating the skin dimpling by 18-G needle subcision. Reproduced with permission from Wang, C.K. Complications of thread lift about skin dimpling and thread extrusion. *Dermatologic Therapy* 2020; 33(4). Reproduced under a CC BY license [9]

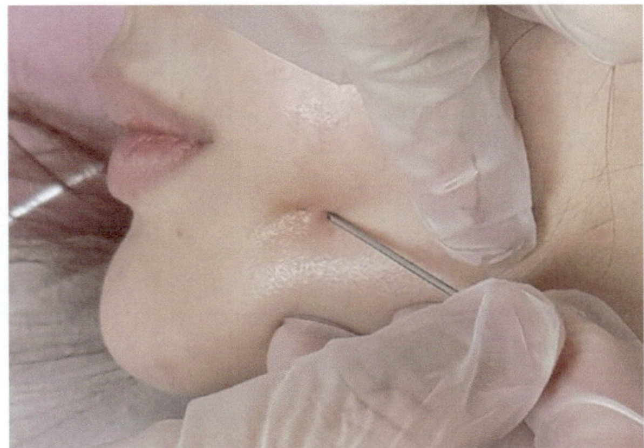

Tips

- Optimal patient selection, including consideration of skin types.
- Selection of the appropriate threads for the procedure, the chosen indication and the treatment area.
- Accurate placement of threads in the correct anatomical layers.
- Diligent care during both insertion and exit of the threads.

Treatment Options

- Manual manipulation and localized massage techniques.
- Cannula dissection for targeted intervention.
- Dermal filler injection to help dislodge the thread.
- Laser therapy.
- Acupotomy.

Asymmetry

Post-treatment asymmetry is a frequently encountered issue, often exacerbated in patients with pre-existing facial asymmetry and can, at times, be attributed to the practitioner's limited experience (Fig. 22.5).

Tips

- Prior to treatment, any existing facial asymmetry should be meticulously documented and communicated to the patient. It's common for patients to scrutinize their facial features more closely after the procedure, potentially noticing pre-existing asymmetries for the first time.
- The paths for thread insertion must be carefully planned to ensure accuracy and symmetry.
- Attention should be paid to the tension of the threads, as differences can contribute to asymmetry.
- Ensure consistent thread placement on both sides of the face to avoid imbalances.
- Avoid both overtreatment and undertreatment by calibrating the procedure to the individual's specific needs and pre-existing conditions.

Treatment Options

- Additional thread lift after swelling has completely subsided
- Adjusting threads that have been overtightened to reduce excessive tension.
- Use of dermal fillers
- Surgery

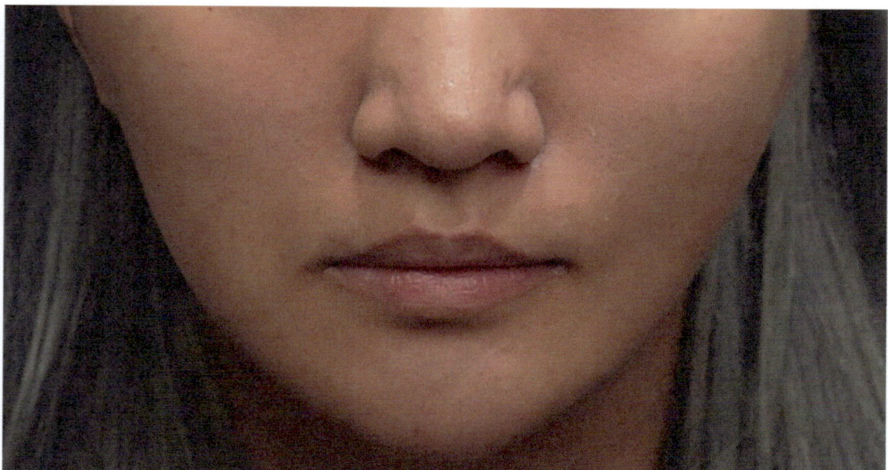

Fig. 22.5 A 35-year-old lady had bilateral PDO thread lifting. One week after the operation, asymmetry is noticeable

Post-inflammatory Hyperpigmentation

Post-inflammatory hyperpigmentation (PIH) typically occurs at the sites of needle insertion or piercing (Fig. 22.6). This dermatological condition results from the cutaneous response to injury, where melanocytes are stimulated to produce excess melanin following trauma inflicted by needles, cannulas, or similar devices used to penetrate the skin. The process is a natural part of the skin's healing mechanism, where increased melanin production is intended to protect the tissue from further damage. However, in the context of aesthetic procedures, this can lead to unwanted pigmentation at the treatment sites. Understanding the pathophysiology of PIH is crucial for practitioners to implement strategies that minimize skin trauma and manage post-procedure pigmentation effectively.

During the initial consultation, it is essential to review any history of post-inflammatory hyperpigmentation (PIH) and a predisposition to keloid formation. Certain skin types, particularly Fitzpatrick skin types III to VI, exhibit a higher propensity for developing PIH, which can adversely affect quality of life. To minimize the risk, it is advised to limit needle insertions and piercings on the face as much as possible during the procedure. Both the practitioner and the patient must ensure diligent post-treatment care of the insertion and exit points to prevent complications.

Tips

- Assess the patient's skin type for vulnerability to PIH and keloids.
- Minimize needle insertions or exits on the face to reduce PIH risk.
- Thoroughly educate patients about PIH and its implications.
- Instruct patients to adhere strictly to aftercare guidelines.

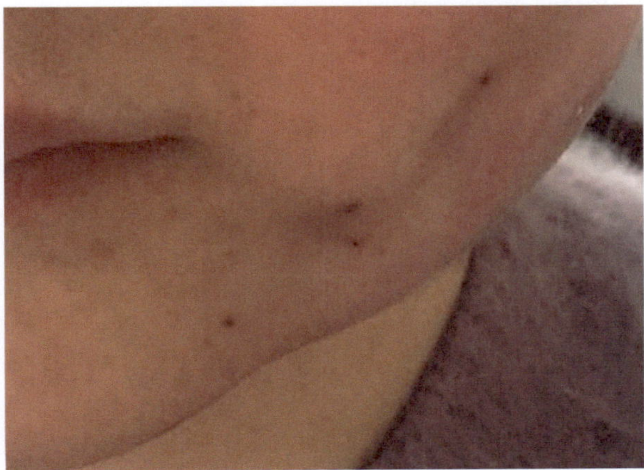

Fig. 22.6 A 45-year-old lady with PIH after retrograde insertion of threads on her face

Treatment Options

Effective topical treatments for PIH include tyrosinase inhibitors (such as hydroquinone, azelaic acid, kojic acid, arbutin, and certain extracts of liquorice), retinoids, mequinol, ascorbic acid, niacinamide, N-acetyl glucosamine, and soy, among others. It's crucial to begin PIH treatment early and educate patients about the condition.

Topical agents should be used with caution to avoid further worsening of hyperpigmentation [10].

While topical agents can be beneficial, they must be used judiciously to prevent exacerbating hyperpigmentation. Combination therapies featuring hydroquinone and retinoids have shown efficacy, and laser and light-based treatments offer additional options for managing PIH [11].

Parotid Gland Injury

Parotid gland or parotid duct injury is one of the most serious complications of thread lifting. Patients would present with rapid onset of swelling and pain (Fig. 22.7). Such symptoms typically result from either rupture of the parotid duct or direct trauma to the parotid gland itself, leading to leakage of saliva. This complication primarily arises from the practitioner's inadequate technique, including incorrect insertion into the facial anatomy's improper layer.

Tips

- Ensure threads are positioned within the correct anatomical layers to minimize risks.
- Review any history of previous surgeries or trauma in the treatment areas to tailor the procedure accordingly.

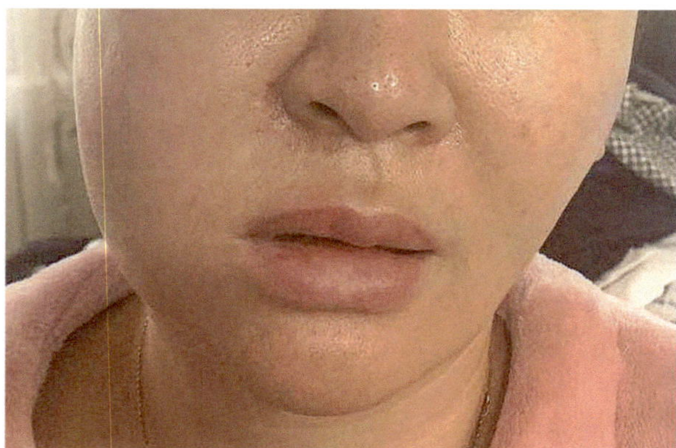

Fig. 22.7 Parotid area swelling 1 day after the procedure

Treatment Options

- Patients experiencing complications from improper thread placement or injury will necessitate surgical intervention for correction. This may include stenting and repair of Stensen's duct to address issues related to parotid gland or duct injuries.

Thread Visibility, Dislocation/Migration, or Exposure

Superficial insertion of the threads can result in thread visibility and/or palpability (Figs. 22.8 and 22.9). Massage therapy may be helpful; however, thread removal is frequently required [2].

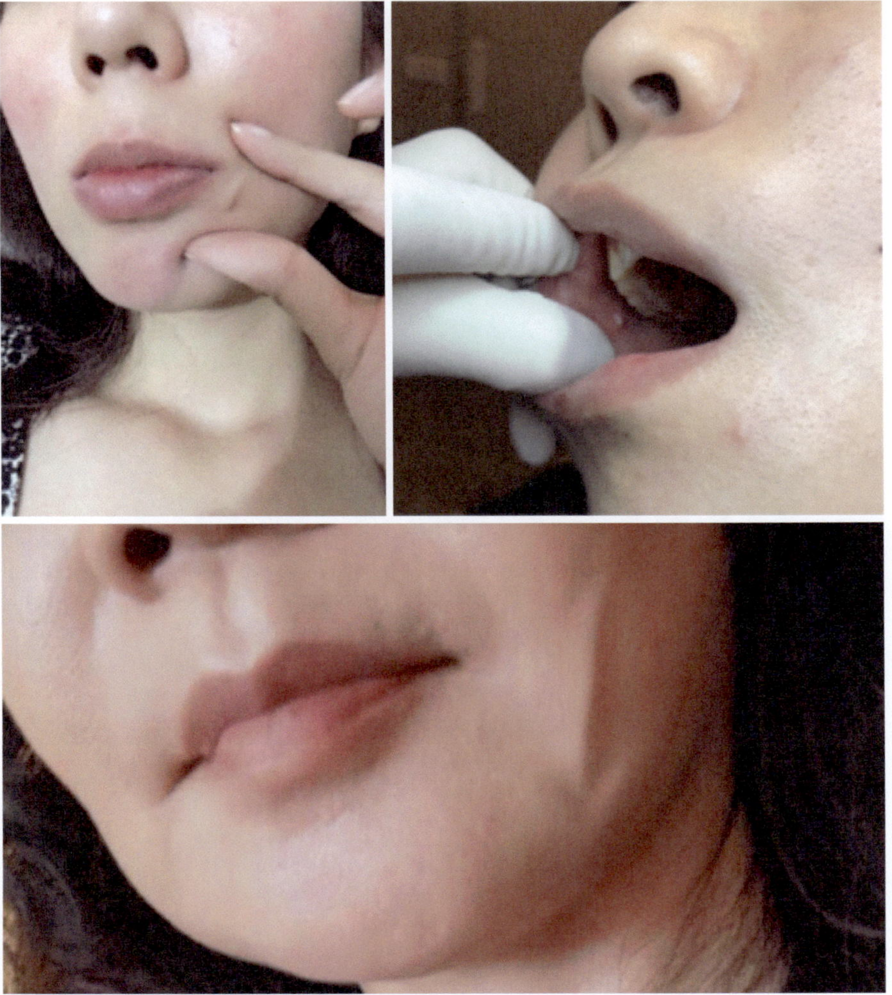

Fig. 22.8 Examples of Thread migration and extrusion 1 week after the procedure

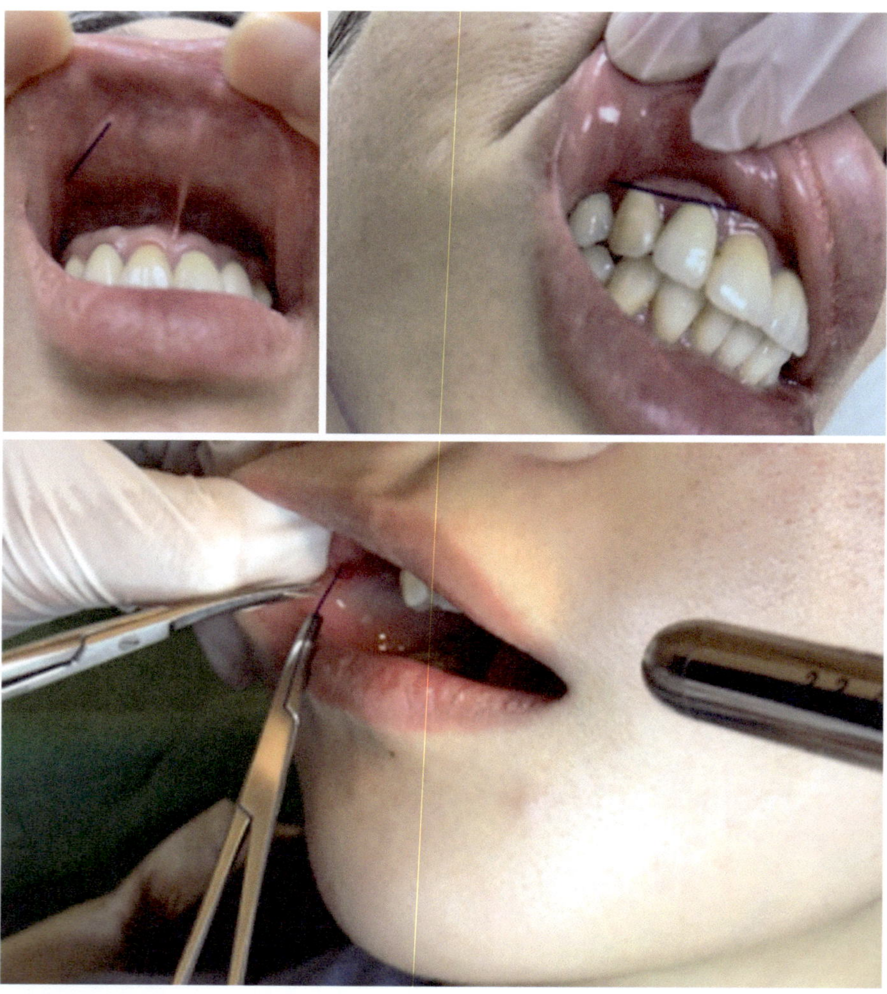

Fig. 22.9 Tread extrusion. Manual therapy can be applied to release the tension of cog threads in the direction opposite that of placement. Thread extraction subsequently in the direction opposite that of placement

Thread migration is a recognized complication, often resulting from the thread moving to a more superficial layer due to repeated inflammatory reactions, thread fracture or separation, foreign body responses, or incorrect placement in the anatomical layers.

Tips

- Ensure threads are placed at the correct depth to minimize migration risk.
- Employ anchoring techniques, such as tying threads together at the same entry point, to enhance stability.

Treatment Options

- For threads that become exposed, removal is necessary and can be achieved with a mosquito clamp following adequate dissection or manual manipulation to safely extract the thread without causing additional tissue damage.

Paresthesia/Nerve Injury

Injury to the facial nerve constitutes a grave complication that may arise from placing threads in an incorrect anatomical layer, the injudicious use of sharp needles, or improper cannula manipulation. Damage to the facial nerve's main temporal branch, for instance, can lead to eyelid sagging and drooping eyebrows, with the zygomatic arch being a high-risk zone due to the soft tissue thickness in this area [12].

There is a lower risk of paresthesia with PDO threads due to their short longevity and hence relief of neural disturbance [13].

Tips

- Placement of threads must be precise, targeting the correct anatomical layers to avoid nerve damage.
- Review the patient's medical history for prior surgeries or trauma in the treatment area, which may affect the procedure.
- Exercise caution and gentleness when manipulating sharp needles or cannulas to prevent tissue and nerve injury.

Treatment Options

- Administration of NSAIDs and corticosteroids to manage inflammation and nerve-related discomfort.
- In cases of persistent and debilitating neurosensory changes, removal of the threads may be necessary.

Hair Loss/Alopecia

Excessive pressure at the needle insertion point can lead to hair follicle damage or poor blood circulation, causing peripheral hair loss. While hair loss typically resolves over time, severe cases have been reported (Fig. 22.10).

Fig. 22.10 Mild hair loss at the insertion point

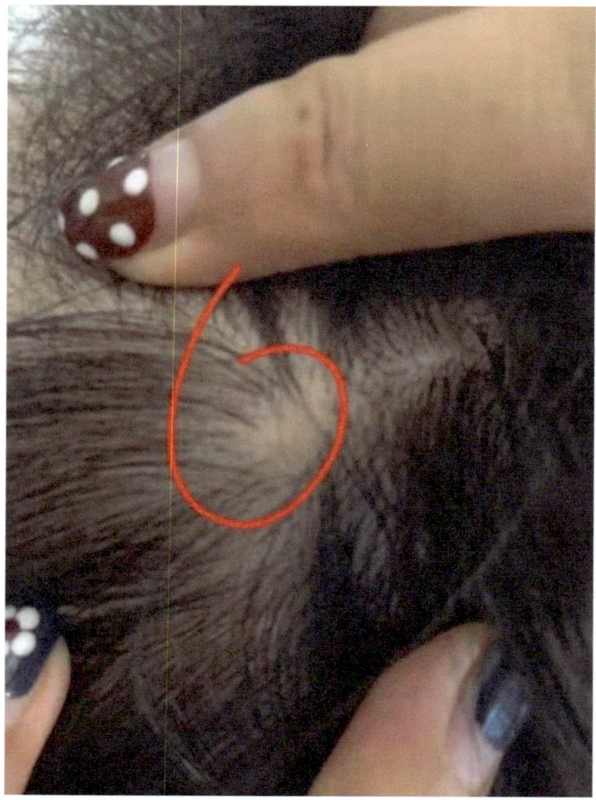

Treatment Options

- Mild cases may not require any treatment.
- Microneedling with growth factors, laser treatments, and hair transplants are potential interventions for more significant hair loss.

Other

Iatrogenic Superficial Temporal Artery Pseudoaneurysm

Following a facial thread-lifting cosmetic procedure, iatrogenic superficial temporal artery pseudoaneurysm was reported [14]. The patient had developed a soft pulsating mass measuring 20 × 20 mm in the left pre-auricular region 3 months post-placement of 4 barb-type threads and required surgical excision. The authors recommended the following prevention measures: [14]

1. Conduct a palpation search for superficial temporal arteries before thread insertion to identify and avoid vascular structures.

2. Take measures to ensure threads do not pierce the superficial temporal arteries, thereby minimizing vascular injury.
3. Implement comprehensive, systematic training for practitioners on thread-lifting techniques to enhance procedural safety and efficacy.

Chronic Inflammatory Reaction

Though rare, chronic inflammatory reactions have been reported, particularly with non-absorbable threads [15].

Conclusion

In conclusion, the technique of thread lifting for facial and neck rejuvenation is increasingly favored among practitioners and patients for its efficacy and minimally invasive nature. A deep understanding of anatomy and careful avoidance of danger zones are crucial to prevent complications. While most side effects are generally mild to moderate and self-resolving, requiring minimal intervention, more serious complications may necessitate surgical intervention. Practitioners must be equipped with the knowledge and skills to manage these complex issues. Importantly, the advent of easily accessible ultrasound imaging has revolutionized pre-procedural planning, allowing for the precise identification of vascular and other critical structures to ensure safer thread placements. Implementing such advanced imaging techniques, alongside the recommended preventive measures, significantly enhances the overall safety and effectiveness of thread-lifting procedures.

References

1. Rachel JD, Lack EB, Larson B. Incidence of complications and early recurrence in 29 patients after facial rejuvenation with barbed suture lifting. Dermatol Surg. 2010;36(3):348–54.
2. Niu Z, Zhang K, Yao W, Li Y, Jiang W, Zhang Q, et al. A meta-analysis and systematic review of the incidences of complications following facial thread-lifting. Aesthet Plast Surg. 2021;1-11
3. Yau B, Lang C, Sawhney R. Mycobacterium abscessus abscess post-thread facial rejuvenation procedure. Eplasty. 2015;15:ic19.
4. Shin JJ, Park JH, Lee JM, Ryu HJ. Mycobacterium massiliense infection after thread-lift insertion. Dermatol Surg. 2016;42(10):1219–22.
5. Joethy J-V, Cheah A, Ang CH. Facial abscess from unlicensed thread lift. Singap Med J. 2020;61(9):498–9.
6. Kasai H, Yashiro K, Kawahara Y. Multiple ulcers on the face due to infection after thread-lifting. J Dermatol. 2018;45(12):e336–e7.
7. Kim B, Oh S, Jung W. Infection. The art and science of thread lifting. Springer; 2019. p. 261–2.
8. Yeo SH, Lee YB, Han DG. Early complications from absorbable anchoring suture following thread-lift for facial rejuvenation. Arch Aesthetic Plast Surg. 2017;23(1):11–6.
9. Wang C-K. Complications of thread lift about skin dimpling and thread extrusion. Dermatol Ther. 2020;33(4):e13446.

10. Davis EC, Callender VD. Postinflammatory hyperpigmentation: a review of the epidemiology, clinical features, and treatment options in skin of color. J Clin Aesthet Dermatol. 2010;3(7):20–31.
11. Taylor S, Grimes P, Lim J, Im S, Lui H. Postinflammatory hyperpigmentation. J Cutan Med Surg. 2009;13(4):183–91.
12. Kim B, Kim B, Oh S, Jung W. The art and science of thread lifting. Springer; 2019.
13. de Benito J, Pizzamiglio R, Theodorou D, Arvas L. Facial rejuvenation and improvement of malar projection using sutures with absorbable cones: surgical technique and case series. Aesthet Plast Surg. 2011;35(2):248–53.
14. Niimi Y, Hayakawa N, Kamei W, Hori K, Niimi Y, Honda T, et al. Superficial temporal artery pseudoaneurysm following midface thread-lift. Plast Reconstr Surg Glob Open. 2021;9(4)
15. Yoo KH, Kim WS, Hong CK, Kim BJ. Chronic inflammatory reaction after thread lifting: delayed unusual complication of nonabsorbable thread. Dermatol Surg. 2015;41(4):510–3.

Part V

Beyond the Face: Body Contouring with Threads

Thread Lifting Techniques for Body Contouring

23

Olga Zhukova and Souphiyeh Samizadeh

Abstract

In aesthetic medicine, the quest for minimally invasive yet effective body contouring techniques is ever-growing. The utilization of threads and tread-lifting techniques for body contouring is an area of growing interest due to its minimally invasive nature. This chapter offers a brief overview of thread lifting for various body regions, focusing on the types of threads and their biological effects, including tissue elevation and collagen stimulation. Initial clinical outcomes and safety considerations are discussed, highlighting the procedure's minimally invasive appeal. This chapter underscores the preliminary nature of current knowledge and experience with these techniques and advocates for continued research in this evolving field.

Keywords

Thread lift · Thread lifting · Thread-lift method · Thread-lift technique · Thread-lift procedure · Facial rejuvenation · Body thread rejuvenation

Introduction

With aging, the skin and subcutaneous tissue lose their turgor and elasticity, and become looser, contributing to the visible signs of aging. These changes may manifest both in the face and the body. A range of surgical and non-surgical options exists to address various aspects of facial and body aging. However, many of these

O. Zhukova (✉)
Moscow Clinical Scientific and Educational Center of Aesthetic Medicine, Moscow, Russia

S. Samizadeh
University College London-Division of Surgery & Interventional Science, London, UK

King's College London-Dentistry, Oral & Craniofacial Sciences, London, UK

Great British Academy of Aesthetic Medicine, London, UK

© Springer Nature Switzerland AG 2024
S. Samizadeh (ed.), *Thread Lifting Techniques for Facial Rejuvenation and Recontouring*, https://doi.org/10.1007/978-3-031-47954-0_23

techniques fall short in delivering significant tissue reinforcement at the dermal level. Thread-lifting methods offer a solution for skin tightening (particularly in relatively young patients) as well as for lifting and/or repositioning soft tissues to achieve a more youthful volume and contour [1, 2].

There has been an increased interest in thread-lifting techniques for lifting and tightening the superficial tissues of the face and body. This interest is due to the simplification of the technique and the excitement caused by the mass media.

I Plastic surgeon Mr. M.A. Sulamanidze innovated and secured a patent for the APTOS Light Lift, which is crafted from a copolymer of lactic acid and caprolactone. This material is entirely biodegradable and has received certification and official approval for cosmetic purposes [2–4].

Absorbable APTOS Excellence Body threads (Fig. 23.1) can be used for tightening the body's superficial tissues. Tightening can be performed to correct aging changes in the areas of the neck, décolletage, inner surface of the shoulders, abdomen, inner surface of the thighs, knees, and female genitals [5]. Ten years of experience with the APTOS procedures was published in 2009 and reported on the ease, safe, and efficacy of APTOS threads and techniques used for face and neck rejuvenation [6]. The advantages of the use of these threads for rejuvenation were reported to be as follows: [6]

- Simplicity, easy, the economy of use
- Minimally invasive nature and low trauma of the procedures
- Reliability and sufficient duration of qualitative lifting
- Possible combination with other interventions and a short rehabilitation period

APTOS Excellence Body threads are made of Lactic acid and caprolactone copolymer. They are multidirectional with specially designed barbs that allow fixing the threads in the soft tissues initiating formation of a new collagen frame. Over time, the threads are completely absorbed by hydrolysis, and a frame of the body's own collagen is formed in their place. The polylactic acid component of the threads ensures an additional rejuvenating effect [7–9].

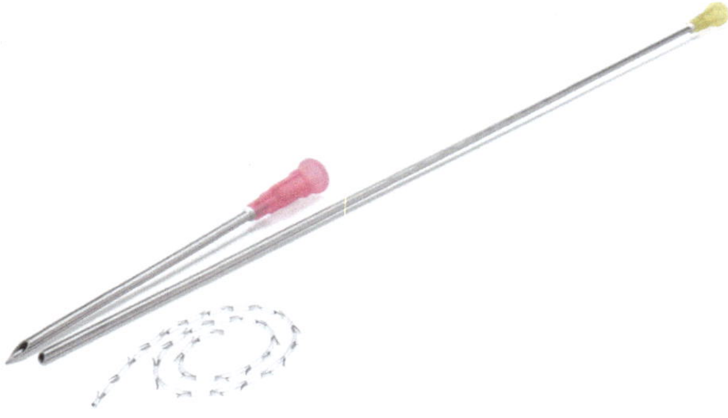

Fig. 23.1 Absorbable threads with barbs for rejuvenation. APTOS threads designed for the Excellence Method are specially tailored for body rejuvenation, taking into account skin texture and the subcutaneous structure. The 20 cm APTOS thread, equipped with barbs, enables doctors to perform 3D armoring in areas with ptotic tissues or where prevention of ptosis is necessary. The procedure strengthens the tissues and makes the skin more elastic and smoother. P(LA/CL) thread with barbs USP 2/0, EP3, 240 mm. Blunt tip needle 19G × 200 mm., straight. Lancet point needle 18G × 40 mm., straight. Removable needle attachment

This absorbable thread with barbs is used to repair and revitalize soft tissues, hence restoring skin structure and elasticity. Subdermally, a mesh of implanted threads creates a robust collagen frame. The outcome is instantly noticeable: the skin is lifted and smoothed. The effect is improved with time and can last up to 2–3 years, depending on the patient's lifestyle and individual characteristics.

Patient Selection

When planning procedures on the body, loose and ptotic skin and subcutaneous tissues should be noted; All types of lipodystrophy (especially during the initial stage) should be noted since this progresses and worsens with ageing.

The contraindications to the thread lift include:

- Inflammation and tumours in the area of the suggested manipulation.
- Tendency to develop keloid or hypertrophic scars.
- Blood disorders (haemophilia), anticoagulant therapy.
- Acute stage of any chronic diseases.
- Pregnancy or lactation.
- Allergies to drugs/medication used.

Preoperative Evaluation

The patient should be informed candidly about potential complications and adverse events during the initial appointment, emphasizing that thread lifting is a surgical procedure, not a 'non-surgical' procedure. The patient should be informed about postoperative pain and discomfort and that there is some downtime [10].

It is critical for the surgeon to understand the patient's desires, wishes, and expectations. Without mutual understanding and agreement, the surgeon may get an ideal result from his or her perspective, but the patient may be disappointed because the outcome does not match their expectations [10].

It is advisable to refrain from using **non-essential** and biologically active food supplements that affect blood clotting for about a week before the procedure.

Prior to the procedure, it is imperative that the patient is thoroughly briefed on the materials to be used, the methodologies employed, the anticipated outcomes, and any possible complications. Following this detailed briefing, the patient is then asked to provide their voluntary informed consent by signing the relevant form, thereby acknowledging their understanding and agreement to proceed with the procedure.

Key stages of the procedure are:

1. Preoperative Marking: Initial demarcation of the target areas is performed to guide the procedure.
2. Aseptic Preparation: The designated correction area is meticulously disinfected using antiseptic solutions to minimize infection risk.
3. Anaesthesia Administration: Local infiltration anaesthesia is employed, utilizing the infiltration technique to adequately numb the treatment area and mitigate the risk of hematoma formation.

4. Thread Insertion: Specialized sutures are carefully introduced into the predetermined marks, adhering to the planned trajectories for optimal lift and tissue engagement.
5. Tension Adjustment and Thread Fixation: The inserted threads are then adjusted for tension and securely fixed, ensuring the desired effect on areas exhibiting skin laxity.
6. Incision Closure: Sterile closure strips are applied to the incision sites for wound protection.

Case Studies

The primary objective is the tightening of superficial tissues, which requires strategic placement of the threads along the natural stretch marks of the skin. The ideal positioning of APTOS threads aligns with Langer's lines, as described by the German anatomist R. S. Langer (1819–1887). Langer's lines represent the skin's natural tension lines, indicating the direction of maximum tension and aligning with the orientation of collagen fiber bundles (Fig. 23.2) [11].

Arm Contouring/Non-surgical Brachioplasty (Figs. 23.3 and 23.4)

Non-surgical brachioplasty is most commonly used to treat flabby sagging skin caused by rapid weight loss, pregnancy/childbirth, ageing, or hormonal changes. Until recently, the only and most common solution to this problem was plastic

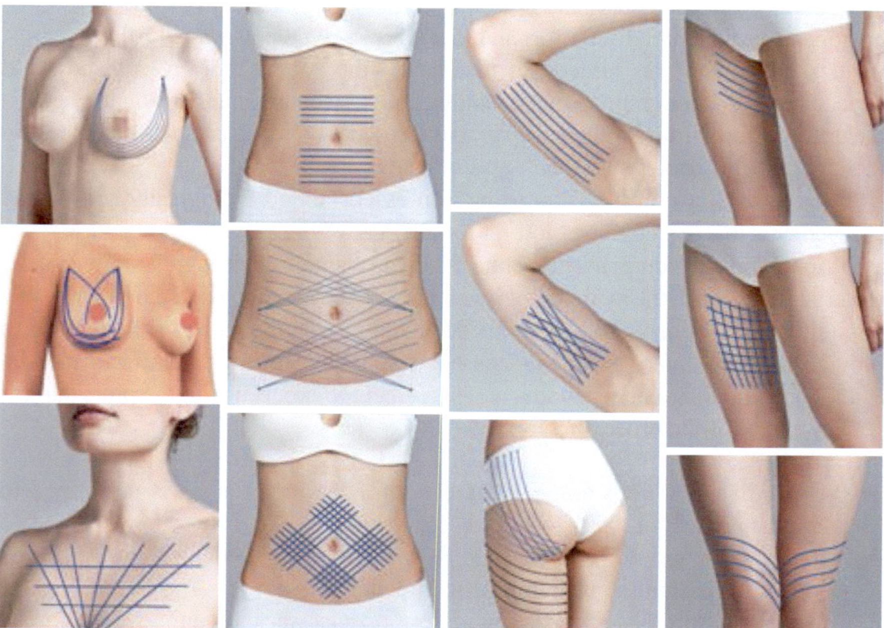

Fig. 23.2 Thread insertion patterns used on various body parts. (by Zhukova O)

Fig. 23.3 Thread insertion pattern

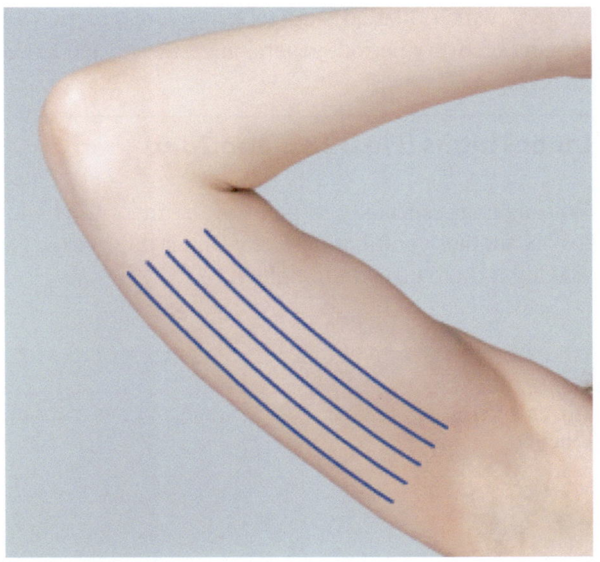

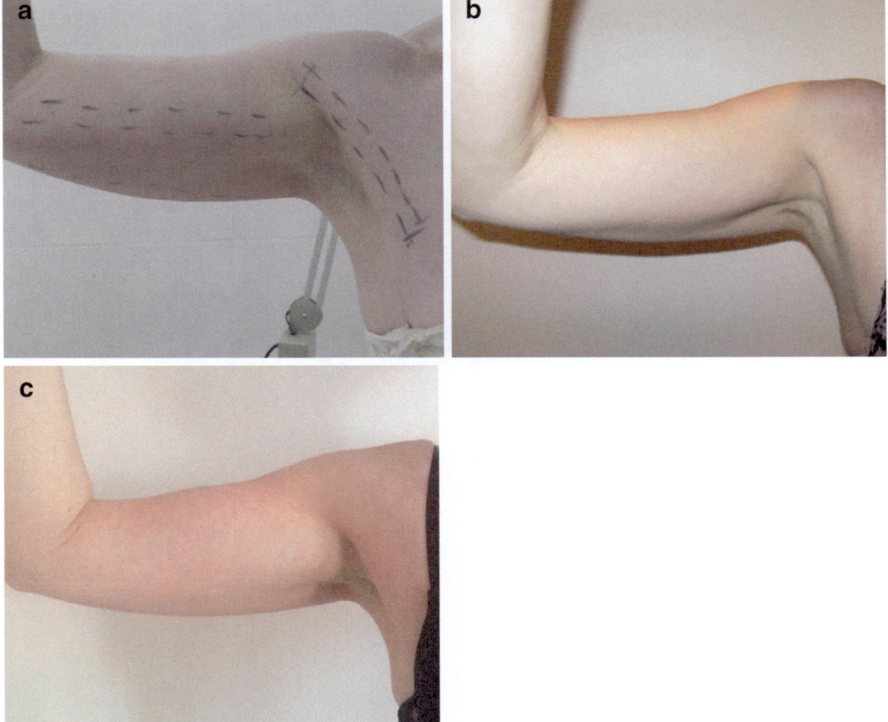

Fig. 23.4 Female, aged 50 years, with dystrophy of superficial tissues of the medial surface of the shoulder and the anterior axillary line. Pronounced tightening and strengthening of the soft tissues can be observed. It should be noted that the effect is more pronounced in 2 years. Before (**a**), after the procedure (in 6 months—**b** and 2 years—**c**)

surgery, which, like all surgical procedures, carries a variety of risks, including a lengthy recovery period, general anaesthesia, and keloid or deep scarring.

Inner Thighs (Figs. 23.5 and 23.6)

With ageing, especially in women, the inner thighs lose firmness. Sudden weight loss is another contributing factor. Inner thighs skin is more delicate and sensitive, making it more difficult to tighten.

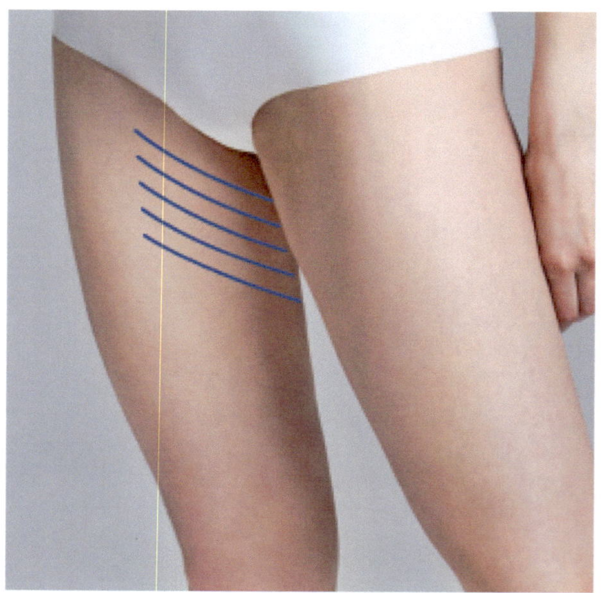

Fig. 23.5 Thread insertion pattern

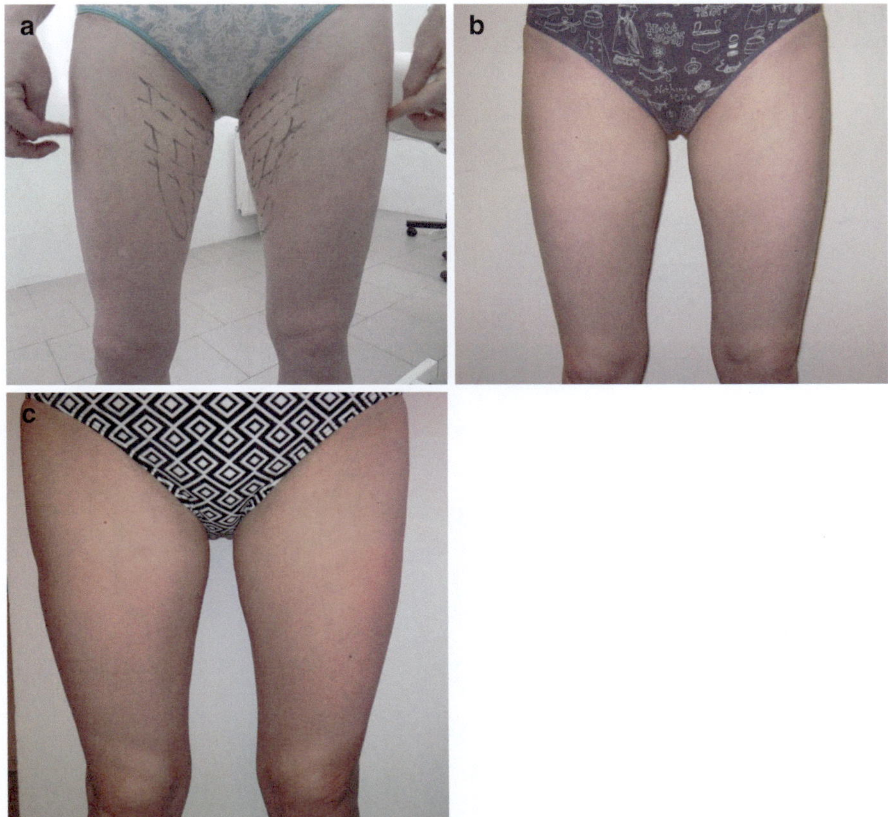

Fig. 23.6 The same patient N, female, aged 50 years, with dystrophy of superficial tissues of the medial surface of the thigh. We can see pronounced tightening and strengthening of the soft tissues. It should be noted that the effect is also more pronounced in 2 years. Before (**a**), after the procedure (in 6 months—**b** and 2 years—**c**)

Above the Knees (Figs. 23.7 and 23.8)

Ageing and sudden weight loss result in deterioration and loss of skin elasticity around the knees. This absorbable thread with barbs is used to repair and revitalize soft tissues, hence restoring skin structure and suppleness. Rejuvenation entails tightening of the skin and enhancement of skin tone and elasticity.

Fig. 23.7 Thread insertion pattern

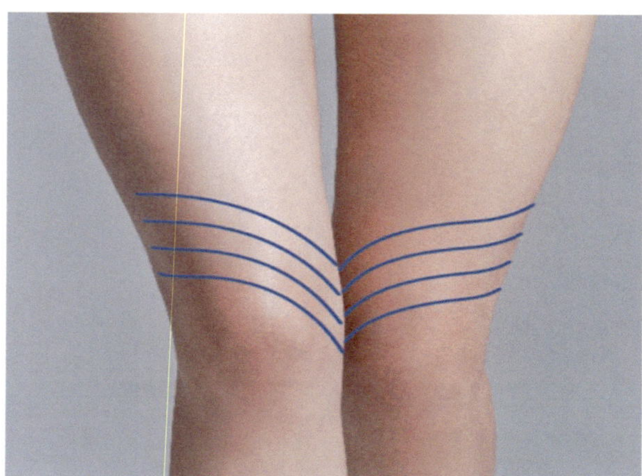

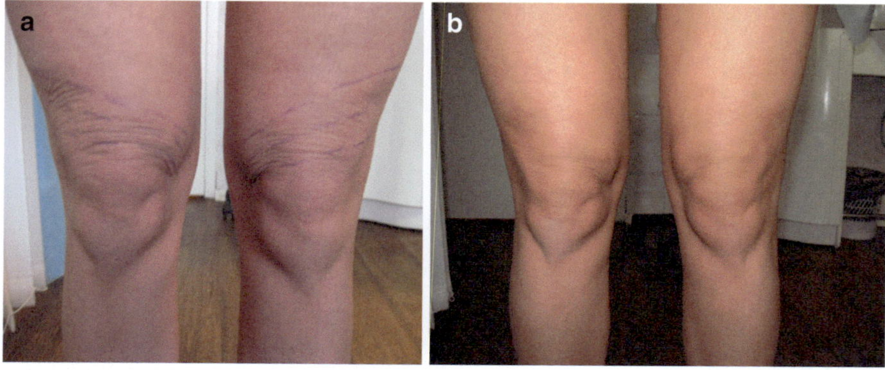

Fig. 23.8 Female aged 35 years. When the patient strains the muscles of the anterior compartment of the thigh, we can see skin folds. Following implantation of only six threads along the lines that cross the observed skin folds, we can see smoothing wrinkles and strengthening of the superficial tissues. Before (**a**), after the procedure (6 months—**b**)

Anterior Abdominal Area

Pregnancy, ageing, weight loss, inadequate diet, and a sedentary lifestyle contribute to the loss of abdominal skin elasticity. Long threads (25 cm) with barbs enable three-dimensional strengthening of body parts where tissues lose elasticity and where ptotic prevention is essential. This process reinforces the tissues and makes the skin elastic, dramatically enhances its quality, and lifts, which is beneficial for patients with flabby skin and cellulite (Figs. 23.9 and 23.10) [12].

For comparison, another option of thread implantation into the abdominal area can be seen below (Figs. 23.11 and 23.12).

Fig. 23.9 Thread insertion pattern

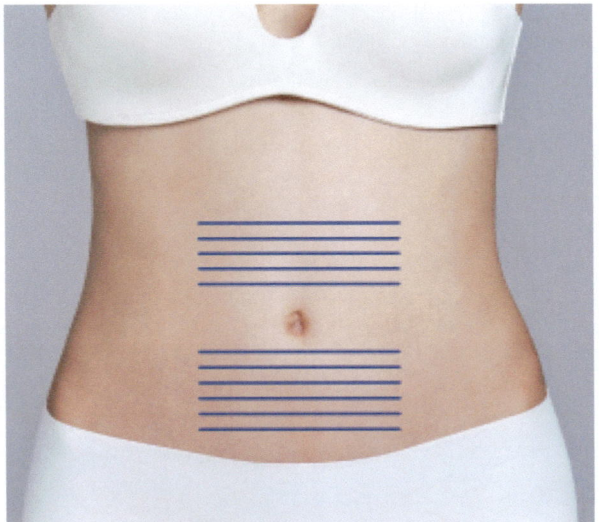

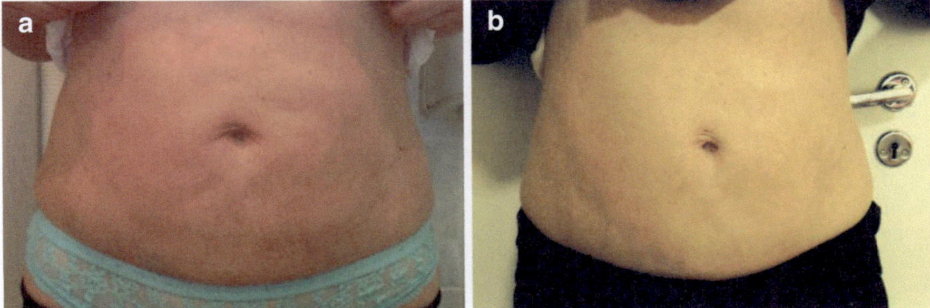

Fig. 23.10 Female, aged 52 years. The patient complained of contour irregularities after the liposuction procedure performed 7 years before. Following implantation of threads, we can see smoothing of the skin. Before (**a**), after the surgery (6 months—**b**)

Fig. 23.11 Thread insertion pattern

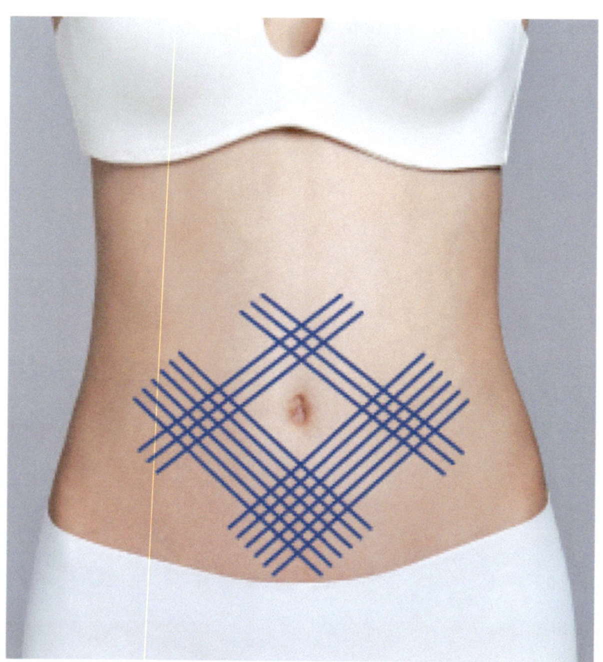

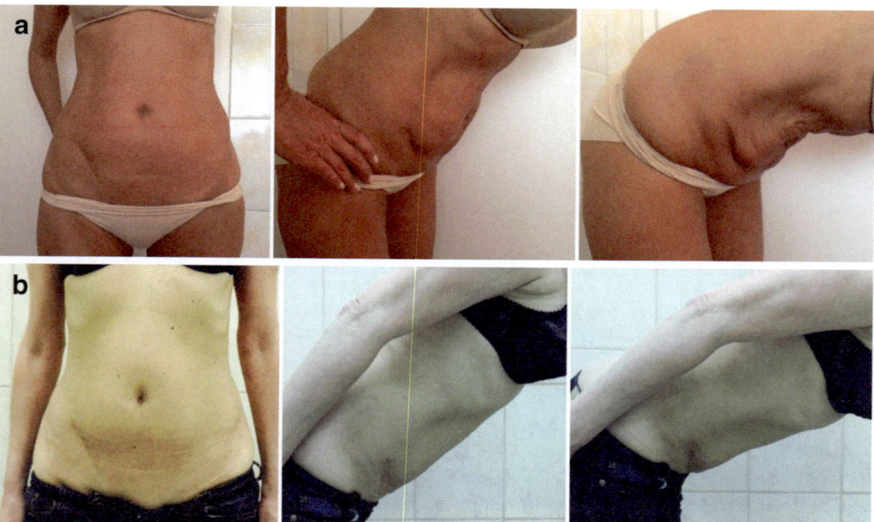

Fig. 23.12 Female, aged 55 years. The photo taken before the procedure shows atrophy of the superficial tissues and loose skin, and subcutaneous fat is noticeable. In the photo taken after the procedure, we can see a significant reduction of the skin and tightening of the superficial tissues. Before (**a**) and 2 years after the procedure (**b**)

Breasts (Figs. 23.13 and 23.14)

Breast ptosis is frequently related to ageing, macromastia, weight loss, pregnancy, and hormonal changes, but it can occur in individuals of any age or size of the breast. Breast ptosis develops naturally over time, beginning with the stretching of the skin envelope, ductal structures, and supporting ligaments. The volume of the breast parenchyma increases, rendering supportive structures inefficient and resulting in skin excess. Ptosis can also occur when the parenchymal volume diminishes, resulting in skin redundancy [13]. Threads can be used in some cases to improve skin quality and for a natural 'lifting' effect [14].

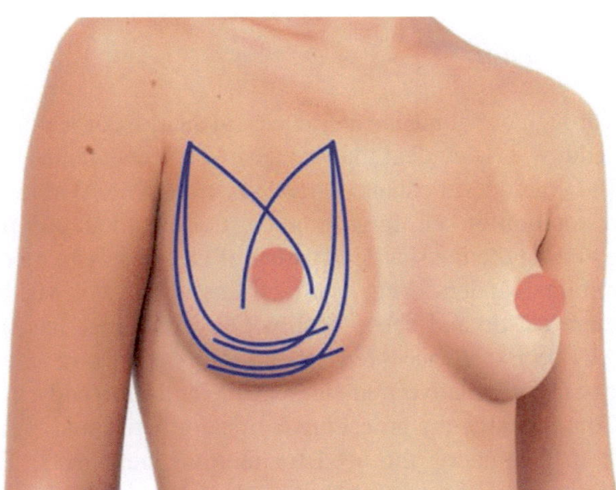

Fig. 23.13 Thread insertion pattern

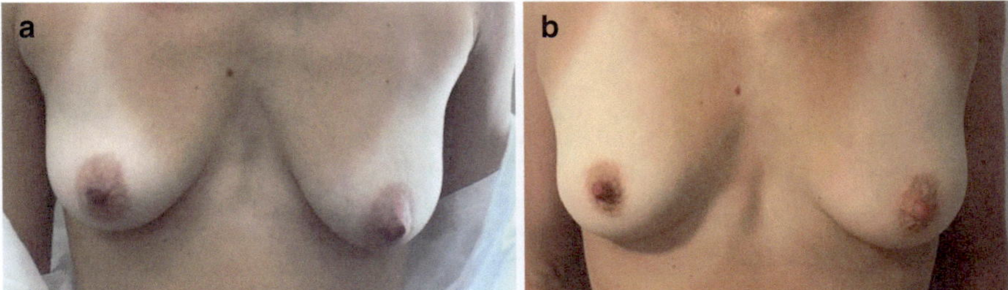

Fig. 23.14 Female aged 50 years. There are clinical signs of breast sagging, reduced skin turgor, sagging and folding of the area around the nipple. The photo demonstrates improvement of the skin turgor, significant smoothing of the skin, and the effect of 'filling' of the soft tissues. Before (**a**) and 6 years after the procedure (**b**)

Avoiding Complications

Complications and adverse events include infection, thread visibility, migration, exposure; linear bleeding along the needle course; skin dimpling; hypo- and hyper-correction; transitory paresthesias; and rarely damage to major arteries and nerve branches. All of them can be prevented with correct patient selection, a thorough understanding of anatomy, aseptic technique, proper thread placement technique and aftercare [10].

Minor bleeding, oedema, asymmetry, and uneven contours (e.g. shallow dimpling at needle insertion sites) are all frequent, temporary problems of all surgical procedures and are therefore not considered complications.

Conclusion

Through our clinical experience and analysis of the outcomes of all performed procedures, it is evident that the desired effects manifest immediately post-procedure and continue to enhance gradually over time. Within a month, there is noticeable restoration of skin turgor and elasticity without any resultant scarring. Moreover, owing to the non-invasive nature of this treatment modality, the recovery period is minimal, underscoring its effectiveness. The skin visibly appears lifted, attaining a more elastic and dense quality. Our experience has shown that Thread lift using APTOS Excellence threads yields long-lasting outcomes and predictable results surpassing alternative non-surgical methods for body contouring and rejuvenation. Consequently, the procedure is transformative and typically requires only one session, eliminating the need for multiple treatments. This underscores the critical importance of comprehensive education, in-depth knowledge, rigorous surgical training, a profound understanding of patient care, and the ability to recognize and effectively manage complications, all while prioritizing patient safety.

References

1. Sulamanidze M, Fournier P, Paikidze T, Sulamanidze G. Removal of facial soft tissue ptosis with special threads. Dermatol Surg. 2002;28(5):367–71.
2. Sulamanidze M, Paikidze T, Sulamanidze G. Lifting of soft tissues: old philosophy, new approach–a method of internal stitching (Aptos needle). Aktuelle Dermatologie. 2004;30(10):82.
3. Sulamanidze M, Sulamanidze G. Facial lifting with Aptos methods. J Cutan Aesthet Surg. 2008;1(1):7–11.
4. Sulamanidze M, Paikidze T, Sulamanidze G, Neigel JM. Facial lifting with "APTOS" threads: featherlift. Otolaryngol Clin N Am. 2005;38(5):1109–17.
5. Агапова МА, Жукова ОГ, Паклина ОВ. Способ коррекции аногенитальной области у женщин; 2017.

6. Sulamanidze M, Sulamanidze G. APTOS suture lifting methods: 10 years of experience. Clin Plast Surg. 2009;36(2):281–306.
7. Sulamanidze G, Sulamanidze M, Sulamanidze K, Kajaia A, Giorgadze S. The subcutaneous tissue reaction on poly (l-lactide-co-caprolactone) based threads. Int J Clin Exp Dermatol. 2018;3:1–9.
8. Fitzgerald R, Vleggaar D. Using poly-L-lactic acid (PLLA) to mimic volume in multiple tissue layers. J Drugs Dermatol. 2009;8(10 Suppl):s5–14.
9. Schierle CF, Casas LA. Nonsurgical rejuvenation of the aging face with injectable poly-L-lactic acid for restoration of soft tissue volume. Aesthet Surg J. 2011;31(1):95–109.
10. Sulamanidze M, Sulamanidze G, Vozdvizhensky I, Sulamanidze C. Avoiding complications with Aptos sutures. Aesthet Surg J. 2011;31(8):863–73.
11. Rubin LR. Langers lines and facial scars. Plast Reconstr Surg. 1948;3(2):147–55.
12. Жукова ОГ, Циноева ФИ. Малоинвазивный способ укрепления и сокращения кожи и подкожной клетчатки передней брюшной стенки человека; 2017.
13. Martinez AA, Chung S. Breast ptosis. StatPearls [Internet]; 2021.
14. Sulamanidze M, Sulamanidze G, Sulamanidze K. Mastopexy–how to reach consistent results–new methods. Miniinvasive Face and Body Lifts: Closed Suture Lifts or Barbed Thread Lifts. 2013:241–7.

Index

© Springer Nature Switzerland AG 2024

S. Samizadeh (ed.), *Thread Lifting Techniques for Facial Rejuvenation and Recontouring*,
https://doi.org/10.1007/978-3-031-47954-0

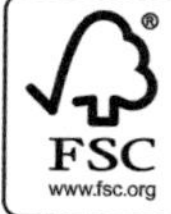